VETERINARY IMMUNOLOGY

An Introduction

Third Edition

IAN TIZARD

PhD., B.Sc., B.V.M.S., M.R.C.V.S.

Professor and Head
Department of Veterinary
Microbiology and Parasitology

Texas A & M University
College of Veterinary Medicine
College Station, TX

1987

W.B. SAUNDERS COMPANY

Philadelphia   London   Toronto
Sydney   Tokyo   Hong Kong

Saunders Company: West Washington Square
Philadelphia, PA 19105

Library of Congress Cataloging-in-Publication Data

Tizard, Ian R.
  Veterinary immunology.

1. Veterinary immunology.   I. Title.

SF757.2.T59   1987   636.089′6079   86–17829

ISBN 0–7216–2098–1

Listed here are the latest translated editions of this book together with the language of the translation and the publisher.

Spanish (*2nd Edition*)–Neuva Editorial Interamericana, Mexico City, Mexico
German (*1st Edition*)–Verlag Paul Parey, Berlin, West Germany
Portuguese (*2nd Edition*)–Livraria Roca Ltda., Sao Paulo, Brazil

Editor: Darlene Pedersen
Developmental Editor: David Kilmer
Designer: Dorothy Chattin
Production Manager: Bill Preston
Manuscript Editor: Susan Short
Illustration Coordinator: Walt Verbitski

Veterinary Immunology   ISBN   0–7216–2098–1

Last digit is the print number: 9   8   7   6   5   4   3   2

To Claire, Robert and Fiona

Preface to the
Third Edition

In writing this book I have tried to provide a text that demonstrates the scope of veterinary immunology in such a way that students and veterinarians can readily comprehend it while at the same time appreciating its complexity. The book is, as its title states, an introductory text. It is not designed to be exhaustively comprehensive nor is it designed to serve as a manual of clinical treatment. I have therefore avoided, as far as possible, giving precise clinical instructions.

Because veterinary students and practitioners are very busy people, a deliberate effort has been made to summarize and consolidate the huge amount of information available. Unfortunately, the developments in immunology over the past five years have necessitated the addition of five new chapters. On the credit side, however, much of the increase has resulted from the addition of many new illustrations and diagrams. These illustrations will, I believe, help in making many complex concepts more clear.

Some of the new information that has been added includes recent information on the role of macrophages, dendritic cells and B cells in antigen presentation, the structure of the T cell receptor, the functions of the interleukins and the functional role of the antigens of the major histocompatibility complex.

Some newer diagnostic procedures, especially the immunoperoxidase techniques and western blotting, and the use of monoclonal antibodies have become commonplace. Less dramatic advances have occurred in our understanding of immunity to infectious agents, although the increased use of gene splicing and cloning techniques has begun to lead to the introduction of genetically engineered vaccines. The growing use of immunostimulants and immunosuppressive drugs has also influenced many areas of veterinary medicine.

Few "new" immunological diseases have appeared, although periodic opthalmia and equine polyneuritis have joined the ranks of undoubted autoimmune diseases, and the list of confirmed immunodeficiency diseases of domestic animals continues to grow.

I am well aware that errors or inaccuracies may have crept into the text, and I have rarely hesitated to state my own opinions. I, therefore, continue to solicit comments, suggestions and opinions from all readers for improvements and corrections. Only with such input can the book fulfil its intended function.

Finally, I must express my sincere thanks to my colleagues Drs. J. Caldwell, F. C. Heck, D. McMurray, S. Reynolds, R. B. Simpson, G. C. Wagner and G. N. Woode, who took the time to review and improve many chapters and provided me with much sound advice. The chapters they reviewed are readily recognized by their quality. I must also thank the secretarial staff in the department of Veterinary Microbiology and Parasitology, especially Mses. J. Canter, J. Mayo, B. L. Suehs and S. Torres, for their help in producing the manuscript and Ms. A. Miley for redrawing all the illustrations with consummate skill. Most importantly, I must express my appreciation to my wife Claire for her help, encouragement and tolerance while the manuscript was in preparation.

IAN TIZARD

Contents

III
PROTECTIVE IMMUNITY

12
Immunity at Body Surfaces................................. 159

13
Immunity in the Fetus and Newborn...................... 171

14
General Principles of Vaccination and Vaccines 185

15
Resistance to Bacteria and Related Organisms............ 201

16
Resistance to Viruses.................................... 219

17
Immunity to Parasites................................... 233

Glossary

Active immunity Immunity that is generated by an animal's own immune response following exposure to foreign antigen.

Acute phase proteins Serum proteins whose levels rise significantly and rapidly following injury, infection or inflammation.

ADCC (Antibody-dependent cellular cytotoxicity) Lysis of target cells through the actions of antibody and neutrophils, macrophages or null cells.

Adjuvant Material that, when given with antigen, enhances the normal immune response.

Affinity A measure of the binding strength between an antibody-combining site and an epitope. It is derived through the law of mass action and is expressed in liters per mole.

Agammaglobulinemia The absence of all serum immunoglobulins.

Agglutination The clumping of particulate antigens such as bacteria or erythrocytes by antibody.

Allele One of two genes at a single locus.

Allergen An antigen that stimulates the production of reaginic antibodies.

Allergy A term that now encompasses any immunologically mediated adverse consequences of exposure to antigens, but which should be restricted to describing immediate (type I) hypersensitivity.

Alloantibody An antibody directed against antigens from a member of the same species as the animal making the antibody. This used to be called an isoantibody.

Allogeneic Genetically dissimilar but of the same species.

Allograft A graft between allogeneic animals. The term homograft was once employed in this respect.

Allotype Genetically controlled antigenic determinants found on protein molecules from some individuals of a species.

Anamnestic response A secondary immune response. The term is generally applied to a secondary response occurring some considerable time after the first exposure to an antigen.

Anaphylactoid reaction A shock syndrome that superficially resembles anaphylaxis but is not immunologically mediated.

Anaphylaxis A form of immediate (type I) hypersensitivity mediated by reaginic antibodies and resulting from the acute release of pharmacologically active agents from mast cells or basophils. The reaction may be local or systemic.

Anergy Absence of a cell-mediated immune reaction (usually a delayed hypersensitivity reaction in the skin) in an animal that has been sensitized.

Antibody Immunoglobulins formed in response to the introduction of material into the body that is recognized by the body as foreign. Their characteristic property is to combine under physiological conditions with the inducing material (antigen).

Antigen Material that can induce an immune response.

Antigenic determinant See *Epitope*.

Antiglobulin test A test that employs an antibody directed against immunoglobulins to agglutinate particles carrying nonagglutinating antibody on their surface. This is also called the Coombs' test, after the veterinarian who developed it.

Arthus reaction A local immune complex-mediated (type III hypersensitivity) inflammatory reaction in the skin.

Atopy A term used to describe the inherited tendency to develop immediate (type I) hypersensitivity found in some humans and dogs.

Attenuated Rendered less virulent for a specific host.

Autoantibody Antibody directed against epitopes on an animal's own tissues.

Autogenous vaccine A vaccine prepared from the organisms causing disease in an individual or herd and subsequently used in that same individual or herd in order to confer protection. This type of vaccine may be useful when immunity is highly strain-specific.

Autoimmune disease Disease caused by an immune response directed against an animal's own tissues.

Avidity A confusing term used by some to describe a property of antibody that determines the rate at which the antibody reacts with antigen, but used by others to refer to the strength of combination of an antiserum with an antigen. The term is best avoided.

Bacterin A preparation of killed bacteria used for immunization.

Bence-Jones proteins Proteins found in the urine of individuals with a myeloma. They precipitate on heating the urine to about 60°C and redissolve at higher temperatures. Bence Jones proteins are usually immunoglobulin light chains.

Blast cell A cell, usually a lymphocyte, that is enlarged prior to cell division. The nucleus is swollen, and the cytoplasm may be abundant.

Blastogenesis The production of dividing cells.

Blocking antibody A noncytotoxic, noncomplement-fixing antibody that can protect cells by coating them against cell-mediated destruction.

Capping The aggregation of cell membrane molecules at a restricted region of a cell surface.

Carrier An immunogenic molecule to which a hapten is bound.

Chemotaxis The movement of cells or organisms under the influence of an external chemical stimulus. It may be either positive or negative.

Chimera An animal that has been successfully populated either naturally or artificially by allogeneic cells.

Clone A population of identical cells or organisms derived from a single precursor cell or organism.

Complement A complex linked-enzyme and self-aggregating protein system that is activated by a number of factors, particularly antigen-antibody interaction, and that results in a wide variety of biological consequences such as cell membrane lysis and opsonization.

Conglutinin   A constituent of bovine serum, unrelated to immunoglobulins, that combines with fixed third component of complement. If this fixed C3 is attached to a particle such as an erythrocyte, then conglutinin will cause the erythrocyte to aggregate in a reaction known as conglutination.

Coombs' test   See *Antiglobulin test*

Cross-reaction   The reaction between an antibody and a different antigen that is different from the antigen that provoked the appearance of the antibody.

Cytophilic antibodies   Immunoglobulins that are able to bind to cell receptors by virtue of a specific site on their Fc region.

Delayed hypersensitivity   A cell-mediated skin reaction to injected antigen. So-called because the reaction does not reach maximal intensity until 24 to 48 hours after administration of antigen. An example of this is the tuberculin reaction.

Domains   Well defined regions of protein molecules.

Effector cell   A cell performing a specific function.

Endocytosis   The uptake of material by a cell.

Endotoxin   A lipopolysaccharide component of gram-negative bacterial cell walls that possesses nonspecific toxic activity.

Enhancement   The prolongation of allograft survival or promotion of tumor growth brought about by blocking antibodies.

Epitope   A site on an antigen molecule that stimulates an immune response and binds to antibody; an antigenic determinant.

Exotoxin   Soluble proteins, either secreted by living bacteria or released from the cytoplasm of dead organisms, that have a specific toxic effect. They are usually produced by gram-positive organisms.

Flocculation   A form of precipitation reaction seen when horse serum is used as a source of antibody, in which the precipitate appears as floccules and in which the ratio of antigen-antibody mixtures that give a precipitate is relatively restricted.

Gamma globulins   The group of plasma proteins that have the slowest electrophoretic mobility. It is within this group that antibodies (immunoglobulins) are found.

Globulins   Proteins precipitated by the addition of an equal volume of a saturated solution of ammonium sulfate to serum.

Gnotobiotic animal   An animal that is either germ-free or contaminated with a known bacterial population.

Hapten   A nonprotein molecule that can combine with specific antibody-combining sites but cannot, by itself, initiate an immune response.

Hemadsorption   The attachment of red blood cells to the surface of cultured animal cells following infection with certain viruses.

Hemagglutination   The bringing together of red blood cells by antibody or virus.

Hemagglutination inhibition   Inhibition of viral hemagglutination mediated by specific antibody against the virus.

Heterophile antigens   Epitopes found widely distributed in nature, e.g., on bacteria, plants and several species of animal.

Histocompatible   With identical transplantation antigens.

Histocompatibility antigens   Antigens found on the surface of nucleated cells, which are characteristic of an individual and which provoke allograft rejection and regulate immune reactions.

Homocytotropic antibodies   A term that includes cytophilic antibodies and all antibodies that attach specifically to cells in the same species as that in which they are made. By convention, use of this term is confined to those antibodies that bind to mast cells or basophils and mediate Type I Hypersensitivity—i.e., reaginic antibodies.

Homology region   See *Domain*.

Humoral   Found in body fluids. In immunology this refers specifically to antibodies and complement.

Hybridoma   A cultured cell line formed by fusion of myeloma cells with antibody-producing B cells.

Idiotope   One of the epitopes that makes up an idiotype.

Idiotype   Antigenic variability of a population of protein molecules within an individual animal. This type of variation is seen in immunoglobulins and is associated with the different amino acid sequences of the antibody-combining sites.

Immediate hypersensitivity   Reaginic antibody-mediated hypersensitivity in which the administration of antigen produces a detectable response within seconds or minutes.

Immune complex   An antigen-antibody complex.

Immunization   Strictly speaking, the administration of antigen to an animal with the intention of producing protective immunity. However, the term is now commonly used to describe the procedure for inducing an immune response.

Immunoconglutinins   Autoantibodies directed against fixed third or fourth components of complement. When these complement components are fixed to particles, the presence of immunoconglutinins may cause them to clump. This is called immunoconglutination.

Immunogen   A substance that is able to elicit an immune response.

Immunoglobulins   The class of proteins that have antibody activity.

Immunological tolerance   A form of immune response in which an animal becomes specifically unresponsive to an antigen and in which neither antibodies nor effector lymphocytes are produced.

Incomplete antibodies   Antibodies that, although they may bind to antigenic particles, are unable to link them together to cause agglutination. A preferable term is nonagglutinating antibodies. They may be detected by means of an antiglobulin test.

Interferons   A family of proteins that possess the ability to interfere with viral replication and regulate immune reactivity.

Isoantibody   See *Alloantibody*

Isogeneic   See *Syngeneic*

Isotype   Antigenic variability between related proteins found in all animals of the same species.

K cells   Non-T, non-B lymphocytes that can destroy target cells by ADCC.

Lectins   Proteins, usually of plant origin, that bind to specific monosaccharides. Most lectins used in immunology stimulate lymphocyte proliferation when they bind to cell membrane sugars.

Lymphokines   Lymphocyte-derived glycoproteins that control the activities of other cells. In this way they serve to regulate many aspects of the immune responses.

Lysosomes   Cytoplasmic vacuoles containing hydrolytic enzymes.

Lysozyme   An enzyme found in neutrophils, macrophages, tears and so forth that destroys the mucopeptides of bacterial cell walls.

Major histocompatibility complex (MHC)   A set of genes located close together on one chromosome and coding for histocompatibility antigens and some complement components.

Mitogen   A substance that stimulates cells to proliferate.

Mixed vaccine   A vaccine containing a mixture of different antigens. Used with the intention of promoting immunity against a number of microorganisms or toxins by a single injection. For instance, the vaccines for canine distemper, infectious hepatitis and *Leptospira* may be satisfactorily combined as a mixed vaccine.

Monoclonal antibody   Homogeneous immunoglobulin molecules secreted by a single clone of cells.

Monokines   Protein products of mononuclear phagocytes that influence the activities of other cell populations.

Myeloma   A tumor of plasma cells.

Natural antibodies   Antibodies found in serum in the absence of a known antigenic stimulus.

Natural killer (NK) cells   Ill-defined lymphoid cells found in normal animals that are capable of destroying tumor- or virus-infected cells.

Null cells   Lymphocytes that lack recognizable T or B cell surface markers.

Opsonin   A substance that binds to particles and facilitates their phagocytosis.

Passive hemagglutination test   A hemagglutination test brought about by antibody directed against an antigen artificially bound to the surface of erythrocytes. This may also be called indirect hemagglutination.

Passive immunity   Immunity conferred by administration of preformed antibodies.

Pathogenic microorganism   A microorganism that has the ability to cause disease in susceptible animals.

Phagocytosis   Eating by cells. The term encompasses a number of processes, including chemotaxis, adherence, ingestion and digestion of particles.

Pinocytosis   Literally, drinking by cells. A term used to indicate the engulfing of fluid droplets at the cell surface.

Precipitation   The bringing together of soluble antigen molecules by antibody to produce a visible precipitate. The visible precipitate will contain both antigen and antibody.

Premunition   A form of immunity seen in protozoan and some helminth infections that is dependent upon the continued presence of the parasite. Superinfection is prevented as long as parasites persist in the host, but the immunity disappears rapidly after parasite elimination.

Prozone   The absence of detectable immunological reaction in a test system in the presence of low dilutions of high-titered antiserum. This may be due to gross antibody excess or to inhibition of agglutination by complement or nonagglutinating antibody.

Pyrogen   A substance that causes fever.

Pyroninophilic   Stained by the pink dye pyronin. Pyronin has an affinity for RNA and thus detects ribosomes in cell cytoplasm. Since ribosomes are associated with protein synthesis, a cell with a pyroninophilic cytoplasm is a protein-synthesizing cell.

Reaginic antibody   Antibody that mediates Type I Hypersensitivity, i.e., IgE and some IgG subisotypes.

Rheumatoid factor   An autoantibody directed against normal immunoglobulin. It is found in many autoimmune diseases, especially rheumatoid arthritis and systemic lupus erythematosus.

Serology   The science of detection of antigens and antibodies.

Serovar   A strain within a group of organisms that can be identified by its distinctive serological properties. The term is synonymous with serotype.

Serum   The clear, yellow fluid expressed when blood has clotted and the clot has been permitted to contract.

Schwartzman reactions   Toxic reactions to bacterial endotoxins in which either a local or a systemic intravascular coagulation occurs. The reaction is precipitated by activation of the alternate pathway of complement.

Syngeneic   Genetically identical.

Titer   A measure of the number of antibody units per unit volume of serum. It is usually expressed as the reciprocal of the dilution of serum in the last tube in a series of increasing dilutions that shows the desired effect.

Tolerance   The failure of the immune system to respond to a specific antigen.

Toxoid   The modification of a toxin in such a way that its toxicity but not its immunogenicity is destroyed. This is usually done by treating the toxin with formaldehyde.

Vaccination   The administration of an antigen (vaccine) to an animal with the intention of stimulating a protective immune response

Viral hemagglutination   The clumping of red blood cells that occurs in the presence of certain viruses as a result of attachment of virus to the red blood cells.

Virulence   This term is used to quantitate the disease-producing power of a pathogenic organism.

Xenograft   A graft between xenogeneic individuals (i.e., individuals of different species).

1

General Features of the Immune Responses

Humoral Immune Responses
Cell-Mediated Immune Responses
Tolerance
Mechanism of the Immune Responses

When epidemics of diseases such as smallpox and plague spread through early human societies, most of those affected died but a few individuals would recover. It was rarely noticed that these recovered individuals never caught the disease again during subsequent epidemics. However, as early as 2650 BC, the Chinese had observed that individuals who recovered from smallpox were resistant to further attacks of this disease. Being practical people, they therefore deliberately infected infants with smallpox by rubbing the scabs from infected individuals into small cuts in their skin. Those infants that survived the resulting disease were protected from smallpox in later life. The risks inherent in this procedure were acceptable in an era of high infant mortality. On gaining experience with the technique it was found that the least severe reactions were obtained by using material from the mildest smallpox cases. As a result, mortality due to "inoculation" or "variolation," as it was called, was eventually reduced to about 1 per cent as compared with a mortality of about 20 per cent in clinical smallpox cases. Knowledge of inoculation spread westward to Europe in the early eight-

eenth century, and soon came to be widely employed.

Severe rinderpest outbreaks had been a common occurrence in cattle throughout western Europe since the ninth century and inevitably killed huge numbers of cattle. Since none of the traditional remedies appeared to work, and the skin lesions in affected cattle resembled those seen in smallpox, it was suggested in 1754 that inoculation might help. This involved soaking a piece of string with the nasal discharge from an animal with rinderpest and then inserting the string into an incision in the dewlap of the animal to be protected. The resulting disease was usually milder than the natural infection. The process proved very popular, and skilled inoculators travelled throughout Europe inoculating cattle and branding them to show that they were protected against rinderpest.

In 1798, Edward Jenner, an English physician, confirmed the suggestion of one of his patients, a dairy maid, that material from cowpox lesions could be substituted for smallpox in variolation. Since cowpox does not cause severe disease in humans, its use reduced the risks incurred in protecting against smallpox to insignificant levels. The effectiveness of this technique was such that it was used to eradicate smallpox from the world.

Once the general principles of inoculation were accepted, attempts were made to utilize a similar procedure to prevent animal diseases. Some of these were relatively successful. Thus, material derived from sheep-pox was successfully used to protect sheep in a process called ovination that was widely employed across Europe. On the other hand, administration of cowpox material to the nose of puppies to prevent canine distemper, although widely employed, was generally considered to be a failure. Attempts to utilize inoculation techniques persisted, as farmers tried to save at least some of their animals from diseases such as pleuropneumonia and hog cholera. Unfortunately, it soon became clear that these attempts generally resulted in the spread of the disease rather than its control.

The general implications of Jenner's observations on cowpox and the importance of reducing the ability of an immunizing organism to cause disease were not realized until 1879, when Louis Pasteur in France began to study the resistance of chickens to fowl cholera, a disease caused by a bacterium now known as *Pasteurella multocida* (Fig. 1–1). Pasteur had a culture of this organism that was accidentally allowed to "age" on a laboratory bench while his assistant went on holiday. When the assistant returned and tried to infect chickens with this aged culture, the birds failed to contract the disease. Being short of funds, Pasteur kept these same chickens for a second experiment in which they were challenged again, this time with a fresh culture of *P. multocida* known to be capable of killing chickens. To Pasteur's surprise the birds were resistant to the infection and did not die. On further investigation, Pasteur recognized that this phenomenon was similar in principle to Jenner's use of cowpox. He therefore called the process vaccination (*vacca* is Latin for "cow"). In vaccination, exposure of an animal to a strain of an organism that will not cause disease (an avirulent strain) can provoke an immune response that will protect the animal against a subsequent infection by a disease-producing (virulent) strain of the same, or closely related, organism. Having established the general principle of vaccination, Pasteur first applied it to anthrax. He rendered anthrax bacteria avirulent by growing them at an unusually high temperature.

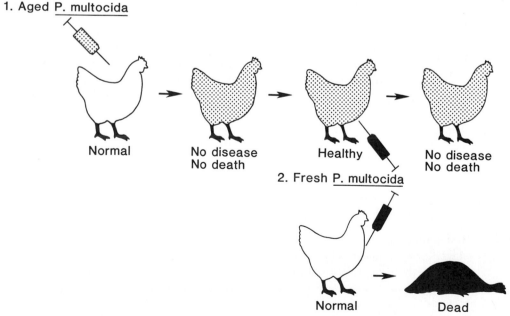

Figure 1–1. Pasteur's fowl cholera experiment. Birds inoculated with aged *P. multocida* did not die. When they were subsequently inoculated with fresh *P. multocida* they were found to be protected.

These "attenuated" organisms were then used to protect sheep against challenge with virulent anthrax bacteria. Pasteur also developed a successful rabies vaccine by allowing spinal cords taken from rabies-infected rabbits to dry, and then using the dried cords as his vaccine material. The drying process effectively rendered the rabies virus avirulent.

Although Jenner and Pasteur both used avirulent living organisms in their vaccines, it was not long before Salmon, working in the United States, demonstrated that a heat-sterilized culture of a bacterium called *Salmonella choleraesuis* (then known as *Bacillus suipestifer* and believed to be the cause of hog cholera) could protect pigeons against the disease caused by that organism, and Von Behring and Kitasato showed that filtrates taken from cultures of the tetanus bacillus (*Clostridium tetani*) could be used to give effective protection against tetanus.

HUMORAL IMMUNE RESPONSES

After Pasteur had discovered that it was possible to produce immunity to infectious agents by vaccination, it was soon recognized that the substances that provided this resistance could be found in blood serum. For example, if serum is obtained from a horse that has been vaccinated against tetanus toxin and is then injected into a normal horse, the normal horse will become resistant to tetanus for several weeks. Serum derived from immune horses in this way is known as tetanus immune globulin or tetanus antitoxin and is widely used for the prevention of tetanus.

The protective factors found in the serum of an immunized animal are known as antibodies. Antibodies against tetanus toxin are not found in normal horse serum but are produced by the horse as a result of exposure to tetanus toxin. Tetanus toxin is an example of a foreign substance that stimulates antibody production. The general term for such substances is antigen. If an antigen is injected into an animal, then antibodies will be produced that can combine with that antigen. Antibodies usually only combine with the antigen that stimulates their production. For example, the antibodies produced by exposure to tetanus toxin react only with tetanus toxin. If serum containing these antibodies is mixed in a test tube with a solution of tetanus toxin, then a visible precipitate will develop as a result of the combination of antibody with the toxin. In addition, the antibody neutralizes the toxin so that it is no longer toxic for animals. In this way antibodies protect animals against the lethal effects of tetanus toxin.

The time course of the immune response to tetanus toxin can be followed by bleeding a horse at intervals after vaccination (Fig. 1–2). The blood is allowed to clot and, once the clot has contracted, the clear serum is removed. The amount of antibody in the serum may be estimated either by measuring the amount of precipitate formed on adding toxin or, alternatively, by measuring the ability of the serum to neutralize a fixed amount of toxin. Both methods yield approximately the same results. Following a single injection of toxin (or its chemically neutralized derivative, tetanus toxoid) into a horse that has never been previously exposed to it, no antibody is detectable for several days. This is known as the lag period. Antibodies first become detectable about one week after the injection, and their level in serum then climbs to reach a peak by 10 to 14 days before declining and disappearing within a few weeks. The amount of antibody formed, and hence the amount of protection conferred, during this first or "primary" response is relatively small.

If, sometime later, a second dose of toxin is injected into the same horse and the antibody response again followed, then the lag period lasts for no more than two or three days. The amount of antibody in serum then rises rapidly to a high level before declining slowly. Antibodies may be detected for many months or years after this injection. A third dose of toxin given to the same animal results in an immune response characterized by an even shorter lag period and a still higher and more prolonged antibody response. The stimulation of resistance to disease through the use of repeated injections of antigen in this way forms the basis of current vaccination techniques employed against infectious diseases.

As we have seen, the response of an animal

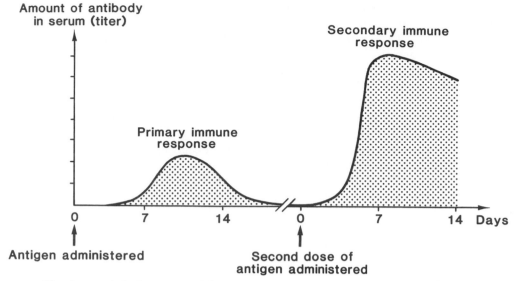

Figure 1–2. The characteristic time course of the immune response to an antigen as measured by serum antibody levels. Note the differences between a primary and a secondary immune response.

to a second dose of antigen is very different from the first in that it occurs much more quickly, antibodies reach very much higher levels, and it lasts for much longer. This "secondary" response is specific in that it can be provoked only by an antigen identical to that given first. A secondary response may be provoked many months or years after the first injection of antigen, although its magnitude does tend to decline as time passes. A secondary response can also be induced even though the response of the animal to the first injection of antigen was so weak as to be undetectable. These features of the secondary response indicate that the antibody-forming system possesses the ability to "remember" previous exposure to an antigen. For this reason, the secondary immune response is sometimes known as an anamnestic response (*anamnesko* is Greek for "recollection").

If a second dose of antigen is given to an animal that still has serum antibodies remaining after its primary immune response, then the level of these antibodies may drop for a few days before the secondary immune response gets under way. This "negative phase" occurs as a result of the injected antigen binding and removing antibodies from the circulation. It should also be noted that re-

peated injections of antigen do not lead indefinitely to greater and greater immune responses. The total level of antibodies in serum is relatively well controlled, so that they tend to plateau, at a constant level, even after multiple doses of antigen or exposure to many different antigens.

CELL-MEDIATED IMMUNE RESPONSES

If a piece of living tissue such as skin is surgically removed from one animal and grafted onto another of the same species, it usually survives only for a few days before being destroyed by the recipient. This process is significant, not so much for the difficulties it presents to the transplantation surgeon but because it demonstrates the existence of a mechanism whereby foreign cells, differing only slightly from an animal's own normal cells, are rapidly recognized and eliminated. Even cells with minor structural abnormalities may be recognized as foreign by the immune system and eliminated though they are otherwise apparently healthy. These abnormal cells include old red cells, virus-infected cells and cancer cells. The immune response to foreign cells as shown by graft rejection may therefore be considered to indicate the existence of a surveillance system that identifies and removes abnormal cells.

If a piece of skin is transplanted from one dog to a second, unrelated dog, it will survive for about 10 days. The grafted skin will initially appear to be healthy, and blood vessels will develop between the graft and its host. By about one week, however, these new blood vessels will begin to degenerate, the blood supply to the graft will be cut off and the graft will eventually die and be shed. This slow rejection process is known as a first-set reaction (Fig. 1–3). If a second graft is taken from the original donor and placed on the same recipient, then that second graft will survive for no longer than one or two days before being rejected. This rapid rejection process is known as a second-set reaction. Thus the rejection of a first graft is relatively weak and slow and analogous to the primary antibody response, whereas a second graft stimulates very rapid and powerful rejection similar in many ways to the secondary antibody response. Graft rejection, like antibody formation, is specific, in that a second-set reaction occurs only if the second graft is from the same donor as the first. Like antibody formation, the graft rejection process also possesses a memory, since a second graft may be rapidly

rejected many months or years after loss of the first.

The graft rejection process is, however, not entirely identical to the process involved in protection against tetanus toxin, since it cannot be transferred from a sensitized to a normal animal by means of serum antibodies. The ability to mount a second-set reaction to a graft can only be transferred between animals by means of living cells. The cells that can do this are known as lymphocytes and can be found in the spleen, lymph nodes or peripheral blood. We must therefore conclude that the process of graft rejection is mediated primarily by lymphocytes and not by serum antibodies.

TOLERANCE

In order to provoke an immune response, an antigen such as tetanus toxin or a graft from another animal must be recognized as being foreign. It is an absolute corollary to this that the immune system must be able to recognize its own cells as being not-foreign, and it must not mount an immune response against them. In other words, the immune system must be tolerant to self-antigens. If this tolerance breaks down, then disease will occur (autoimmune disease) as either antibodies or lympho-

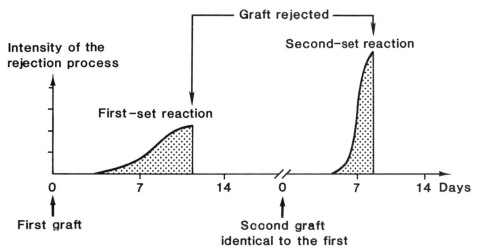

Figure 1–3. The characteristic time course of the rejection of a foreign skin graft. Notice how similar this diagram is to Figure 1–2.

cytes destroy normal cells in an attempt to eliminate the offending antigen. Tolerance occurs in both the cell-mediated and antibody-mediated immune systems and can be considered another form of normal immune response. For example, tolerance, as shown by an inability to react to a specific antigen, may be induced by an appropriately administered dose of that antigen. Tolerance is specific for the inducing antigen and, like other forms of the immune response, may be boosted only by re-exposure to that same antigen. If an animal is not re-exposed to that antigen, then tolerance is gradually lost.

The immune responses may therefore be considered to consist of three general types, the antibody-mediated responses, the cell-mediated responses and tolerance.

If we consider why an immune system is needed, it is apparent that its primary task must be the protection of the body against invasive organisms. Indeed, if the immune system fails to develop, or if it is destroyed by a virus (such as happens in AIDS), then an animal will rapidly succumb to severe recurrent infections. It has been pointed out earlier, however, that it is important to identify and eliminate abnormal cells through self-surveillance. It is tempting to suggest therefore that the cell-mediated immune responses are active in surveillance whereas the antibody-mediated responses protect against invasion by micro-organisms. Such a distinction is not absolute, however, since antibodies may contribute to graft rejection and cell-mediated immune responses can participate in resistance to many infectious diseases. Tolerance, on the other hand, represents an essential protective mechanism that serves to prevent an animal from being damaged by an indiscriminate immune response.

MECHANISM OF THE IMMUNE RESPONSES

In some ways the immune system may be compared to a totalitarian state in which foreigners are expelled and citizens who behave themselves are tolerated, but those who "deviate" are eliminated. While this analogy must not be pursued too far, it is apparent that such regimes possess a number of characteristic features. These include border defenses and a police force that keeps the population under surveillance and promptly eliminates dissidents. Organizations of this type also tend to develop a pass system, so that foreigners not possessing certain identifying features are rapidly detected and dealt with.

Similarly, when a foreign antigen enters the body, it first must be trapped and processed so that it can be recognized as being foreign. If so recognized, then this information must be conveyed either to the antibody-forming system or to the cell-mediated immune system. These systems must then respond promptly by the production of specific antibody or cells that are capable of eliminating the antigen. The immune system must also remember this event so that on subsequent exposure to the same antigen, its response will be faster and more efficient. In our totalitarian state analogy, the information would be filed away for future use.

We can therefore consider the basic requirements of the immune systems to include four components (Fig. 1–4). First, a method of trapping and processing antigen. Second, a mechanism for reacting specifically to the antigen or, in other words, antigen-sensitive cells. Third, cells to produce antibodies or to participate in the cell-mediated immune responses. Fourth, cells to retain the memory of the event and to react specifically to the antigen in future encounters. All of these components can be recognized within the body, and each is associated with a specific type of cell. Antigen is trapped, processed and eventually eliminated by cells known as macrophages. Lymphocytes are able to recognize this processed antigen and are thus antigen-sensitive cells. Lymphocytes also function as memory cells and therefore initiate a secondary immune response. The cells that mediate the cell-mediated responses are also identified as lymphocytes, while antibody-producing cells are derived from lymphocytes and are known as plasma cells.

In subsequent chapters we will examine each of these basic components of the immune system in turn.

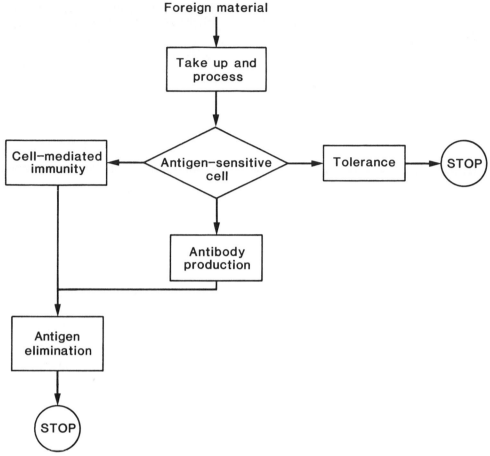

Figure 1–4. A simple flow diagram showing the essential features of the immune responses.

WHERE TO GO FOR ADDITIONAL INFORMATION

Immunology

Basic Immunology Texts Describing the Immune System in Detail

Barrett JT. 1983. Textbook of Immunology, 4th Ed. C.V. Mosby Company, St. Louis. A very readable standard immunology text.

Hood LE, Weissman IL, Wood WB and Wilson WB. 1984. Immunology. Benjamin Cummings, Menlo Park, California. A text focusing on the molecular and cellular aspects of immunology.

Klein J. 1982. Immunology. The Science of Self Non-self Discrimination. John Wiley and Sons, New York. A highly acclaimed general text.

Nisonoff A. 1984. Introduction to Molecular Immunology. Sinauer Associates, Sunderland, MA. Introductory coverage of immunochemistry.

Paul WE. 1984. Fundamental Immunology. Raven Press, New York. An advanced text with a sophisticated treatment of contemporary immunology.

Roitt I, Brostoff J and Male D. 1985. Immunology. C.V. Mosby Company, St. Louis. A text characterized by the extensive use of colored diagrams.

Tizard I. 1984. Immunology, An Introduction. CBS College Publishing, Philadelphia. A very basic immunology text.

Clinical Immunology Texts

Bellanti JA. 1985. Immunology III. W.B. Saunders Company, Philadelphia. An excellent account of the application of immunology to clinical problems.

Dixon, FJ and Fisher DW. 1983. The Biology of Immunologic Diseases. Sinauer Associates, Sunderland, MA. A beautifully produced text.

Stites DP, Stobo JD, Fudenberg HH, and Wells JV. 1984. Basic and Clinical Immunology. Lange Medical Publications, Los Altos, California. A very comprehensive text.

Series in Immunology

Advances in Immunology. Academic Press, New York.

Immunological Reviews. Munksgaard, Copenhagen.

Progress in Allergy. S. Karger, Basel.

Journals

If you can afford only one general immunology journal, then Immunology Today is probably the most useful and current. Other important journals include: Cellular Immunology, Clinical and Experimental Immunology, Infection and Immunity, Immunology, Journal of Experimental Medicine, Journal of Immunology, Parasite Immunology as well as Science and Nature.

Veterinary Immunology

Many recent review articles will be found cited at the end of each chapter. However, major reviews on veterinary immunology as a whole can be found in:

Veterinary Clinics of North America (1978) 8:4, W.B. Saunders Company, Philadelphia.

Advances in Veterinary Science and Comparative Medicine (1979) 23, Academic Press, New York.

The Ruminant Immune System (1981) Adv. Exp. Med. Biol. 137, Butler J.E. ed., Plenum, New York.

Colloquium on Clinical Immunology (1982) JAVMA 181, 181, 962. (November 16 issue.)

Journals

Veterinary Immunology research is effectively covered in Veterinary Immunology and Immunopathology. However, many veterinary journals carry articles of interest to immunologists. Some of the most important are Acta Veterinaria Scandinavica, American Journal of Veterinary Research, Australian Veterinary Journal, British Veterinary Journal, Canadian Journal of Comparative Medicine, Journal of the American Animal Hospital Association, Journal of the American Veterinary Medical Association, Journal of Comparative Pathology, Research in Veterinary Science, Veterinary Bulletin, Veterinary Pathology and The Veterinary Record.

I

THE IMMUNE SYSTEM

2
Trapping and Processing Foreign Material

Animals are faced with the task of permitting the free access of nutrients and oxygen to the body while at the same time excluding potentially dangerous organisms such as bacteria, parasites and viruses. In order to do this, several different protective mechanisms have developed, especially at body surfaces (Chapter 12). In addition, systems have evolved within the body to trap and then eliminate any material that succeeds in getting through the outer defenses. These trapping systems act through cells that are able to bind, ingest and destroy foreign material through a process known as phagocytosis (Greek for "eating by cells"). The phagocytic cells of mammals belong to two complementary systems. One system, the myeloid system, consists of cells that act rapidly but are incapable of sustained effort. The second system, the mononuclear-phagocytic system, consists of cells that act more slowly but are capable of repeated phagocytosis. The cells of the mononuclear-phagocytic system process antigen for the immune response.

THE MYELOID SYSTEM

The major cell type in the myeloid system is the polymorphonuclear neutrophil granulocyte (otherwise known as the neutrophil). Neutrophils are formed in the bone marrow and migrate to the blood stream, where they spend about 12 hours before moving on into the tissues. Their total life-span is only a few days. Neutrophils constitute about 60 to 75 per cent of the blood leukocytes in man and carnivores but only about 20 to 30 per cent in ruminants.

Structure of Neutrophils

When suspended in blood, neutrophils are round cells about 12μm in diameter. They possess a finely granular cytoplasm at the center of which is a sausage-like or segmented nucleus (Fig. 2–1). Within the cytoplasm are two distinct types of granules (Table 2–1). The primary, or azurophil, granules are electron-dense structures that contain microbicidal enzymes such as myeloperoxidase and lysozyme, neutral proteases such as elastase, and acid hydrolases such as β-glucuronidase and cathepsin B. The secondary, or specific, granules contain enzymes such as lysozyme and collagenase and the iron binding protein lactoferrin. Neutrophils possess a small Golgi apparatus and some mitochondria but no ribosomes or rough endoplasmic reticulum.

Functions of Neutrophils

Phagocytosis

The major function of neutrophils is the destruction of foreign material through the process of phagocytosis. This process is best described by arbitrarily dividing it into stages: chemotaxis, adherence, ingestion and digestion (Fig. 2–2). The first stage in the phagocytic process is the directed movement of neutrophils under the influence of external chemical gradients. This movement is called chemotaxis. When exposed to such a gradient,

Table 2–1 THE CONTENTS OF NEUTROPHIL GRANULES

Primary granules	Myeloperoxidase
	Lysozyme
	Elastase
	Cathepsin G
	Acid hydrolases
Secondary granules	Lysozyme
	Collagenase
	Lactoferrin

neutrophils become polarized and migrate toward the highest concentration of the attractant. Neutrophils are attracted by many bacterial products, by factors released by damaged cells, by metabolites of arachidonic acid known as leukotrienes (Chapter 19), by a peptide generated by activation of the complement system known as C5a (Chapter 10) and by mast cell–derived factors (Chapter 20).

Once a neutrophil encounters a foreign particle, it must bind it firmly. This adherence may not happen spontaneously, since both cells and particles suspended in body fluids have a negative charge (the zeta potential) and hence repel each other. It is therefore necessary to neutralize the negative charge by coating the particle with a positively charged protein. Examples of such proteins include antibody molecules and a protein called C3 (the third component of complement—Chapter 10). Particles coated by antibody or C3 therefore have a reduced zeta potential, enabling them to make close contact with negatively charged neutrophils. Neutrophils also

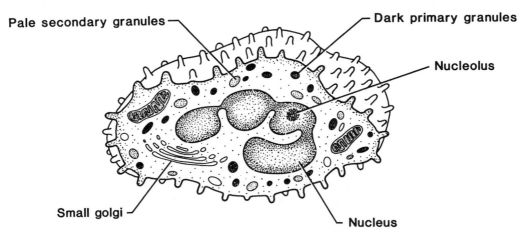

Figure 2–1. The major structural features of a polymorphonuclear neutrophil granulocyte.

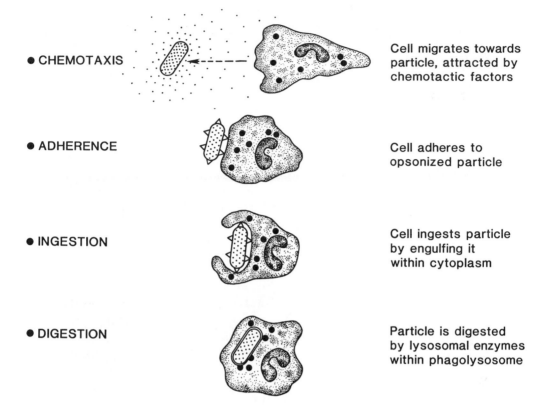

● CHEMOTAXIS — Cell migrates towards particle, attracted by chemotactic factors

● ADHERENCE — Cell adheres to opsonized particle

● INGESTION — Cell ingests particle by engulfing it within cytoplasm

● DIGESTION — Particle is digested by lysosomal enzymes within phagolysosome

Figure 2–2. Different stages in the process of phagocytosis.

carry specific receptors for both antibody and C3 on their surface. As a result, particles coated with these molecules will bind to neutrophils by these receptors.

Another mechanism that assists in promoting contact between particles and neutrophils is trapping. Normally, particles are free to float away when they encounter a neutrophil in blood plasma. If a particle is lodged in tissues however, it may be trapped between a neutrophil and another surface and thus prevented from escaping. This process is known as surface phagocytosis.

Once attached firmly to the neutrophil membrane, an adherent particle stimulates local infolding of the cell membrane as a result of contraction of actin and myosin filaments attached to cytoplasmic microtubules. The particle is therefore drawn into the cell and enclosed in a vacuole called a phagosome (Fig. 2–3). The ease with which this engulfment is accomplished depends, in part, on the nature of the particle surface. In general, it is es-

sential that the particle be more hydrophobic than the cell. Highly hydrophobic bacteria such as *Mycobacterium bovis* are spontaneously taken into cells. In contrast, *Streptococcus pneumoniae*, which possesses a hydrophilic carbohydrate capsule, is poorly phagocytosed. Fortunately, antibodies and C3 can coat *S. pneumoniae* and render it hydrophobic, so that it may then be readily engulfed. Substances such as antibodies and C3 that promote attachment and engulfment of particles in this way are known as opsonins (*opson* is Greek for "food preparation").

Destruction of the ingested particle occurs through two distinct mechanisms. Once the particle is attached to the neutrophil membrane, the primary granules (or lysosomes) rapidly migrate through the cytoplasm, fuse with the phagosome and release their enzymes. (The complete vacuole is then known as a phagolysosome.) The enzymes contained in these granules can digest bacterial walls and can kill most microorganisms, but, as

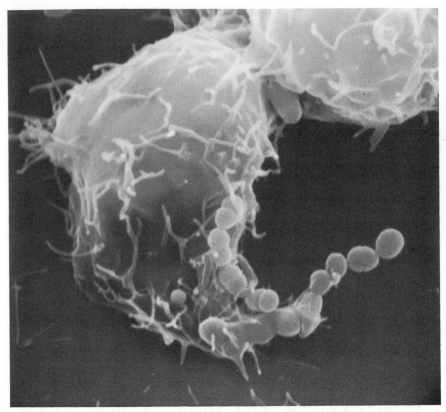

Figure 2–3. A scanning electron micrograph of a bovine milk neutrophil ingesting *Streptococcus agalactiae*. Note how a film of neutrophil cytoplasm appears to flow over the surface of the bacterium. × 5000.

might be expected, variations in susceptibility are observed. Gram-positive organisms susceptible to lysozyme are rapidly destroyed. Gram-negative bacteria such as *Escherichia coli* survive somewhat longer, since their outer wall is relatively resistant to digestion. Some organisms such as *Brucella abortus* and *Listeria monocytogenes* are so resistant to the lethal effects of the lysosomal enzymes that they may multiply within phagocytic cells.

The Respiratory Burst

Of more importance in protecting animals are the oxidative bactericidal mechanisms of the cell (Fig. 2–4). When a particle attaches to the surface of a neutrophil it activates the enzyme NADPH oxidase which is found on the cell surface. This enzyme catalyzes the conversion of NADPH (the reduced form of NADP, nicotinamide adenine dinucleotide phosphate) to NADP. When this happens electrons are released. One of these electrons first combines with a molecule of oxygen to form superoxide anion thus:

$$NADPH + 2O_2 \rightarrow NADP^+ + H^+ + 2O_2^-$$

The NADP generated by the NADPH oxidase accelerates the hexose monophosphate shunt, a metabolic pathway that converts sucrose to a pentose and CO_2, and releases energy for use by the cell. The superoxide anion is destroyed by the enzyme, superoxide dismutase, gaining a second electron and reacting with hydrogen ions to form hydrogen peroxide (H_2O_2).

$$O_2^- + O_2^- + 2H^+ \rightarrow H_2O_2 + O_2$$

The hydrogen peroxide is converted to highly potent bactericidal compounds through the action of the enzyme myeloperoxidase. The myeloperoxidase system is believed to be the most important bactericidal system in neutrophils. The enzyme is found in large amounts in the primary granules. It catalyzes several oxidative reactions but the most important one is that between hydrogen peroxide and intracellular chloride ions thus;

$$H_2O_2 + Cl^- \rightarrow H_2O + OCl^-$$

The hypochloride ions (OCl^-) kill bacteria by oxidizing their proteins and they also enhance the bactericidal activities of the lysosomal enzymes.

A second important bactericidal pathway is activated by the reaction of superoxide with hydrogen peroxide. This reaction generates hydroxyl radicals and singlet oxygen.

$$H_2O_2 + O_2^- \rightarrow 2OH^\cdot + \cdot O_2$$

The hydroxyl radical is very unstable and reacts with lipids to form bactericidal hydroperoxides. Singlet oxygen is a form of oxygen in which one electron is shifted into a high energy orbit. Because of its distorted electron shell, singlet oxygen is very unstable and also

reacts with bacterial lipids to form toxic hydroperoxides. The importance of the respiratory burst is shown by the observation that animals deficient in either superoxide dismutase or in myeloperoxidase suffer from severe recurrent bacterial infections (Chapter 26).

The Fate of Neutrophils

Neutrophils possess a limited reserve of energy, which cannot be replenished. Therefore, although neutrophils may be very active immediately after release from the bone marrow, they are rapidly exhausted and are usually capable of undertaking only a limited number of phagocytic events. Thus, neutrophils may be considered a first line of defense, moving rapidly toward foreign material and destroying it promptly but being incapable of sustained effort. Fortunately, a second line of defense is available—the mononuclear-phagocytic sys-

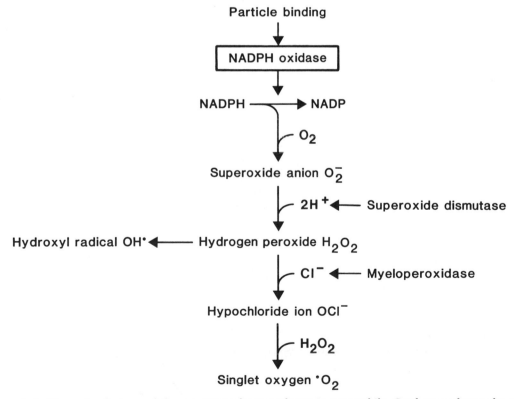

Figure 2–4. The major features of the respiratory burst pathway in neutrophils. Catalase performs the same function as myeloperoxidase within macrophages.

tem. Since neutrophils usually destroy all ingested foreign material, they cannot process antigen in preparation for presentation to antigen-sensitive cells.

Eosinophils

The second major cell type of the myeloid system is the eosinophil, so-called because its cytoplasmic granules stain intensely with eosin, a red dye. Eosinophils develop within the bone marrow before migrating into the blood stream, where they circulate with a half-life of only 30 minutes. (For every circulating eosinophil there is a reserve of about 500 stored in the tissues.) They subsequently migrate into the tissues, where they have a half-life of about 12 days. The proportion of eosinophils among the blood leukocytes varies with the parasite burden of an animal but ranges from 2 per cent in dogs to about 10 per cent in cattle.

Eosinophils are less efficient than neutrophils at phagocytosis, but they do possess cytoplasmic granules and mount a marked respiratory burst when appropriately provoked. Their large granules contain an arginine-rich basic protein, a peroxidase, a lyso-

phospholipase and a cationic protein. All of which are able to kill the larvae of some parasitic helminths by disrupting their cuticles (Chapter 17). Eosinophils can be activated by products of T-lymphocytes (Chapter 7) so that their ability to destroy invading parasites is enhanced.

Basophils

Basophils are the least numerous myeloid cells in the blood of domestic animals, constituting about 0.5 per cent of blood leukocytes. Their cytoplasmic granules stain intensely with basophilic dyes such as hematoxylin. Basophils function in the same way as mast cells (Chapter 20)—namely, to provoke acute inflammation at sites of antigen deposition.

THE MONONUCLEAR-PHAGOCYTIC SYSTEM (Fig. 2–5)

If an animal is injected intravenously with a suspension of carbon particles such as those found in India ink, these particles are taken up from the blood stream by cells throughout the body. Aschoff, the German scientist who

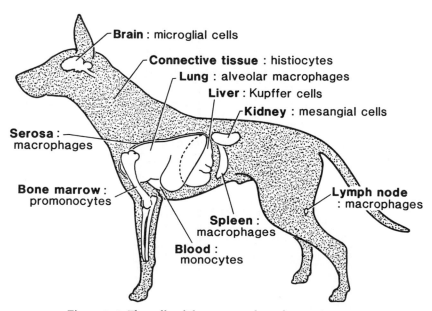

Figure 2–5. The cells of the mononuclear-phagocytic system.

discovered this phenomenon, considered that these cells collectively constituted a body system, which he named the reticuloendothelial system. It is now clear, however, that some of the cells that take up carbon only do so inadvertently and that this is not their prime function. These cells include epidermal cells, intestinal epithelial cells and vascular endothelial cells. The cells whose major function is the removal of foreign material and cell debris are but one component of Aschoff's original reticuloendothelial system, and they are now considered to belong to the mononuclear-phagocytic system. The mononuclear-phagocytic system consists of cells called macrophages, each containing a single, rounded nucleus. In contrast to neutrophils, the macrophages of the mononuclear-phagocytic system are capable of sustained phagocytic activity, they do process antigen in preparation for the immune response and they make a direct contribution to the repair of tissue damage by removing dead, dying and damaged tissue.

Macrophages are widely distributed throughout the body. Immature macrophages found in the blood stream are called monocytes. They normally constitute about 5 per cent of the total leukocyte population. Mature macrophages may be found in connective tissue, where they are known as histiocytes; they may be found lining the sinusoids of the liver, where they are called Kupffer cells. The macrophages of the brain are called microglia, and those of the lung are called alveolar macrophages. Large numbers of macrophages are found in the spleen, bone marrow

and lymph nodes in close association with sinusoidal endothelium. Nevertheless, irrespective of their name or location, they are all macrophages and they are all part of the mononuclear-phagocytic system.

Structure of Macrophages

Because of their various habitats, macrophages occur in a wide variety of shapes. When in suspension, however, they are round cells, about 14 to 20 μm in diameter. They possess abundant cytoplasm, at the center of which is a single, round, bean-shaped or indented nucleus (Figs. 2–6 and 2–7; see also Fig. 7–7). The perinuclear cytoplasm contains mitochondria, large numbers of lysosomes, some rough endoplasmic reticulum and a Golgi apparatus, indicating an ability to synthesize and secrete protein (Table 2–2). The peripheral cytoplasm is usually devoid of organelles, and in living macrophages appears to be in continuous movement, forming and reforming veil-like ruffles. Macrophages adhere tenaciously to glass surfaces, on which they spread by sending out long, thin cytoplasmic filaments. Some macrophages show variations from this basic structure. Thus, peripheral blood monocytes tend to have round nuclei, which elongate as the cells mature; alveolar macrophages rarely possess rough endoplasmic reticulum, but their cytoplasm tends to be full of granules. The microglia of the central nervous system have rod-shaped nuclei and possess very long,

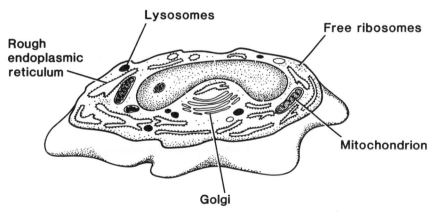

Figure 2–6. The major structural features of a macrophage.

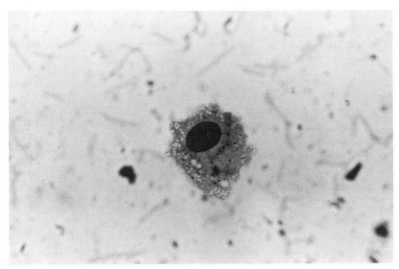

Figure 2–7. A bovine alveolar macrophage containing phagocytosed *Pasteurella hemolytica*. × 900. (From a specimen kindly provided by Dr. B. N. Wilkie.)

cytoplasmic processes that are lost when the cell is stimulated into activity by tissue damage.

As a result of the cell-mediated immune response to certain organisms, macrophages may enlarge and their lysosomes increase greatly in number (see Fig. 7–7). These are then known as activated macrophages. When foreign material persists for long periods within the body, macrophages may accumulate in large numbers around the persistent material, giving an epithelium-like appearance on histological examination. These cells are therefore referred to as epithelioid cells (Chapter 23). Epithelioid cells are usually packed closely together and hence are polygonal in shape. They possess abundant cytoplasm containing many lysosomes and much endoplasmic reticulum. Epithelioid cells may fuse together to form multinucleated giant cells when attempting to enclose large particles that cannot be ingested by a single cell.

Life History of Macrophages

All of the cells of the mononuclear-phagocytic system arise from bone marrow stem cells known as promonocytes. Promonocytes develop into monocytes, which enter the blood stream, where they remain for only a few days (three days in rodents) before entering tissues and developing into macrophages. Under some circumstances and in some species, macrophages may divide to yield daughter macrophages. Tissue macrophages are relatively long-lived cells, replacing themselves at a rate of about 1 per cent per day unless called upon to ingest foreign particles. Their life-span in that case depends upon the nature of the ingested material. If, for instance, the ingested particles are easily digested by lysosomal en-

Table 2–2 THE SECRETIONS OF MACROPHAGES

Enzymes	Lysozyme
	Neutral proteases
	Acid hydrolases
Complement components	C1, C2, C3, C4, C5, I, B, P
Transferrin	
Fibronectin	
Reactive oxygen metabolites	
Prostanoids	Leukotrienes
	Prostaglandins
	Platelet activating factor
Monokines	Interleukin 1
	Interferon α
	Fibroblast stimulating factors
Enzyme inhibitors	α2-macroglobulin
	α1-protease inhibition

zymes, the macrophage life-span may be unaffected. Some ingested particles, such as the carbon injected in tattoo marks, may be chemically inert. In this case, macrophages may survive for a long time with the inert particle inside, although they may fuse to form giant cells in a further attempt to eliminate the foreign material. In some circumstances, such as after intravenous injection of India ink, macrophages may carry the particles to the lung or intestine and from there into the bronchiolar or intestinal lumen whence they are eliminated from the body. In contrast, other particles, although readily phagocytosed, are toxic to macrophages. For example, asbestos particles kill macrophages after phagocytosis and so must be rephagocytosed repeatedly. This continuing destruction of macrophages leads to excessive release of lysosomal enzymes and reactive oxygen metabolites and results in chronic tissue destruction, inflammation and granulation tissue formation (Chapter 19).

Functions of Macrophages

The major functions of macrophages are to promote the defense of the body by mediating phagocytosis, fever, inflammation and immunity, and to promote the healing of tissues (Fig. 2–8.) Thus in addition to being phagocytic, macrophages secrete factors that cause a fever and which influence the inflammatory response and they process foreign material in such a way that it can provoke an immune response.

Phagocytosis

Phagocytosis by macrophages is a very similar process to that described previously for neutrophils. Macrophages are chemotactically attracted not only to microbial products and the products of immune reactions, but also to factors released by damaged cells, especially damaged neutrophils. Neutrophils thus not only reach and attack foreign material first, but in dying serve to attract macrophages to the site of invasion. Macrophages possess receptors for C3 and for antibodies (immunoglobulins). As a result, particles opsonized with either of these can bind firmly to macrophages. Antigen is destroyed within macrophages in a manner similar to the process in neutrophils. However, the respiratory burst is much less intense within macrophages. Mature macrophages do not contain myeloperox-

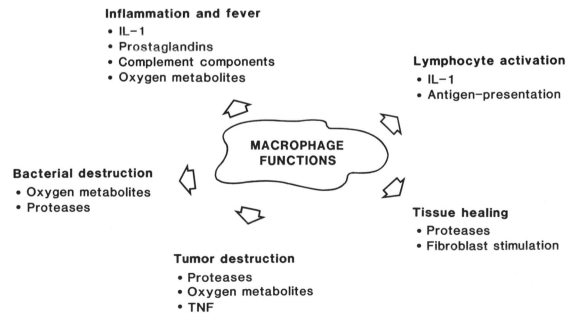

Inflammation and fever
- IL–1
- Prostaglandins
- Complement components
- Oxygen metabolites

Lymphocyte activation
- IL–1
- Antigen–presentation

Bacterial destruction
- Oxygen metabolites
- Proteases

MACROPHAGE FUNCTIONS

Tissue healing
- Proteases
- Fibroblast stimulation

Tumor destruction
- Proteases
- Oxygen metabolites
- TNF

Figure 2–8. The many different functions of macrophages.

idase, but they do contain catalase, which may have an equivalent function.

Macrophages, Fever and the Body's Response to Injury

When macrophages are stimulated by bacteria and their products or by tissue damage, they secrete a protein called interleukin 1. Interleukin 1 is responsible for stimulating a general response to injury. Thus it provokes a fever, it mobilizes neutrophils and it alters the body's metabolic pathways, mobilizing resources to fight off invasion. The functions of interleukin 1 are discussed in detail in Chapter 19.

Macrophages and Inflammation

Macrophages are active participants in the inflammatory process. They are attracted to sites of microbial invasion and in addition to helping to eliminate the invaders, they secrete factors such as the complement components, C2, C3, C4 and C5 (Chapter 10), the enzymes lysozyme (Chapter 15), collagenase, elastase and plasminogen activators, hormones such as cyclic AMP and pharmacologically active agents such as the prostaglandins, leukotrienes and platelet activating factor. They are also important in the healing process, since they influence the activities of fibroblasts. Inflammation is discussed in detail in Chapter 19.

Antigen Processing by Macrophages

If all foreign material were totally ingested, digested and destroyed by phagocytic cells, there would be no necessity and no stimulus for the immune responses. It is clear, therefore, that at least some intact antigen must persist in order to stimulate antigen-sensitive cells. When the fate of radioactively labeled antigen is closely followed, it is found that, although most antigen is digested and destroyed, a few molecules remain intact within some macrophages and may be found on the cell surface membrane. The subpopulation of macrophages that process antigen in this way possess characteristic surface proteins. These proteins are called the class II histocompatibility antigens and are discussed in Chapter 8. Antigen molecules may persist on the macrophage surface for a very long time. In that location they are able to effectively stimulate antigen-sensitive cells.

The processing of antigen by macrophages regulates the amount of foreign material that can reach antigen-sensitive cells. If antigen evades the macrophages and reaches the antigen-sensitive cells directly, then either tolerance will develop or the resulting immune response will be considerably poorer than normal.

Dendritic Cells

Throughout the body, but especially in lymphoid organs and in the skin, there exists a population of macrophage-like cells that are characterized by possessing an extensive array of long, filamentous cytoplasmic processes, lobulated nuclei and a clear cytoplasm containing, in some cases, characteristic granules called Birbeck granules. They are collectively known as dendritic cells. (In lymphoid organs these cells are called dendritic cells or interdigitating cells; in the skin they are called Langerhans cells [Fig. 2–9].) Dendritic cells have complement and antibody receptors but are poorly phagocytic. They can, however, adsorb antibody to their processes in such a way that it remains free to attach to antigen. As a result, dendritic cells coated with antibody form an extensive antigen-trapping web. Antigen trapped by dendritic cells is a very potent stimulant for antigen-sensitive cells, being about ten thousand times more efficient in this respect than unbound antigen. (This is because these cells have large amounts of class II histocompatibility antigens on their surface. See Chapter 8.) Since the presence of antibody is required for effective antigen trapping by these cells, the dendritic cell system can only process antigen after some antibody has been formed. The enhanced immune responses that occur following a second or subsequent dose of antigen are probably due, at least in part, to the efficiency of the dendritic cell system.

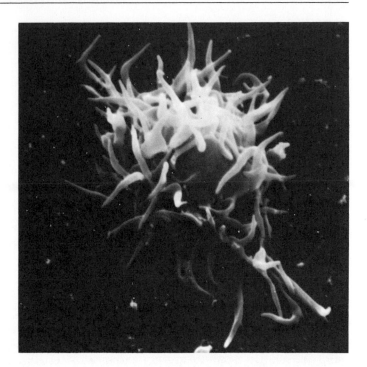

Figure 2–9. A scanning electron micrograph of what is believed to be a dendritic cell from a guinea pig lymph node. × 4000. (From Tizard IR and Holmes WJL. 1975. Proc Reticuloendothel Soc *17* 333–341. Used with permission.)

THE FATE OF FOREIGN MATERIAL

Particulate Antigens Given Intravenously

If colloidal particles, such as the carbon particles of India ink or those of a bacterial suspension, are injected intravenously, they will circulate for a period of time but will be progressively trapped and removed by the macrophages that line the blood sinusoids of the liver, spleen and bone marrow. Large viruses or bacteria may be cleared completely by a single passage through the liver. The spleen is a more effective filter than the liver but, being a much smaller organ, is quantitatively less important. Some of the injected particles may also be trapped in the capillary bed of the lung as they pass through that organ. The rate of clearance of particles from the circulation is regulated by the presence of opsonins. The most important nonspecific opsonin in the blood stream is a protein called fibronectin. If fibronectin levels drop, as happens after severe trauma, then clearance of bacteria from the blood stream is impaired. If an animal is injected intravenously with a very large dose of colloidal carbon, then fibronectin will be depleted and other particles (such as bacteria) will not be cleared from the blood stream. In this situation, the mononuclear-phagocytic system is said to be blockaded. Blockade as a result of depletion of fibronectin by massive numbers of bacteria may be a significant factor in reducing the resistance of animals suffering from a severe bacteremia.

Clearance from the blood stream is greatly enhanced if antibodies directed against the bacteria are also present, since opsonization increases the trapping efficiency of the sinusoidal macrophages (Fig. 2–10). If antibodies are absent or if the bacteria possess an antiphagocytic polysaccharide capsule, then the rate of clearance is decreased.

Some compounds such as bacterial endotoxins, estrogens and simple lipids stimulate macrophage activity and therefore also increase the rate of bacterial clearance. Drugs, such as steroids, that depress macrophage activity also depress the clearance rate.

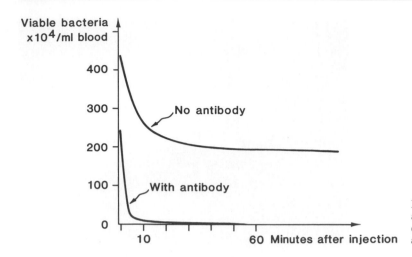

Figure 2–10. The blood clearance of bacteria. In the absence of antibody, bacteria are slowly and incompletely removed.

Soluble Antigens Given Intravenously

Unless very carefully treated, protein molecules in solution tend to aggregate spontaneously. If a solution of a soluble protein antigen is injected intravenously, these aggregates are rapidly removed by macrophages. The unaggregated molecules remain in solution and are distributed evenly through the animal's blood. If the molecules are sufficiently small (≤100,000 daltons), they are also distributed through the extravascular tissue fluids. Once distributed, the antigen is treated like other body proteins and catabolized, re-

sulting in a slow but progressive decline in antigen concentration. Within a few days, however, the animal begins to mount an immune response to the antigen. Antibodies are produced that combine with the antigen to form immune complexes. These immune complexes are rapidly cleared from the circulation by the sinusoidal macrophages. In this way all the antigen is rapidly and completely eliminated (Fig. 2–11).

This triphasic clearance pattern of distribution, catabolism and immune-elimination may be modified under certain circumstances. For example, if the animal has not been previously exposed to the antigen, then the immune

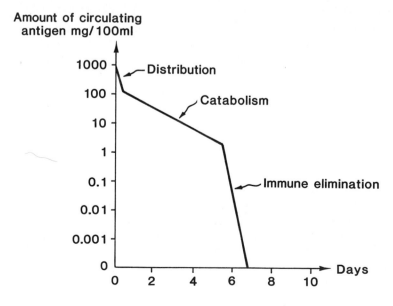

Figure 2–11. The clearance of soluble antigen from the blood stream.

response will be a primary one. In this case, it takes between five and ten days before antibodies are produced and immune-elimination occurs. If, on the other hand, the animal has been previously primed by exposure to the antigen, then a secondary immune response will be mounted in two to three days, and the stage of progressive catabolism is therefore relatively short. If antibodies are already circulating in the animal at the time of antigen administration, then immune-elimination will occur immediately and no phase of catabolism is seen. If the injected material is not antigenic or if the immune response does not occur, owing to either tolerance or immunosuppression, then the phase of progressive catabolism will continue until all the material is eliminated.

Fate of Antigen Administered by Other Routes

If insoluble or aggregated antigen is injected into a tissue, some slight damage is bound to occur. As a result of this, phagocytic cells (first neutrophils and then macrophages) migrate toward the injection site under the influence of chemotactic factors released from the damaged tissue. These cells phagocytose and process the injected material, eventually stimulating an immune response. Antibodies and complement (Chapter 10) interact with the antigen, generating more chemotactic factors that attract still more macrophages and in this way hasten the final elimination of the offending material.

If soluble antigen is injected into a tissue, it is redistributed by the flow of tissue fluid through the lymphatic system and eventually reaches the blood stream; its final fate is thus similar to intravenously injected material. Any aggregated material present is phagocytosed either by tissue macrophages or by the macrophages and dendritic cells of lymph nodes through which the tissue fluid flows.

Normally, antigens passing through the intestinal tract are catabolized by the digestive enzymes to nonantigenic molecules such as amino acids and monosaccharides. However, some antigenic molecules usually do remain intact and pass through the intestinal epithelium. Bacterial polysaccharides and those antigens that associate with lipids are especially effective in this respect, since they are absorbed in chylomicrons. Antigens that succeed in entering the blood stream from the intestine in this way are promptly removed by the Kupffer cells of the liver, whereas those entering the intestinal lymphatics are trapped in the mesenteric lymph nodes. The relatively large size of these nodes in many species testifies to their activity in this respect.

The fate of inhaled antigenic particles depends in large part on their size (see Fig. 12–1). Relatively large particles (greater than 3 μm diameter) are deposited on the mucus layer overlying the respiratory epithelium from the trachea to the terminal bronchioles. These particles are then removed from the respiratory tract by the flow of mucus toward the pharynx or by coughing. Particulate antigens that succeed in reaching the alveoli are mainly ingested by alveolar macrophages that carry them back to the bronchioalveolar junction, where they are also removed from the lung by the flow of mucus. Nevertheless, some antigens may be absorbed from the alveoli and diffuse into the intra-alveolar tissue. Small particles absorbed in this way are cleared to the draining lymph nodes, whereas soluble antigens tend to enter the blood vessels and are therefore distributed throughout the body. When very large quantities of particles are inhaled, as occurs in workers exposed to industrial dusts and to a lesser extent in cigarette smokers, the alveolar macrophage system may be temporarily blockaded and the lung rendered more susceptible to invasion by microorganisms.

ADDITIONAL SOURCES OF INFORMATION

Baggiolini M and Dewald B. 1985. The Neutrophil. Int. Archs. Allergy Appl. Immunol. 76 suppl. 1 13–20.

Bertram TA. 1985. Neutrophil leukocyte structure and function in domestic animals. Adv. Vet. Sci. Comp. Med. 30 91–129.

Boxer GJ, Curnutte JT and Boxer LA. 1985. Polymorphonuclear leukocyte function. Hosp. Pract. 20 69–90.

Brownlow MA. 1982. Mononuclear phagocytes of peritoneal fluid. Equine Vet. J. *14* 325–328.

Eagleson JS and Moriarty KM. 1984. Neutrophils, oxidative killing mechanisms and chemiluminescence. N.Z. Vet. J. *32* 41–43.

Gennaro R, Dolzani L and Romeo D. 1983. Potency of bactericidal proteins purified from the large granules of bovine neutrophils. Infect. Immun. *40* 684–690.

Geisow M. 1980. Pathways of endocytosis. Nature *288* 434–436.

Ginsburg I and Lahav M. 1983. Are bacterial cells degraded by leukocytes in vivo? An enigma. Clin. Immunol. Newsletter *4* 147–153.

Goodell EM, Blumenstock DA and Bowes WE. 1985. Canine dendritic cells from peripheral blood and lymph nodes. Vet. Immunol. Immunopathol. *8* 301–309.

Gray GD, Knight KA, Nelson RD and Herron MJ. 1982. Chemotactic requirements for bovine leukocytes. Am. J. Vet. Res. *43* 757–759.

Grey HM and Chestnut R. 1985. Antigen processing and presentation to T cells. Immunol. Today *6* 101–106.

Nathan CF, Murray HW and Cohn ZA. 1980. The macrophage as an effector cell. N. Engl. J. Med. *303* 622–626.

O'Donnell RT and Anderson BR. 1982. Characterization of canine neutrophil granules. Infect. Immun. *38* 351–359.

Snyderman R and Goetzl EJ. 1981. Molecular and cellular mechanisms of leukocyte chemotaxis. Science *213* 830–837.

Tew JG, Thorbecke JG and Steinman RM. 1982. Dendritic cells in the immune response: characteristics and recommended nomenclature. J. Res. *31* 371–380.

Unanue ER. 1980. Cooperation between mononuclear phagocytes and lymphocytes in immunity. N. Engl. J. Med. *303* 977–985.

Van Furth R. 1985. Cellular biology of pulmonary macrophages. Int. Arch. Allergy Appl. Immunol. *76* supp. 1 21–27.

Washburn M, Klesius PH and Ganjam VK. 1982. Characterization of the chemiluminescence response of equine phagocytes. Am. J. Vet. Res. *43* 1147–1151.

3

Antigens and Antigenicity

Although neutrophils and the cells of the mononuclear-phagocytic system trap and phagocytose foreign material, not all this foreign material is subsequently able to stimulate an immune response. In fact, there are strict limitations on the nature of substances that can do so. The two most important of these limitations are first, physicochemical restrictions on the types of molecules involved and, second, the nature of the foreign material, which must be such that it can be recognized as not being a normal body constituent.

ESSENTIAL FEATURES OF ANTIGENICITY (Table 3–1)

Physicochemical Limitations

In order to be antigenic, molecules must be large, stable and chemically complex. Large molecules are better antigens than small molecules. For example, serum albumin, with a molecular weight of over 60,000 daltons, is an effective antigen, while angiotensin, with a molecular weight of 1031 daltons, is an extremely poor antigen, and a single amino acid such as phenylalanine (molecular weight 165 daltons) is never antigenic by itself. Macromolecules of complex structure such as the proteins are considerably better antigens than simple large polymers with identical repeating subunits. For this reason, lipids, carbohydrates and nucleic acids, as well as monoamino acid polymers, are relatively poor antigens. As will be described later, the immune system responds to characteristic stereochemical shapes on the surface of macromolecules, and as a result of this response, compounds that have a very flexible structure (i.e., those not able to assume a stable configuration) cannot be easily recognized and hence are

Table 3–1 ESSENTIAL FEATURES OF ANTIGENICITY

Feature	Property
Size	Larger is better
Complexity	Simple polymers may be poor antigens
Stability	Structural stability is mandatory
Degradability	Very unstable molecules are poor antigens
	Totally inert molecules are poor antigens
Foreignness	The more "foreign" the better

poorly antigenic. An example of this type of molecule is gelatin, a protein well known for its structural instability, which is a weak antigen unless stabilized by the incorporation of tyrosine or tryptophane molecules. Similarly, flagellin, a protein component of bacterial flagellae, is structurally unstable, so that its antigenicity is greatly enhanced by polymerization.

One other physicochemical limitation on antigenicity is degradability. Because the immune response is an antigen-driven process, it follows that if molecules are very rapidly destroyed in the body, insufficient quantities may be available to stimulate antigen-sensitive cells. Conversely, large inert organic polymers such as the plastics are not antigenic because they are metabolically inert, and cannot be degraded and processed by macrophages to a form suitable for initiation of an immune response. A practical consequence of this is seen in the use of glutaraldehyde-treated pig heart valves in human heart surgery. The glutaraldehyde "fixes" the valve protein, rendering it metabolically inert and thus non-antigenic.

Foreignness

The second major requirement for antigenicity is foreignness. Antigen-sensitive cells do not respond to material that is not recognized as foreign. This discrimination results from the early elimination or "turning off" of cells that may react to self-antigens. The lack of response to self-antigens is brought about by exposure of antigen-sensitive cells to these antigens early in fetal life. If this exposure does not occur, then self-tolerance does not occur. For example, certain cells such as those in the testes are not in immediate contact with the blood circulation and therefore do not encounter the cells of the immune system. If their isolation is broken down by trauma or infection of the testes, then the testicular cells may encounter antigen-sensitive cells that regard them as foreign and so stimulate an immune response. On a smaller scale, the mitochondria of normal cells are also removed from direct contact with the circulation. As a result, if extensive cell destruction occurs in

organs such as the liver or heart, antimitochondrial antibodies may be detected in the serum several weeks later.

EPITOPES

While complex particles such as bacteria, nucleated cells or erythrocytes can stimulate the immune response, they are obviously composed not of single antigenic molecules but a complex mixture of proteins, glycoproteins, polysaccharides, lipopolysaccharides, nucleic acids and lipids. When we observe an immune response against such a particle, we are really observing several simultaneous immune responses directed against each of the antigenic molecules on these particles.

On a smaller scale, single protein molecules are not, in themselves, single antigens. Macromolecules have areas on their surface against which the immune response tends to be directed and with which antibodies bind. These areas are called epitopes or antigenic determinants. The epitopes found on protein molecules usually consist of about four to six amino acids and are located on exposed or prominent areas on the surface of the molecule (Fig. 3–1). (In general, the number of epitopes on a molecule is directly related to the molecule's size. There is about one epitope for each 5000 daltons.)

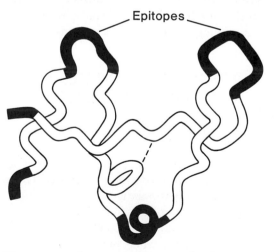

Figure 3–1. A diagram of a protein molecule, showing the location of epitopes on prominent surface features.

We can therefore narrow our definition of foreignness to the recognition of those epitopes not recognized as self. When animals encounter a large, complex antigenic molecule such as a protein, they make antibodies only against the epitopes, and much of the molecule is therefore nonantigenic. Different animals may respond against different epitopes on the same molecule. The selection of epitopes by the immune system is controlled by genes known as immune response genes. These genes code for regulatory proteins located on the surface of cells of the immune system and are called class II histocompatibility antigens (Chapter 8). The epitopes are also selected by the way in which the antigen is presented to the antigen-sensitive cells. Epitopes also differ in the type of immune response that they stimulate. Some epitopes stimulate antibody formation, others stimulate cell-mediated immune responses, and some epitopes may provoke tolerance by stimulating cells that suppress the immune response. The immune response stimulated by a large molecule is therefore a complex mixture of responses. The final result depends upon the nature of all the epitopes that are found on the surface of the molecule.

Cross-Reactions

Identical epitopes may be found on a number of different antigenic molecules. As a result, antibody directed against one antigen may be found to react unexpectedly with antigen from an apparently unrelated source. This is known as a cross-reaction (Fig. 3–2). For example, antibodies against some bacteria also cross-react with some animal red cells because they each possess surface epitopes in common. Thus, pigs of blood group O develop antibodies that react with red cells from pigs of blood group A. These antibodies arise not as a response to previous immunization with group A red cells, but in response to the cross-reacting antigens that originate in feed or in the bacterial flora and are absorbed from the intestine.

Another example of cross-reactivity occurs between *Brucella abortus* and some strains of

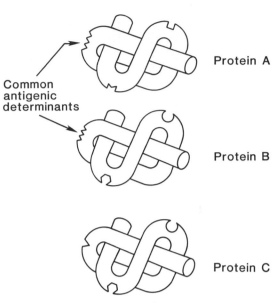

Figure 3–2. A diagram of three related protein molecules, showing how cross-reactions may occur. An antiserum to protein A also reacts with protein B because they each possess a common epitope (antigenic determinant). Similarly, an antiserum to protein B will react with both A and C, and an antiserum to protein C also reacts with B.

Yersinia enterocolitica. Y. enterocolitica, a relatively unimportant organism, may provoke cattle to make antibodies that cross-react with *B. abortus*. Since brucella-infected animals are detected by testing for the presence of serum antibodies, a Yersinia-infected animal may be wrongly thought to carry *B. abortus* and so be killed.

Cross-reactivity occurs between the virus of feline infectious peritonitis (FIP) and the virus of pig transmissible gastroenteritis (TGE). It is very difficult to grow the FIP virus in the laboratory. TGE virus, on the other hand, is readily propagated. By detecting antibodies to TGE in cats, it is possible to diagnose FIP without having to culture the FIP virus.

The degree of cross-reactivity between two antigens is a reflection of their shared epitopes and their structural similarity. This principle may be used to determine relationships between molecules or between species of animals or plants. Thus, in the example given in Figure 3–3, it is apparent that, on the basis of antigenic cross-reactivity, goats and sheep are more closely related to cattle than are pigs or chickens.

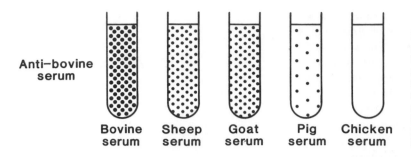

Anti–bovine serum

Bovine serum | Sheep serum | Goat serum | Pig serum | Chicken serum

Figure 3–3. The relative amount of immune precipitate formed when antibodies to bovine serum albumin are allowed to react with serum from several different species. Thus, sheep and goat serum give a stronger reaction than pig serum. Chicken serum does not react with anti-bovine serum.

Haptens and Carriers

Although we have already stated that antigens must be large molecules, it has also been pointed out that epitopes are relatively small. It is therefore possible to generate artificial epitopes by chemically linking small organic molecules to macromolecules. If an antigen is modified in this way and used to immunize an animal, antibodies will be formed against any unaltered epitopes on the macromolecule, and against the new epitope formed by the small organic molecule.

Since small molecules by themselves are not capable of stimulating an immune response, they are not immunogenic. Nevertheless, because they can become so when linked to larger molecules and because they can combine with antibodies generated as described above, they must be considered to be antigenic. Molecules used in this fashion are known as haptens, and the macromolecules to which they are attached are generally called the carriers. By using haptens of known chemical structure, it is possible to study in great detail the factors that influence the specificity of the reaction between an antibody and an epitope. For example, the ability of an antiserum to bind to one hapten may be compared with its ability to bind to structurally related haptens. By means of this simple technique it can be shown that any change in the hapten's charge, its size or its surface configuration will severely reduce its ability to bind to antibodies directed against the unmodified molecule. This means that the antibodies produced against an epitope are highly specific for that epitope alone, and implies that the antibody

binding site must have a configuration that is very specific for the shape of a specific epitope. Purely chemical changes, which do not alter the shape or the charge distribution on the hapten, do not influence its ability to combine with specific antibody. Nevertheless, even very minor chemical changes usually result in significant alterations in molecular shape and hence affect the ability of an antibody to combine with a hapten (Fig. 3–4). As a result, it has been suggested that an animal must be able to generate an enormously large variety of different antibody molecules in order to account for their ability to combine with all potential haptens.

When the properties of epitopes are studied in more detail, it is apparent that antibodies prefer to bind to the more mobile portions of protein molecules. By binding to flexible epitopes, the fit between antigen and antibody does not have to be perfect. Because of this flexibility as well as structural similarities and overlaps, the actual number of different epitopes that can stimulate an immune response is probably only about 10 million.

The response of animals to hapten-carrier conjugates has also served to indicate that the epitopes recognized by the antibody-producing system and the cell-mediated immune system are not identical. Antibodies may be produced that are specific for a given hapten and that can combine with that hapten irrespective of the carrier molecule to which it is attached. In contrast, if a cell-mediated immune response is mounted against a hapten-carrier conjugate, it is found that this response is directed against the hapten only if it remains bound to the original carrier. Sensitized lym-

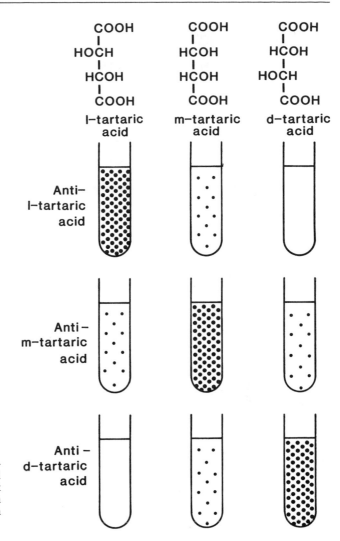

Figure 3–4. The remarkable specificity of antibodies. Antisera against the three optical isomers of tartaric acid will give the strongest reaction with the hapten that induced them and will only respond weakly, if at all, with the other optical isomers.

phocytes will not react to the hapten if it is bound to an unrelated carrier molecule. For this reason the cell-mediated immune response is said to be "carrier specific."

The concept of haptens and carriers not only provides a basis for much of our knowledge about the specificity of the immune response but is also of clinical importance. Thus, many drugs can combine with proteins and so form hapten-carrier conjugates *in vivo*. Penicillin, for instance, is a small molecule that by itself is nonantigenic. When being degraded in the body, however, a reactive penicilloyl group can be formed, which may bind to serum proteins to form penicilloyl-protein conjugates (Fig. 3–5). These conju-

gates, not being normal constituents of the body, are recognized as foreign and therefore induce the formation of antipenicilloyl antibodies, which may participate in hypersensitivity reactions to penicillin (Chapter 20). Another example of a naturally occurring reactive chemical that binds to body proteins and hence acts as a hapten is the toxic component of poison ivy, called urushiol. On contact with skin, urushiol penetrates and binds to dermal proteins and cells. These modified cells are consequently regarded as foreign and attacked in a manner akin to the rejection of a skin graft. The resulting inflammatory reaction is known as allergic contact dermatitis (Chapter 23).

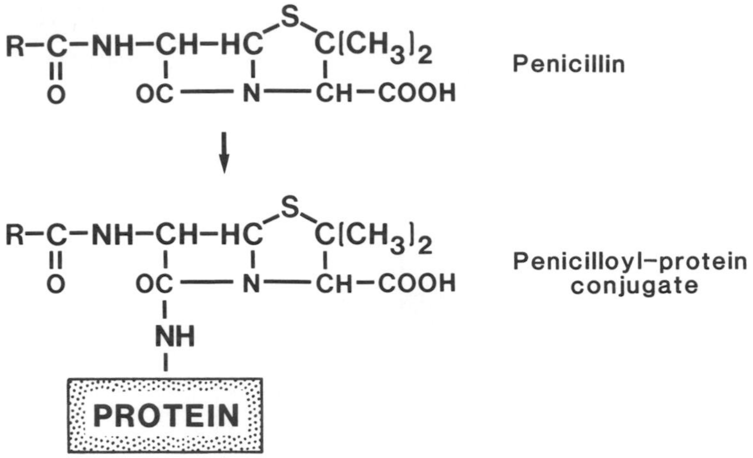

R–C–NH–CH–HC$\overset{\text{S}}{\diagdown}$C(CH$_3$)$_2$ Penicillin
‖ | | |
O   OC — N — CH–COOH

↓

R–C–NH–CH–HC$\overset{\text{S}}{\diagdown}$C(CH$_3$)$_2$
‖ | | |
O   OC — N — CH–COOH   **Penicilloyl–protein**
              | **conjugate**
             NH
              |
        [PROTEIN]

Figure 3–5. Penicillin as a hapten. Penicillin can break down *in vivo* by several different pathways. The most important derivative is a penicillenic acid that combines with protein amino groups to form a penicilloyl-protein conjugate. This conjugate may provoke an immune response and result in penicillin allergy.

SOME SPECIFIC ANTIGENS

Whereas many different antigens will be discussed in subsequent chapters, some general comments on antigens may be made here. As mentioned earlier, proteins are usually the best antigens because of their size and structural complexity. Almost all proteins with molecular weights over 1000 daltons are antigenic, although some, like the interferons, are of such uniform structure and so widely distributed among mammals that it is difficult to make good antisera against them. Many of the major antigens of micro-organisms, such as the clostridial toxins, bacterial flagellae, virus capsids and protozoan cell membranes, are all proteins. Others include snake venoms, serum and milk proteins and even antibodies themselves when injected into another species.

Polysaccharides are poorer antigens than proteins simply because they tend to consist of structurally mobile polymers containing only a small number of different types of monosaccharide subunits. This is particularly true of the simpler molecules such as starch or glycogen. However, other more complex carbohydrates (particularly those linked to proteins) are of immunological importance. These include the major cell wall antigens of gram-negative organisms and the blood group antigens present on erythrocytes. Many of the so-called natural antibodies found in the serum of unimmunized animals are directed against polysaccharide epitopes and probably arise as a result of exposure to antigens derived from the normal intestinal flora or from food.

Lipids, like polysaccharides, are poor antigens because of their relative simplicity. Nevertheless, if linked to proteins or polysaccharides, they may be fully antigenic. Naturally occurring lipid antigens are uncommon. In syphilis, however, antibodies may be produced against cardiolipin, a phospholipid hapten found in heart muscle. The Forsmann antigen, an important cell membrane antigen found in many species of animal, also is a glycolipid (Chapter 21). The cell walls of gram-negative bacteria are composed of complex lipopolysaccharides, but the immune response against these tends to be directed largely against the polysaccharide component.

Because of their relative simplicity and flexibility and also because they are very rapidly degraded, nucleic acids such as DNA or RNA are relatively poor antigens. Nevertheless, it is possible to produce antinucleic acid antibodies after artificially stabilizing and linking them to an immunogenic carrier. In certain diseases, such as systemic lupus erythematosus in man and dogs (Chapter 25), relatively high levels of antibodies to nucleic acids and nucleoproteins may be found in serum.

ADDITIONAL SOURCES OF INFORMATION

Atassi MZ. 1978. Precise determination of the entire antigenic structure of lysozyme. Immunochemistry 15 909–936.
Green N, Alexander H, Olson A et al. 1982. Immunogenic structure of the influenza virus hemagglutinin. Cell 28 477–487.

Katz ME, Maizels RM, Wicker L et al. 1982. Immunological focussing by the mouse major histocompatibility
complex: mouse strains confronted with distantly related lysozymes confine their attention to very few
epitopes. Eur. J. Immunol. *12* 535–540.

Landsteiner K. 1945 (reprinted 1962). The Specificity of
Serological Reactions. Dover Publications, New York.

Marx JL. 1984. Do antibodies prefer moving targets?
Science *226* 819–821.

Tizard I. 1982. Antigen structure and immunogenicity.
JAVMA *181* 978–982.

Wilson IA, Niman HL, Houghten RA et al. 1984. The
structure of an antigenic determinant in a protein. Cell
37 767–778.

4

Antibodies

Antibodies are protein molecules produced by plasma cells as a result of the interaction between antigen-sensitive B lymphocytes and specific antigen (Chapter 6). They have the ability to bind specifically to antigen and hasten its destruction or elimination. Antibodies are found in many body fluids but are present in highest concentrations and are most easily obtained from blood serum.

NATURE OF ANTIBODIES

Antibody molecules, like other proteins, may be classified on the basis of their solubility in strong salt solutions, their electrostatic charge, their molecular weight and their antigenic structure.

Solubility in Salt Solutions

Many years ago when biochemistry was in its infancy, it was found that some of the proteins in serum were precipitated when mixed with an equal volume of a saturated solution of ammonium sulfate, while others remained in solution. Those proteins that precipitate in this way are called globulins; those that remain in solution are called albumins. Antibodies are precipitated from serum by ammonium sulfate and so are classified as globulins. This very simple technique can be readily adapted to provide a method of determining whether antibodies are present in serum, and so may be employed to determine whether a young animal has suckled or not (Chapter 13).

Electrostatic Charge

Since protein molecules consist of chains of assorted amino acids, some of which are basic and some acidic, the overall charge on a protein molecule depends on its amino acid composition and is characteristic for that protein. A mixture of proteins may therefore be separated into its constituents by subjecting it to an electrical potential, causing the more positively charged molecules to migrate toward the cathode while negatively charged molecules migrate toward the anode at a rate dependent on their charge. If this technique, known as electrophoresis, is performed on a semisolid matrix such as agar, cellulose acetate or starch gel, then it is possible to fractionate and identify individual proteins in a mixture. When whole serum is treated in this way, it consistently separates into four fractions. The most negatively charged of these consists of a single protein called serum albumin. (It also

happens not to be precipitated by strong salt solutions.) The other three fractions are all globulins and are divided according to their electrophoretic mobility into α, β and γ globulins (Fig. 4–1). The α globulins are the most negatively charged of these and therefore migrate towards the anode just behind the albumin. They consist of proteins with various nonimmunological functions; these proteins include α_1-antitrypsin and α_2-macroglobulin, both of which are inhibitors of proteases. The β globulins are slower, migrating just behind the α globulins. They contain some antibody molecules as well as many of the proteins of the complement system (Chapter 10). The γ globulins are the most positively charged serum proteins. They move the shortest distance from the origin and contain most of the antibodies.

Because antibody molecules are globulins, they are generally known as immunoglobulins (which may be abbreviated to Ig). The term

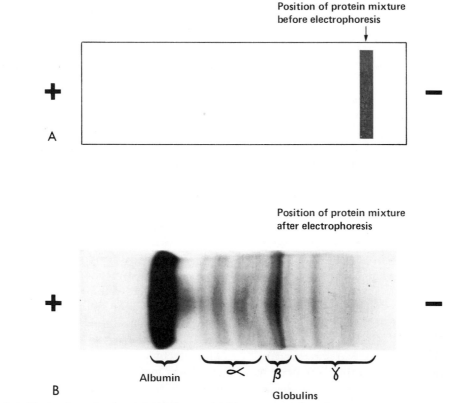

Figure 4–1. Electrophoresis of a protein mixture, in this case normal mink serum, on a strip of cellulose acetate. (Courtesy of Dr. S. H. An.)

immunoglobulin is used to describe all proteins with antibody activity as well as some proteins that have the characteristic molecular structure of antibody molecules but do not have known antibody activity.

Molecular Weight

In addition to their charge, proteins may also be characterized by their molecular weight. When the molecular weights of immunoglobulins are estimated they are found to be heterogeneous. Most serum antibodies have a molecular weight of around 180,000 daltons, but about 20 per cent have a molecular weight of 900,000 daltons. The major immunoglobulin in intestinal and respiratory secretions has a molecular weight of 360,000 daltons; the antibody responsible for classical allergies has a molecular weight of 200,000 daltons.

One method of estimating the size of a protein molecule is by ultracentrifugation. Each molecule has a "sedimentation coefficient," which is proportional to its molecular weight and which can be determined by analytical ultracentrifugation. This coefficient is expressed as an S value. Thus the 180,000 MW molecule has a sedimentation coefficient of 7S. The 200,000 MW molecule is 8S, the 360,000 MW molecule is 11S and the 900,000 MW molecule is 19S.

Antigenic Structure

As proteins, immunoglobulins are excellent antigens when injected into animals of a different species; consequently, antisera can be made that react with immunoglobulin molecules. By using these antisera (known as antiglobulins) it is possible to show that immunoglobulins are antigenically heterogeneous and fall into a number of different isotypes or classes. The five major isotypes detected in this way are called immunoglobulins M, G, A, E and D, and each possesses unique epitopes, called μ, γ, α, ε and δ respectively. The basic characteristics of each of these immunoglobulin isotypes are shown in Table 4–1.

STRUCTURE OF IMMUNOGLOBULINS

Immunoglobulin G (IgG) is the immunoglobulin found in highest concentration in serum, and its structure can serve as a model for the other immunoglobulins. IgG has a molecular weight of 180,000 daltons and a sedimentation constant of 7S. On electron microscopy it can be seen to be a Y-shaped molecule, and the "arms" of the Y are capable of binding antigen. If the molecule is treated with chemicals that break disulfide (-S-S-)bonds, it falls apart into four separate polypeptide chains. Two of these chains are "heavy," since they are of about 50,000 daltons. The other two chains are "light," since they each have a molecular weight of about 25,000 daltons. Additional information on the overall structure of IgG can be obtained by studying the effect of proteolytic enzymes on the molecule (Fig. 4–2). Papain, for example, can break the molecule into three approximately equal-sized fragments, which correspond to the two arms and

Table 4–1 BASIC CHARACTERISTICS OF THE MAJOR IMMUNOGLOBULIN ISOTYPES IN THE DOMESTIC ANIMALS

| Property | Immunoglobulin Isotype | | | | |
	IgM	IgG	IgA	IgE	IgD
Most usual sedimentation coefficient	19S	7S	11S	8S	7S
Molecular weight (daltons)	900,000	180,000	360,000	200,000	180,000
Electrophoretic mobility	β	γ	β-γ	β-γ	γ
Heavy chain antigen	μ	γ	α	ε	δ
Largely synthesized in	Spleen and lymph nodes	Spleen and lymph nodes	Intestinal and respiratory tracts	Intestinal and respiratory tracts	Spleen and lymph nodes

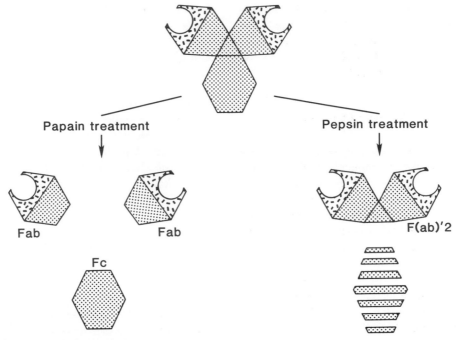

Figure 4–2. The effect of treating IgG with the proteolytic enzymes, pepsin and papain. Papain cleaves the molecule into three large fragments. Pepsin cleaves the molecule into one large fragment and many small ones.

the tail of the Y-shaped molecule. The two fragments from the arms of the molecule are identical and can still bind antigen; they are called the Fab fragments. The third fragment, from the tail, cannot bind antigen but is crystallizable and so is called the Fc fragment. Another proteolytic enzyme, pepsin, can destroy the Fc fragment but leaves the two Fab fragments joined together to form a fragment known as F(ab)'$_2$. All these observations may be synthesized into a model of IgG structure, seen in Figure 4–3.

Primary Structure of Immunoglobulins

The immunoglobulins found in serum are a complex mixture of antibodies directed against

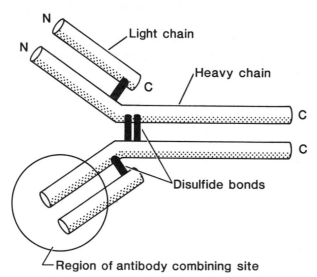

Figure 4–3. A simple model of an IgG molecule. The "correct" shape of this molecule is much more complex than this and approximates the shape seen in Figure 4–4.

a very wide spectrum of epitopes. Because of this heterogeneity, it is impossible to analyze their structure in more than the general terms already described. However, B cells occasionally become neoplastic, with the result that a clone of cancerous plasma cells arises from a single precursor cell. Because of their "monoclonal" origin, all these plasma cells synthesize and release a single molecular form of immunoglobulin, which appears in the serum of affected individuals in high concentrations. This plasma cell tumor is known as a myeloma or a plasmacytoma and its immunoglobulin product is called a myeloma protein (Chapter 26). Myeloma proteins are absolutely homogeneous immunoglobulin molecules. As a result they may be purified and their chemical and antigenic structure analyzed in detail. In this way each immunoglobulin molecule can be shown to consist of variable regions in the arms of the Y, through which the immunoglobulin binds to antigen; a hinge region where the arms join the tail, which confers flexibility on the molecule; and constant regions in both arms and the tail, which determine the biological properties of the molecule.

Variable Regions

When the amino acid sequences of a large number of IgG myeloma proteins are compared, it is found that their polypeptide chains, both light and heavy, can be divided into two distinct regions. The portion of the chains situated at the C-terminal end (the end of the peptide chain with a free carboxyl group) has a constant amino acid sequence when different myeloma proteins of the same isotype are compared. In contrast, the N-terminal portion (the end with a free amino group) of each chain is found to be highly variable, so that the amino acid sequence differs greatly between different myeloma proteins. These variable regions are each about 110 amino acid residues long and constitute about half of each light chain and about a quarter of each heavy chain (Fig. 4–4).

When the variable regions are further examined and their degree of variability measured, it can be shown that the amino acid sequences in certain areas within these regions vary considerably more than others. These areas are called hypervariable regions. Between these hypervariable regions are located relatively constant segments in which the amino acids remain relatively unchanged. When the three-dimensional structure of the variable regions is examined, it is found that the chain is folded in such a way that these hypervariable positions lie close to each other on the surface of the molecule (Fig. 4–5). The hypervariable regions on each light and heavy chain act together to form a single antigen-binding site. Because there is an antigen-binding site on each Fab region, each IgG molecule is functionally bivalent.

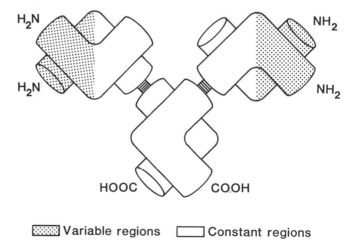

Figure 4–4. A model of an IgG molecule, showing its major regions.

▒▒ Variable regions ☐ Constant regions
≡ Hinge regions

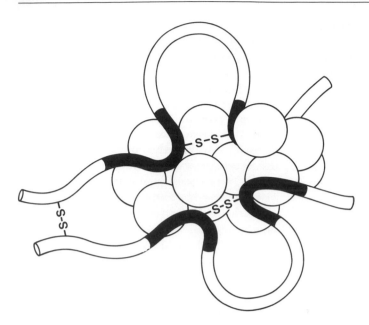

Figure 4–5. The way in which the hypervariable regions come together to form the antigen binding site on an immunoglobulin molecule is shown. The structure located between the two immunoglobulin chains is an epitope. The black areas are the hypervariable regions.

The specificity of the interactions between an antibody and an epitope may be explained on the basis that the various amino acid sequences in the hypervariable regions give rise to a uniquely shaped peptide chain. As a result there is a region on the surface of an immunoglobulin molecule that has a unique conformation. The antibody molecule will only bind to epitopes whose shape exactly matches the conformation of its own binding site.

By screening myeloma proteins for antibody activity against a very large number of potential antigens, it has been possible to determine their specificity, and it has been found that some myeloma proteins may bind equally well to several apparently unrelated epitopes. This may be explained by the fact that the antigen-binding site on an immunoglobulin is considerably larger than a single epitope, and may be considered to consist of a number of closely associated binding sites for unrelated antigens. When an immune response is mounted against a single epitope, many different antibody molecules are produced with a single feature in common—the ability to bind the inducing epitope. These molecules will also be able to bind other unrelated epitopes but, since activity against any one of these unrelated epitopes will be present on only a few molecules, it

will remain undetected and the antiserum will appear to be specific.

The binding forces between an antigen and its antibody are noncovalent interactions. In classic chemical reactions, molecules are assembled through the establishment of firm, nonreversible covalent bonds. In biological systems, however, these bonds may be insufficiently flexible or adaptable for the body's purposes. In contrast, the formation of noncovalent bonds provides a rapid and reversible way of forming complexes and permits reuse of antibody molecules in a way that covalent bonding does not allow. Noncovalent bonds are generally formed over relatively small intermolecular distances and as a result are only established when two molecules can approach very closely (Fig. 4–6). Thus, the strongest binding between antigen and antibody occurs when the shape of the epitope and the shape of the antibody-combining site conform very closely. This requirement for a close fit has been likened to the specificity of a key for its lock.

One of the most obvious of the forces that bind antigen to antibody is the electrostatic (ionic) interaction between the negatively charged aspartic or glutamic acids on one molecule and the positively charged lysine, arginine and histidine side-chains on the other. The significance of electrostatic bonding is not completely clear, however, since most biological interactions occur in solutions of relatively high salt concentration, which may neutralize these charges.

The major noncovalent force that contributes to antigen-antibody interaction is hydrophobic bonding. Many nonpolar–side-chains of amino acids are hydrophobic, and they tend to come together in such a way that by excluding water they form a stable bond. These hydrophobic interactions are but one example of the mutual attraction of very closely approximated atoms that occur as a result of Van der Waals' forces.

The third group of noncovalent forces that contribute to antigen-antibody bonding are hydrogen bonds. Hydrogen bonds develop when a hydrogen ion attached to one electronegative atom interacts with a second electronegative atom and thus links the two. Hydrogen bonds commonly form between many side-chain groups of proteins, and although a single hydrogen bond is relatively weak, collectively they can develop considerable strength.

All the interactions discussed here require that the antigen and antibody approach each other extremely closely before firm bonding can occur and, in fact, the strength of the bonds so formed will be an indication of this closeness of fit. The strength of binding between an epitope and an immunoglobulin molecule is termed affinity and may be calculated using the Law of Mass Action, since the reaction is reversible. As well as being a measure of the strength of the interaction between antigen and antibody, affinity is also a reflection of the specificity of the antibody. An antibody that binds strongly to a specific epitope is likely to bind fairly well to other structurally related epitopes and therefore will appear to be relatively nonspecific. In contrast, an antibody that possesses a low affinity for an epitope probably will interact even less strongly with structurally related epitopes, and if this cross-reaction cannot be detected, then that weak antibody will appear to be highly specific. During the course of an immune response, the affinity of antibodies for antigen climbs progressively, but as a result of this there is an apparent simultaneous decrease in antibody specificity. Because serum contains a complex mixture of different antibody molecules, it is not correct to use the term affinity to describe the strength of reaction of an antiserum with antigen; the term avidity is preferable in this context.

Hinge Region

On electron microscopy of IgG molecules it can be seen that the Fab regions (the arms of the Y) are mobile and can swing freely around the center of the molecule as if they are hinged. When the amino acid sequence in this part of the molecule is investigated, it is found to contain an unusually large number of proline residues. Because of its unique shape, proline produces a right-angle bend in polypeptide chains, and since polypeptide chains can rotate freely around peptide bonds, the effect of several linked prolines is to produce a "universal joint" around which the polypeptide chains may swing freely (Fig. 4–7). Pro-

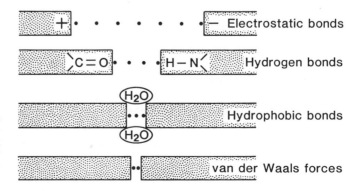

Figure 4–6. The four major noncovalent bonds responsible for the binding of antigen to its antibody. The most important are the hydrophobic bonds that act by excluding water from the gap between the epitope and the antigen binding site.

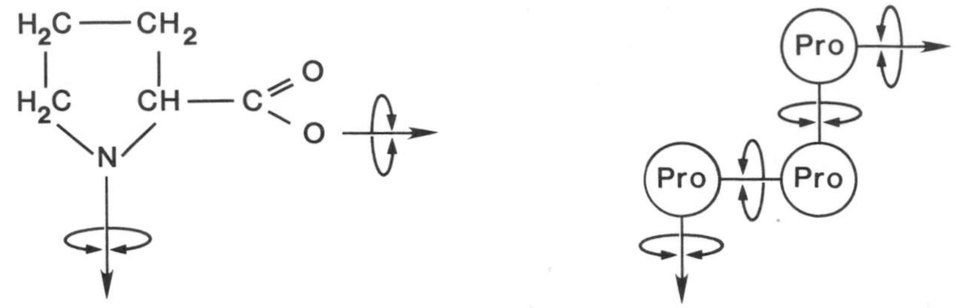

Proline molecule

Figure 4–7. The structure of the amino acid proline, when inserted in a peptide chain, produces a right-angle band. Because peptide bonds are free to rotate, three prolines therefore act as a "universal joint."

line also tends to "open up" the arrangement of the polypeptide chains, which is why proteolytic enzymes can attack the molecule in this region. Finally, the disulfide bonds that link the heavy and light chains are also found in the hinge region. This region therefore plays a very significant role in determining the biological activities of the immunoglobulin molecule.

Constant Regions

The amino acid sequence in the C-terminal half of each light chain and the C-terminal three quarters of each heavy chain remains unchanged between different IgG molecules. The constant region of the light chains (C_L) is about 110 amino acid residues long, whereas the constant region of each heavy chain (C_H) is 330 residues long. When the C_H region of IgG is sequenced, it is found to consist of three similar subunits, or domains, called C_H1, C_H2 and C_H3 (IgM and IgE possess a fourth domain in their heavy chains, called C_H4). Each constant domain in both light and heavy chains possesses a single intrachain disulfide bond, which folds the chain into a loop. (Similar loops are also seen in the variable regions where they bring the hypervariable regions close together to form the antigen-binding site.)

C_L **Regions.** Light chains are divided into two types on the basis of their constant region structure. These types are called kappa (κ) and lambda (λ). Any single immunoglobulin molecule has a pair of identical light chains, that is, both kappa or both lambda. The proportion of κ and λ light chains varies greatly between species. Dogs, cats, cattle and sheep have 90 per cent λ chains, whereas mice, rabbits and rats have 90 per cent κ chains. Pigs have equal amounts of each type, whereas horses and mink have only λ light chains.

C_H **Regions.** In addition to binding to specific antigen, immunoglobulins possess a number of other biological activities, most of which are initiated after the immunoglobulin binds to an epitope. These biological activities include activation of the complement cascade (Chapter 10) and binding of immune complexes to phagocytic cells preparatory to ingestion (opsonization). These and other functions are mediated through sites on the constant region of immunoglobulin heavy chains (Fig. 4–8). Thus, a small area found on the C_H2 domain of IgG is responsible for the initiation of the complement cascade, whereas a site on the C_H4 domain of IgM performs the same function in that molecule. The catabolic rate of IgG is also controlled by a site on C_H2, whereas adherence to macrophages is mediated through a site on C_H3. Placental transfer of IgG (in humans) and antibody-dependent cell-mediated cytotoxicity (Chapter 7) are also controlled by sites on the heavy chain in the Fc region but probably not by a single domain.

Immunoglobulin Isotypes

Immunoglobulin G

IgG is the immunoglobulin isotype found in highest concentration in blood (Table 4–2), and for this reason it plays the major role in antibody–mediated defense mechanisms. It

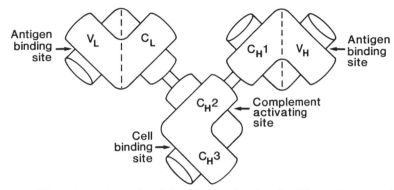

Figure 4–8. The major regions of an IgG molecule, showing the different function of each.

has a molecular weight of 180,000 daltons and γ epitopes on its heavy chains. Because of its relatively small size, IgG can escape from blood vessels more easily than can the other immunoglobulin molecules. Therefore, it readily participates in the defense of tissue spaces and body surfaces. IgG can opsonize, agglutinate and precipitate antigen (Chapter 11), but it can activate the complement cascade only if sufficient molecules have accumulated in a correct configuration on the antigen surface (Chapter 10).

Immunoglobulin M

IgM is the immunoglobulin found in second highest concentration in the serum of most animals. It is a 19S molecule with a molecular weight of 900,000 daltons, and is made up of five identical, 180,000 dalton, subunits. Each of these subunits is structurally similar to the basic Y-shaped immunoglobulin molecule, except that they possess four, rather than three, C_H domains and they carry μ epitopes. The

IgM monomers are linked by disulfide bonds in a circular fashion to form a star, and a small cysteine-rich polypeptide called the J chain (15,000 daltons) links two of the units (Fig. 4–9). IgM molecules are secreted intact by plasma cells, and the J chain must therefore be considered to be an integral part of this molecule.

IgM is the major immunoglobulin isotype produced in a primary immune response. It is also produced in a secondary response, but this tends to be masked by the predominance of IgG. Although produced in a relatively small quantity, IgM is considerably more efficient (on a molar basis) than IgG at complement activation, opsonization, neutralization of viruses and agglutination. Because of their very large size, IgM molecules are usually confined to the blood stream and are therefore probably of little importance in conferring protection in tissue fluids or body secretions. IgM monomers are found on the surface of B cells and aligned in such a way that they function as receptors for antigen (Chapter 6).

Table 4–2 SERUM IMMUNOGLOBULIN LEVELS IN DOMESTIC ANIMALS AND MAN

| Species | Immunoglobulin Levels (mg/100 ml) | | | | | |
	IgG	IgM	IgA	IgG(T)	IgG(B)	IgE
Horse	1000–1500	100–200	60–350	100–1500	10–100	–
Cattle*	1700–2700	250–400	10–50	–	–	–
Sheep	1700–2000	150–250	10–50	–	–	–
Pig	1700–2900	100–500	50–500	–	–	–
Dog	1000–2000	70–270	20–150	–	–	2.3–42
Chicken	300–700	120–250	30–60	–	–	–
Human	800–1600	50–200	150–400	–	–	0.002–0.05

*Cattle show very significant seasonal differences in serum immunoglobulin levels.

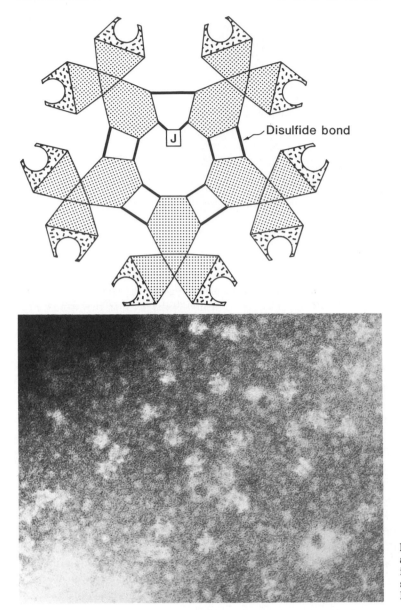

Disulfide bond

Figure 4–9. The structure of IgM and an electronmicrograph of this immunoglobulin from bovine serum. × 240,000. (Courtesy of Drs. K. Nielsen and B. Stemshorn.)

Immunoglobulin A

IgA is a carbohydrate-rich immunoglobulin of conventional structure. It tends to form polymers so that dimers, trimers and higher polymers are found in addition to the basic molecule (see Fig. 12–3). The most common form of IgA is a dimer, consisting of two monomers joined by a J chain. While IgA is the second most concentrated immunoglobulin in human serum, it is usually only a minor component in animal serum (Table 4–2). However, IgA is the major immunoglobulin isotype in the external secretions of nonruminants. As such, it is of critical importance in protecting the intestinal, respiratory and urogenital tracts, the mammary gland and the eyes against microbial invasion. IgA does not activate the complement cascade nor can it act as an opsonin. It can, however, agglutinate particulate antigen and neutralize viruses. It is thought that the major mode of action of IgA is to prevent the adherence of antigens to the body surfaces. Because of its importance, IgA is dealt with in greater detail in Chapter 12.

Immunoglobulin E

IgE is a typical Y-shaped, four-chain immunoglobulin, with an additional domain in the heavy chain near the hinge region. As a result, it has a molecular weight of 196,000 daltons. This immunoglobulin is found in extremely low concentrations in the serum of many species (for example, 20 to 500 ng/ml in humans) but is, nevertheless, of major importance in that it mediates type I hypersensitivity reactions (allergies and anaphylaxis) (Chapter 20). It is also associated with the immune response to many helminth infestations (Chapter 17). IgE possesses a unique Fc region that enables it to bind to mast cells and basophils, and together with antigen it mediates the release of vasoactive agents from these cells. IgE is also unique among immunoglobulins in that it is destroyed by heating to 56°C for 30 minutes.

Immunoglobulin D

IgD is an immunoglobulin found mainly on the surface of some B lymphocytes, where it functions as an antigen receptor. Its molecular weight is 180,000 daltons. IgD has been demonstrated in man, pigs, laboratory animals and chickens. It has not yet been shown to be present in the other domestic mammals although they almost certainly possess it.

The Immunoglobulin Superfamily

Structural studies on the proteins involved in various aspects of the immune response have revealed that many appear to share a basic common structural unit. This structural unit is related to a single immunoglobulin domain, consisting of about 110 amino acids and a single intrachain disulfide bond. It has been suggested that this structure provides the body with a useful "building block" and as a result it is a common component of many other important molecules. These immuno-globulin-related molecules include β_2-microglobulin, a small molecule that is an integral part of all class I histocompatibility antigens and is thus found on all nucleated cells (Chapter 8). The amino acid sequence of β_2-microglobulin is so similar to that of an immunoglobulin constant domain that it can fix complement and also bind to the Fc receptors of macrophages. Other members of the immunoglobulin superfamily include C-reactive protein, a protein that is found in the serum of animals suffering from infection, tissue damage or severe inflammation (Chapter 19); Thy-1 antigen, a cell-surface protein found on brain cells and thymus-derived lymphocytes; class I and class II histocompatibility antigens, immunoregulatory proteins found on lymphocyte membranes (Chapter 8); and the receptor for IgA on intestinal epithelial cells, which contributes to the structure of secretory component (Chapter 12).

Immunoglobulins as Antigens

Immunoglobulins are proteins and are therefore antigenic when taken from one animal and inoculated into an unrelated species. When the resulting anti-immunoglobulin antibodies are analyzed, several major categories of epitope may be recognized.

First, as described earlier, some of these antibodies are directed against major epitopes on the immunoglobulin heavy chains—i.e., against γ, μ, α, δ, or ϵ epitopes—and these antibodies can thus delineate immunoglobulin isotypes. However, closer examination of these antibodies shows that these major isotypes may be subdivided (Table 4–3). For example, bovine IgG is a mixture of two antigenically distinct subisotypes or subclasses, called IgG1 and IgG2. Not only are these two subisotypes antigenically different, but IgG1 has a faster electrophoretic mobility than IgG2 and so can be readily distinguished from it by immunoelectrophoresis (Chapter 11). The importance of these immunoglobulin subisotypes lies in the fact that they are involved in different biological activities; for example, bovine IgG2 agglutinates particulate antigen, whereas IgG1 does not. This can be

Table 4–3 IMMUNOGLOBULIN ISOTYPES AND SUBISOTYPES OF
DOMESTIC ANIMALS AND MAN

| Species | Immunoglobulin Isotypes | | | | |
	IgG	IgA	IgM	IgE	IgD
Horse	Ga, Gb, Gc, G(B), G(T)a, G(T)b	A	M	E	?
Cattle	G1, G2 (G2a, G2b?)	A	M	E	?
Sheep	G1 (G1a?), G2, (G3?)	A1, A2	M	E	?
Pig	G1, G2, G3, G4	A1, A2	M	E	D
Dog	G1, G2a, G2b, G2c	A	M	E	?
Cat	G1, G2	A	M	E	?
Chicken	G1, (G2, G3?)	A	M	?	D
Human	G1, G2, G3, G4	A1, A2	M	E	D

of significance in the immunological diagnosis of infectious diseases such as brucellosis (Chapter 15). Some IgG subisotypes may bind to mast cells and therefore participate in type I hypersensitivity (Chapter 20).

The second group of epitopes recognized by anti-immunoglobulin sera are those found on the constant regions of the light and heavy chains in the immunoglobulins of some, but not all, animals of a species. These epitopes, which arise as a result of inherited variations in amino acid sequences, are inherited by individuals in mendelian fashion and are known as allotypes (Fig. 4–10). Allotypes are stable genetic markers that can be of use in identifying animals in cases of disputed paternity.

The third group of epitopes are those found within the variable regions. These are known as idiotopes. Each variable region contains several different idiotopes found both inside and outside the antigen-binding site. The col-

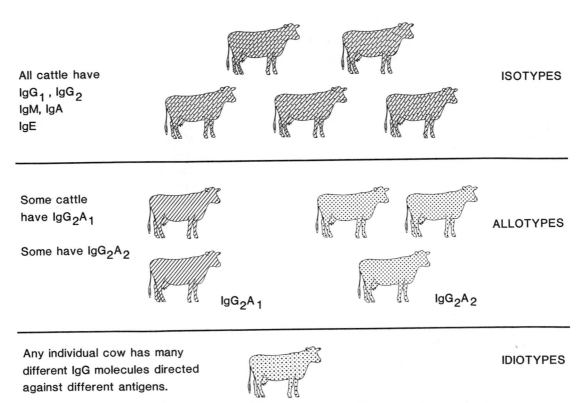

All cattle have
IgG$_1$, IgG$_2$
IgM, IgA
IgE

ISOTYPES

Some cattle
have IgG$_2$A$_1$

Some have IgG$_2$A$_2$

IgG$_2$A$_1$

IgG$_2$A$_2$

ALLOTYPES

Any individual cow has many
different IgG molecules directed
against different antigens.

IDIOTYPES

Figure 4–10. The classification of the major epitopes of immunoglobulin molecules.

lective term for the set of idiotopes on a molecule is idiotype. In most cases the antigen-binding site itself forms a major idiotope. Since any one animal possesses a mixture of immunoglobulins directed against a wide variety of epitopes, it must possess an equally wide spectrum of idiotypes. Antisera directed against idiotypes are of great use in investigating the nature of antigen recognition by antigen-sensitive cells.

IMMUNOGLOBULINS OF DOMESTIC ANIMALS

All mammals possess IgG, IgM and IgA, and it is probable that they also possess IgE and IgD (Table 4–3). The basic characteristics of each of these isotypes do not differ among species, and their properties and functions are as described previously. Nevertheless, mammals do differ in the number and types of subisotypes present in each species as well as in the possession of allotypes.

Horse

In the horse there exist five IgG subisotypes— IgGa, IgGb, IgGc, IgG(B) (sometimes called IgB) and IgG(T) sometimes called IgT. IgG(T) is interesting in that it is rich in carbohydrate and, because it is found in high concentrations in body secretions, was originally thought to be the equine homologue of IgA. Its designation T was derived from the observation that it was greatly elevated in horses employed for tetanus immune globulin production. However, analysis of its antigenic structure and amino acid sequence shows that it is closely related to IgG and so is best considered an IgG subisotype. IgG(T) does not fix guinea pig complement and reacts in a precipitation reaction by a rather characteristic flocculation (see Fig. 11–11). Other unclassified immunoglobulins described in the horse include a 10S γ_1 molecule and two immunoglobulins of fast γ mobility. Horses also possess IgM, IgA and IgE.

Cattle

In cattle, as discussed earlier, IgG is divided into two subisotypes, IgG1 and IgG2, on the basis of antigenicity and electrophoretic mobility. There is evidence to suggest that there may be two IgG2 subisotypes, IgG2a and IgG2b, but this is not confirmed. IgG1 constitutes about 50 per cent of the serum IgG and is remarkable for being the predominant immunoglobulin in cow's milk rather than IgA. The structure of its Fc region is responsible for its selective uptake by the mammary gland. IgG2 levels are highly heritable and thus concentrations vary greatly between cattle. The structure of the Fc region of IgG2 is responsible for its selective binding to neutrophil receptors. Allotypes have been reported to occur in cattle. One allotype, known as B1, is found on light chains of some cattle but is relatively uncommon. Several other allotypes have been reported; they include G_2A1 and G_2A2, found on IgG2 heavy chains and inherited as autosomal dominants, and G_1A1 found on IgG1 heavy chains. IgE has also been identified in cattle.

Sheep

The immunoglobulins of sheep are similar to those of cattle. Sheep possess IgG1, IgG2 and IgG3. Some sheep have been reported to possess an IgG1a, but this is probably an allotype. Sheep also possess a heat labile IgE with a molecular weight of 210,000 daltons.

Pigs

Pigs possess four IgG subisotypes, named IgG1, IgG2, IgG3 and IgG4. In addition, adult pigs may possess a γl, 18S macroglobulin antigenically similar to IgG2, and newborn piglets possess a 5S IgG, which may not have light chains. Four IgG allotypes have been reported in sows, and spontaneously occurring antibodies to these have been found in the serum of young piglets. It is thought that the piglets may become sensitized to the sow's immunoglobulins following neonatal absorption of these from colostrum. IgE and IgD have been reported to occur in the pig.

Dogs and Cats

Dogs possess four IgG subisotypes named IgG1. IgG2a, IgG2b and IgG2c, as well as IgA, IgM and IgE. Cats possess two IgG subisotypes (IgG1 and IgG2), IgM and IgA. An IgM allotype has been reported to occur in the dog.

Chickens

Although the IgG in this species has some unique properties (so much so that it has been named IgY by some workers) it is the functional counterpart of IgG in mammals and will therefore be called that here. Chicken IgG has a molecular weight of 200,000 daltons. Some workers have reported the existence of three subisotypes, termed IgG1, IgG2 and IgG3, although this has not been completely substantiated. Chickens also possess IgA, which is present in secretions and, like its mammalian equivalent, tends to form polymers. Chicken IgM is formed predominantly during the primary immune response, and it contains a J chain. A monomeric IgM can be detected in the amniotic fluid of eggs and in day-old chicks. It is thought to be derived from oviduct secretions in the hen. An avian homologue of IgD has also been identified.

Chickens have at least five immunoglobulin allotypes, two on the C_H1 domain of IgG, two on the IgM heavy chains and one on light chains.

Immunoglobulin N

Some fish, turtles, marsupials, ducks and rabbits have a low molecular weight immunoglobulin that some investigators have called IgN. Duck IgN has a molecular weight of 118,000 and is a 5.7S molecule. It contains two light chains of normal size and two small heavy chains. These heavy chains probably consist of one V_H domain and two C_H domains. This is the predominant immunoglobulin in duck serum and is neither a precursor nor a breakdown product of IgG. IgN does not fix complement. It is not known if it is related to the small immunoglobulin of pigs.

ADDITIONAL SOURCES OF INFORMATION

Barlough JE, Jacobson RH and Scott FW. 1981. The immunoglobulins of the cat. Cornell Vet. *71* 397–407.

Blattner FR and Tucker PW. 1984. The molecular biology of immunoglobulin D. Nature *307* 417–422.

Capparelli R, Rando A, Iannelli D et al. 1985. Age influenced IgG_3 allotype in sheep. Comp. Immunol. Micro. Infect. Dis. *8* 1–8.

Davies DR, Padlan EA and Segal DM. 1975. Three-dimensional structure of immunoglobulins. Ann. Rev. Biochem. *44* 639–667.

Feinstein A. 1979. Immunoglobulins and histocompatibility antigens. Nature (London) *282* 230.

Frieden E. 1975. Non-covalent interactions. J. Chem. Educ. *52* 754–761.

Halliwell REW, Schwartzman RM, Montgomery PC and Rockey JH. 1975. Physiochemical properties of canine IgE. Transplant. Proc. *7* 537–543.

Heddle RJ and Rowley D. 1975. Dog immunoglobulins. Immunochemical characterization of dog serum, parotid saliva, colostrum, milk and small bowel fluid. Immunology *29* 185–195.

Higgins DA. 1975. Physical and chemical properties of fowl immunoglobulins. Vet. Bull. *45* 139–154.

Philips DR, Chappel RJ and Hayes J. 1982. A possible role of $Cu2^+$ ions in bovine antibody-antigen interactions. Res. Vet. Sci. *32* 221–224.

Porter P. 1979. Structural and functional characteristics of immunoglobulins of the common domestic species. Adv. Vet. Sci. Comp. Med. *23* 1–21.

Proposed Rules for the Designation of Immunoglobulins of Animal Origin. 1978. Bull. WHO *59* 815–817.

Suter M and Fey H. 1983. Further purification and characterization of horse IgE. Vet. Immunol. Immunopathol. *4* 545–554.

Trebichavsky I, Zikan J and Travnicek J. 1983. The appearance of an IgD–like molecule on pig lymphocytes during ontogeny. Folia Microbiol. *28* 484–488.

Williams AF. 1984. The immunoglobulin superfamily takes shape. Nature *308* 12–13.

5

The Structure of the Immune System

Although antigen is trapped and processed by the macrophages of the mononuclear-phagocytic system, the mounting of an immune response is a function of lymphocytes. Lymphocytes are the small round cells that constitute the predominant cell type in organs such as the spleen, lymph nodes and thymus (Fig. 5–1). Although their morphology provides few clues as to their function, lymphocytes have been shown to be very complex. Their major functions include the production of antibodies and specific effector cells in response to macrophage-bound antigen. These responses occur within lymphoid organs (Fig. 5–2), which must therefore provide an environment for efficient interaction between lymphocytes, macrophages and antigen. In addition, control systems must be provided in order to regulate the immune responses, and this regulation can occur at two levels. On the first level, the production of lymphocytes must be controlled so that their numbers are appropriate for the tasks involved. In addition, some form of "editing" of these cells must occur so that those produced are reactive only to foreign epitopes and not to "self" antigens. On the second level, the magnitude of the response of each lymphocyte also must be regulated so that it is sufficient but not excessive for the body's requirements.

The tissues of the lymphoid system may therefore be classified on the basis of their roles in generating lymphocytes, in regulating the production of lymphocytes, and in provid-

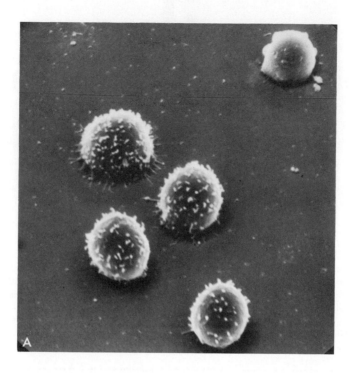

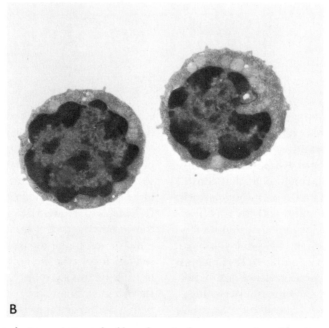

Figure 5–1. *A*, Scanning electron micrograph of lymphocytes from a mouse lymph node. × 1500. *B*, Transmission electron micrograph of lymphocytes from the peritoneal cavity of a mouse. × 3000.

Internal lymphoid tissues

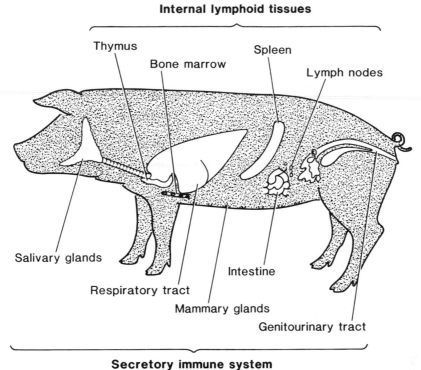

Secretory immune system

Figure 5–2. The lymphoid tissues of animals.

ing a suitable environment for the interaction between processed antigen and antigen-sensitive cells (Fig. 5–3).

SOURCES OF LYMPHOID CELLS

In the very young fetus, lymphoid stem cells are first produced in the primitive omentum and later in the fetal liver and yolk sac (Chapter 13). In older fetuses and in adult animals, the bone marrow serves as the major source of lymphoid cells. The central role of the bone marrow is emphasized by the observation that of all the tissues in the adult animal it alone is able to prevent the death of animals that have been lethally irradiated. Therefore, it is presumably capable of providing all the cells necessary to restore the functions of the other lymphoid organs.

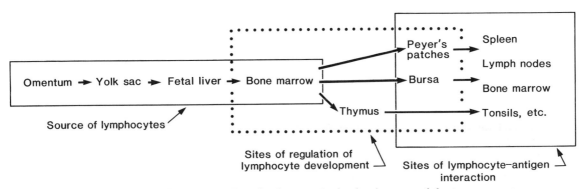

Figure 5–3. The role of the various lymphoid tissues in the development of the immune system.

The bone marrow in adult animals serves two functions. Not only is it a hematopoietic organ, serving as the source of all blood cells, including lymphocytes, but like the spleen, liver and lymph nodes it also contains many mononuclear-phagocytes and thus serves to remove particulate antigens from circulating blood. Because of this dual function, the bone marrow has two compartments, a hematopoietic compartment and a vascular compartment. These two compartments alternate, like slices of cake, in wedge-shaped areas within long bones. The hematopoietic areas contain precursors of all the blood cells as well as macrophages and lymphocytes and are enclosed by a layer of adventitial cells. In older animals these adventitial cells may become so loaded with fat that the hematopoietic tissue is masked, and the marrow may have a fatty yellow appearance. The vascular compartment consists of blood sinuses lined by endothelial cells and crossed by reticular cells and macrophages.

PRIMARY LYMPHOID ORGANS

The organs whose function is to regulate the production and differentiation of lymphocytes are known as primary lymphoid organs. They include the thymus, found in both mammals and birds, the bursa of Fabricius, found only in birds, and Peyer's patches in mammals. These organs arise early in fetal life. The thymus arises from the third and fourth pharyngeal pouches, whereas the bursa develops from the cloaco-dermal junction. The Peyer's patches are of endodermal origin. As they develop, lymphoid stem cells from the omentum, the fetal liver and eventually the bone

marrow migrate into the thymus, bursa and Peyer's patches via the blood stream, and it is in them that recognizable lymphocytes are first observed in the fetus (Chapter 13) (Table 5–1).

Thymus

The thymus is an organ found in the anterior mediastinal space. In horses, cattle, sheep, pigs, and chickens, it also extends up the neck as far as the thyroid gland. The size of the thymus can vary considerably, its relative size being greatest in the newborn animal and its absolute size being greatest at puberty. After puberty, atrophy of the thymic parenchyma occurs and the cortex is replaced by adipose tissue, but remnants of the thoracic thymus may persist in many animals until old age. In addition to this age-related involution, the thymus also atrophies rapidly in response to stress so that the thymus of animals dying after prolonged sickness may be abnormally small.

Structure of the Thymus (Fig. 5–4)

The thymus consists of lobules of loosely packed epithelial cells, each covered by a connective tissue capsule. The outer part of each lobule, the cortex, is densely infiltrated with lymphocytes, but in the inner part, the medulla, the epithelial cells are clearly visible. Within the medulla are round bodies known as thymic (Hassall's) corpuscles, whose function is not known. The corpuscles contain keratin and perhaps represent an abortive attempt at keratinization by the epithelial cells. Occasionally, the remains of a small blood vessel may be observed at their center, and in cattle they may contain high concentra-

Table 5–1 COMPARISON OF PRIMARY AND SECONDARY LYMPHOID ORGANS

	Primary Lymphoid Organ	Secondary Lymphoid Organ
Origin	Ectoendodermal junction or endoderm	Mesoderm
Time of development	Early in embryonic life	Later in fetal life
Persistence	Involutes after puberty	Persists through adult life
Effect of removal	Loss of lymphocytes Loss of immune responses	No effect or only minor consequences
Response to antigen	Unresponsive	Fully reactive
Examples	Thymus; bursa; some Peyer's patches	Spleen; lymph nodes

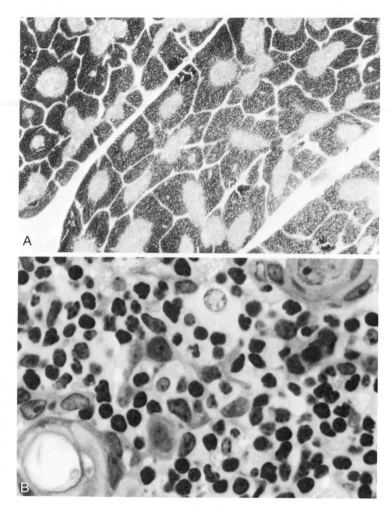

Figure 5–4. *A,* A section of a monkey thymus. Each lobule is divided into a cortex rich in lymphocytes, hence darkly staining, and a paler medulla, consisting mainly of epithelial cells. × 10. *B,* A high-power view of the medulla of a monkey thymus, showing several pale-staining epithelial cells with cytoplasmic processes and many dark-staining, round lymphocytes. × 1000.

tions of IgA (Chapter 12). The blood supply to the thymus is derived from arteries that enter through connective tissue septa and run as arterioles along the cortico-medullary junction. The capillaries that arise from these arterioles enter the cortex and loop back to the medulla. These capillaries are surrounded by an abnormally thick basement membrane and a continuous layer of epithelial cells. This barrier effectively prevents circulating antigens from entering the thymic cortex. No lymphatics leave the thymus.

Function of the Thymus

The functions of the thymus are best demonstrated by studying the effects of its surgical removal in newborn rodents (Fig. 5–5).

Neonatal Thymectomy. Thymectomy performed on mice within a day of birth results in these animals becoming much more susceptible to infection and occasionally failing to grow. Examination of these neonatally thymectomized animals reveals that they have greatly reduced numbers of circulating lymphocytes and their ability to mount some types of immune response is impaired (Table 5–2). In particular, their ability to reject grafts is severely compromised, reflecting a total loss of the cell-mediated immune response. Antibody-mediated immunity is also depressed, but to a lesser extent.

Neonatal thymectomy of domestic animals yields much less dramatic results. This is because the thymus matures earlier in these species and has performed many of its critical

NEONATAL THYMECTOMY

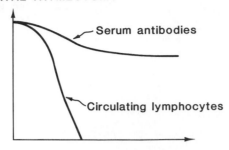

NEONATAL BURSECTOMY

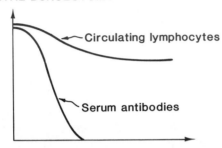

Figure 5–5. The effects of neonatal thymectomy and bursectomy on antibody- and cell-mediated immune responses.

functions well before the animal is born. For details of this see Chapter 14.

Adult Thymectomy. Removal of the thymus from adult animals produces no immediately obvious results. If, however, animals are examined several months after this operation, the numbers of their circulating lymphocytes and their ability to mount cell-mediated immune responses are found to be reduced. These results suggest that, although the adult thymus is still functional, there exists a reservoir of thymus-derived cells that must be

exhausted before the effects of thymectomy become apparent.

The results of thymectomy indicate therefore that the neonatal thymus is a source of many of the circulating blood lymphocytes. These are called thymus-derived lymphocytes or T cells. These thymus-derived lymphocytes actually originate in the bone marrow but are "processed" in the thymus after being attracted there by hormones secreted by thymic epithelial cells. Once within the thymus, these lymphocytes rapidly divide. Of the new cells produced, most die in the thymus, while others (about 5 per cent of the total in rodents and about 25 per cent in calves) emigrate after about 40 to 50 days and colonize the secondary lymphoid organs.

Nurse Cells

The thymus clearly provides an environment in which T cells can mature. In mice, at least some of this maturation may take place inside cells called nurse cells. Nurse cells are very large cells that can engulf up to 50 thymic lymphocytes and eventually release them unharmed. Perhaps it is within these cells that T cells acquire the ability to recognise self-antigens and learn not to respond to them. To the best of my knowledge, nurse cells have not been identified in the thymus of any major domestic animal.

Thymic Hormones. The thymus also functions as an endocrine gland. Several different hormones are secreted by thymic epithelial cells, the most important of which are thymosin (fraction 5), thymic humoral factor, the thymopoietins, thymostimulin, thymulin and

---

Table 5–2 EFFECTS OF NEONATAL THYMECTOMY AND BURSECTOMY ON THE IMMUNE
RESPONSES AND ON LYMPHOID TISSUES

Function	Thymectomy	Bursectomy
Numbers of circulating lymphocytes	↓ ↓ ↓	–
Presence of lymphocytes in thymus-dependent areas	↓ ↓ ↓	–
Graft rejection	↓ ↓ ↓	–
Presence of lymphocytes in thymus-independent areas and germinal centers	↓	↓ ↓ ↓
Plasma cells	↓	↓ ↓ ↓
Serum immunoglobulins	↓	↓ ↓ ↓
Antibody formation	↓	↓ ↓ ↓

interleukin 1 (IL-1) (Chapter 6). While these are distinct factors, their biological activities may be summarized by indicating that they induce the maturation of immature T cells and enhance many T cell functions such as cytotoxicity and helper activity. All the thymic hormones except IL-1, are small peptides.

Thymulin is interesting since it is a zinc-containing octapeptide secreted by the thymic epithelial cells, and it can partially restore T-cell function in thymectomized animals. (Its sequence in the pig is Gln-Ala-Lys-Ser-Glu-Gly-Ser-Asn.) Zinc is an essential mineral for the development of the thymus and of T cells. As a result zinc deficient animals suffer from a significant defect in their cell-mediated immune responses (Chapter 26).

Skin

The skin has the same embryologic origin as the thymus and there is some evidence to suggest that it too can promote T cell maturation. There is, for example, a subpopulation of T cells with a preference for the skin environment. These cells interact with keratinocytes and can undergo some maturation within the epidermis. However, the skin also functions as an effective antigen trapping barrier and these T cells may serve a localized defense function.

Bursa of Fabricius

The bursa of Fabricius (Fig. 5–6) is a lymphoepithelial organ found in birds but not in mammals. It arises from the ectoendodermal junction as a round, sac-like structure just dorsal to the cloaca. Like the thymus, the bursa reaches its greatest size in the chick about one to two weeks after hatching and then undergoes gradual involution.

Structure of the Bursa

Like the thymus, the bursa consists of lymphoid cells embedded in epithelial tissue. This epithelial tissue lines a hollow sac connected to the cloaca by a duct. Inside this sac, large folds of epithelium extend into the lumen, and scattered through these folds are follicles of lymphoid cells. Each lymphoid follicle is divided into a cortex and medulla. The cortex contains lymphocytes, plasma cells and macrophages. At the corticomedullary junction there is a basement membrane and capillary network on the inside of which are epithelial cells. These medullary epithelial cells show frequent mitotic figures, and toward the center of the medulla appear to be replaced by lymphoblasts and lymphocytes, so that the center of the follicle may appear to consist solely of lymphocytes.

Function of the Bursa

The bursa may be removed either surgically or by infecting newborn chicks with a virus that causes bursal destruction (infectious bursal disease). Since the bursa involutes when chicks become sexually mature, premature bursal atrophy may also be provoked by administration of testosterone. When bursectomized, birds produce very little antibody, and antibody-producing plasma cells disappear. Bursectomized birds still possess circulating lymphocytes and can reject foreign skin grafts. Thus bursectomy has little effect on the cell-mediated immune response. These birds are more susceptible than normal to leptospirosis and salmonellosis but not to bacteria against which cell-mediated immunity is important, such as *Mycobacterium avium*.

These results have been interpreted to suggest that the bursa is a primary lymphoid organ whose function is to serve as a maturation and differentiation site for the cells of the antibody-forming system. These cells are therefore called B cells. More recent studies however have suggested other interpretations. For example, it can be shown that spleen cells from a neonatally bursectomized bird, if transplanted into a normal bird, cause the recipient to lose its ability to make antibodies. This is due to the development of a population of cells (suppressor cells) in the bursectomized bird that can suppress antibody formation.

The bursa also functions as a secondary lymphoid organ; that is, it can trap antigen and undertake some antibody synthesis. It also

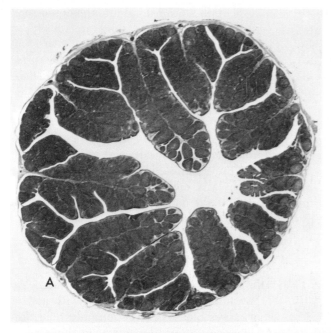

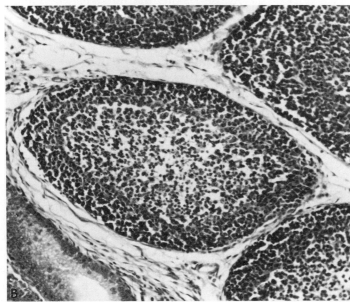

Figure 5–6. Photomicrographs showing the structure of the bursa of Fabricius. *A,* Low-power micrograph showing the bursa of a 14-day-old chick. × 5. *B,* A single follicle. × 360. (From a specimen kindly provided by Dr. S. Yamashiro.)

contains a small focus of T cells just dorsal to the bursal duct opening. It is probable, therefore, that the bursa has a number of different functions and can no longer be considered to be a pure primary lymphoid organ.

Peyer's Patches

In germ-free or newborn animals the lymphoid tissue of the intestine consists of clusters of lymphocytes and macrophages within the mucosa. These clusters are overlaid by a characteristic epithelium. This epithelium is thin, and consists of specialized cells called M cells. These M cells, which are also found in the bursa, are able to transport antigen from the intestinal lumen into the underlying lymphoid tissues. The appearance of this lymphoid tissue is independent of antigenic stimulation, but under the influence of antigen it expands rapidly to form Peyer's patches.

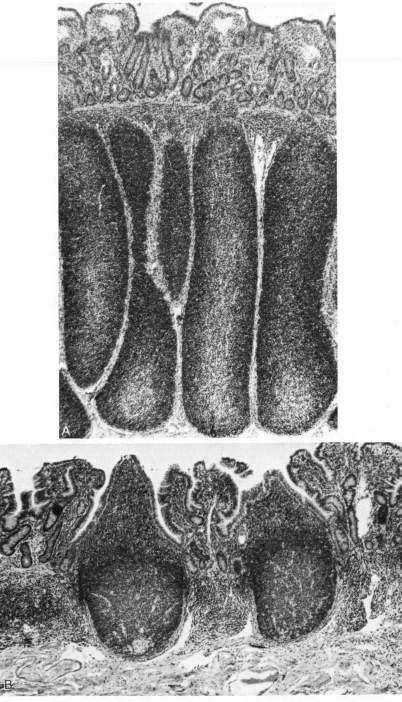

Figure 5–7. The structure of the two different types of Peyer's patch in sheep. *A,* An ileocecal Peyer's patch at 8 weeks of age. *B,* A Peyer's patch from the jejunum, also at 8 weeks. × 32. (From Reynolds JD and Morris B. Eur. J. Immunol. *13* 631, 1983. Used with permission.)

Two distinct types of Peyer's patch (PP) have been described in sheep. One form is found in the jejunum, whereas the other form is found in the ileum and cecum. Jejunal PP persist throughout the animal's lifetime. Ileocecal PP, in contrast, reach their maximum size and maturity before birth at a time when they are shielded from the presence of external antigens. They involute by about 15 months of age and cannot be detected in adult sheep. The two types of PP have very different structures (Fig. 5–7). Ileocecal PP consist of densely packed lymphoid follicles each separated by a connective tissue sheath and containing only B cells. Jejunal PP, however, have pear-shaped follicles separated by extensive interfollicular tissue, and they contain up to 30 per cent T cells. The ileocecal PP collectively form the largest lymphoid tissue in six-week-old lambs, constituting about 1 per cent of total body weight (about the same size as the thymus). It has been calculated that they can produce about 3.6×10^9 lymphocytes per hour but most of these are destroyed and only about 0.2×10^9 lymphocytes per hour are released into the circulation. Nevertheless surgical removal of the ileocecal PP leads to a loss of circulating B cells and a failure of antibody production. The bone marrow of lambs contains many fewer lymphocytes than the bone marrow of laboratory rodents and it is probable that the ileocecal PP are a significant source of B cell production in this species. It has been suggested that the jejunal PP are secondary lymphoid organs. The ileocecal PP, in contrast, are probably primary lymphoid organs (at least in lambs) and serve a similar function to the bursa of Fabricius. The bursa itself may be considered to be no more than a specialized Peyer's patch.

DIFFERENTIATION BETWEEN B AND T CELLS

B cells and T cells look identical, and it is not possible to distinguish between them on the basis of morphology (Figs. 5–1 and 5–8). It is therefore necessary to identify some functional features characteristic of each cell population in order to differentiate them (Table 5–3).

The best method of differentiating lymphocytes is to identify characteristic antigens on their surface. This may be done by preparing specific antisera against lymphocyte sub-populations. For example, thymus cells from one species may be inoculated into an animal of a different species, which then responds by making anti–T cell antibodies. These antibodies can be chemically linked to a fluorescent dye. If lymphocytes are immersed in this fluorescent antiserum, the antibodies will bind only to T cells. If the treated cell suspension is then washed and examined under an ultraviolet microscope, the T cells, having bound fluorescent antibody, will be seen to fluoresce.

This fluorescent antibody technique (which

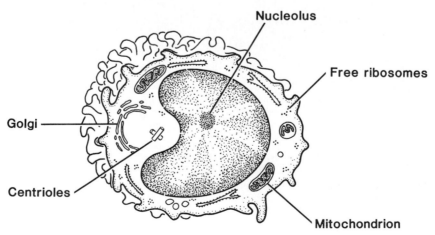

Figure 5–8. The structure of a typical lymphocyte. Remember T cells and B cells look identical.

Table 5–3 THE IDENTIFYING FEATURES OF T AND B LYMPHOCYTES

Property	B Cells	T Cells
Distribution	Lymph node cortex, splenic follicles	Lymph node paracortex, spleen periarteriolar sheath, peripheral blood
Cell surface receptors for		
Antigen	+ + +	+ +
Immunoglobulin Fc	+ + +	+
C3b	+	−
Foreign erythrocytes	−	+ + +
Cell-surface antigens	Immunoglobulin	Thy 1, T1–T11
Divide in response to	Pokeweed mitogen, bacterial lipopolysaccharide	Phytohemagglutinin; concanavalin A; BCG vaccine, pokeweed mitogen
Antigen receptor	Immunoglobulin	Ti–T3
Antigens preferentially recognized	Foreign macromolecules	Foreign macromolecules and MHC antigens
Tolerance induction	Difficult	Relatively easy
Progeny cells	Plasma cells, memory cells	Effector lymphocytes, memory cells
Major secreted products	Immunoglobulins	Lymphokines

is described in greater detail in Chapter 11) may also be used to identify B cells. We know that B cells possess immunoglobulin molecules on their surface. By using a fluorescent anti-immunoglobulin serum made as described previously, it is possible to identify B cells within a cell mixture.

When properly applied, the fluorescent antibody technique is capable of identifying not only T cells and B cells, but also of identifying sub-populations within these groups. T cells, for example, possess many specific cell-surface antigens (T4, T8, T3, etc.) that are found in characteristic patterns among the T cell sub-classes. B cells may be subdivided on the basis of the immunoglobulin isotype (IgM, IgG, IgA, etc.) on their surfaces.

A second group of techniques used to distinguish T cells from B cells involves the demonstration of characteristic cell-surface receptors (Table 5–4). Thus, T cells, but not B cells, possess receptors enabling them to bind to foreign erythrocytes. If mouse T cells and sheep erythrocytes are centrifuged gently together and resuspended, then the sheep erythrocytes stick to the T cells to form "rosettes." B cells, in contrast, do not possess erythrocyte receptors, but they do have receptors for immunoglobulin Fc regions. B cells therefore form rosettes with antibody-coated erythrocytes (Fig. 5–9). It may also be shown by using complement-coated erythrocytes that B cells but not T cells possess receptors for certain complement components (Chapter 10).

A third technique by which T and B cells may be distinguished is by measuring their responses to certain proteins called lectins. Lectins—which come from many different

Table 5–4 IDENTIFICATION OF T AND B CELLS USING SURFACE MARKERS

Cell	Marker	Method Of Detection
T cells	Erythrocyte receptor	Rosette formation
	Thy 1 antigen	Immunofluorescence
	Fc receptor	Rosette formation using antibody-coated red cells
	T cell antigens	Immunofluorescence
B cells	Immunoglobulin	Immunofluorescence
	Complement receptor	Rosette formation using complement-coated red cells
	Fc receptor	Rosette formation using antibody-coated red cells

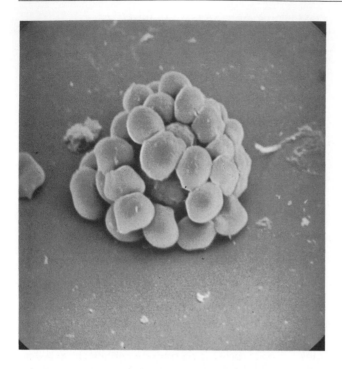

Figure 5–9. Scanning electron micrograph of a "rosette" formed by allowing antibody-coated sheep erythrocytes to come into contact with a mouse lymphocyte. × 2250.

sources, especially plants—have an affinity for cell-surface sugars. Since these sugars may differ between T and B cells, some lectins bind only to T cells, others bind only to B cells, and some bind to both. When lectins bind to lymphocytes they commonly provoke them to divide. Thus, the lectins phytohem-agglutinin, derived from the kidney bean (*Phaseolus vulgaris*) and concanavalin A, from the jack bean (*Canavallia ensiformis*), stimulate T cells (and B cells to a much lesser extent) to divide. Pokeweed mitogen, a lectin from the pokeweed plant (*Phytolacca americana*), stimulates both B and T cells.

Other nonlectin products may also function as lymphocyte mitogens; for example, the bacterial endotoxins stimulate B cells to divide, whereas BCG vaccine stimulates only T cells to divide.

These techniques enable investigators to characterize mixed lymphocyte populations. Thus, about 70 per cent of mouse or human peripheral blood lymphocytes can be shown to be T cells and about 25 per cent B cells. The remaining lymphocytes are neither typical T nor typical B cells. In the absence of characteristic markers, they may be called "null"

cells. Unfortunately, the techniques described above for distinguishing T from B cells were first worked out in mice and subsequently modified for use in humans. The reliability of these techniques in distinguishing T from B cells in the major domestic animals remains unclear (Table 5–5). Most results suggest that the relative proportions of T, B and null cells in the blood of domestic animals are similar to those in man and rodents, although some studies show a higher percentage of null cells. This is probably a reflection of the inadequacies of the techniques presently available.

Table 5–5 THE PERIPHERAL BLOOD LYMPHOCYTES OF DOMESTIC ANIMALS AND MAN

Species	Percentage of T cells	Percentage of B cells
Horse	38–66	20
Cattle	40–70	20–40
Sheep	28–80	15–35
Pig	45–57	26–38
Dog	70	23–30
Cat	50	30–40
Chicken	45	30
Human	65–75	16–28

SECONDARY LYMPHOID ORGANS

In contrast to the thymus and bursa, the other lymphoid organs of the body arise from mesoderm late in fetal life and persist through adult life (see Table 5–1). They are responsive to antigenic stimulation and thus are poorly developed in germ-free animals. This is in marked contrast to the primary lymphoid organs, which do not normally respond to antigen and are thus of normal size in germ-free animals. Removal of a secondary lymphoid organ does not significantly reduce an animal's immune capability. Examples of secondary lymphoid organs include the spleen, the lymph nodes and the lymphoid nodules of the gastrointestinal, respiratory and urogenital tracts. These organs are rich in macrophages and dendritic cells that trap and process antigens and in T and B lymphocytes, which mediate the immune responses. The overall anatomical structure of these organs is therefore designed to facilitate antigen trapping and to provide maximum opportunities for processed antigen to be presented to antigen-sensitive cells.

Lymph Nodes

Structure of Lymph Nodes

Lymph nodes are round or bean-shaped structures strategically placed on lymphatic channels in such a way that they can trap antigen being carried through the lymph. Thus, lymph nodes consist of a reticular network filled with lymphocytes, macrophages and dendritic cells through which lymphatic sinuses penetrate (Figs. 5–10 and 5–11). A subcapsular sinus is located immediately under the connective tissue capsule of the node. Other sinuses pass through the body of the node but are most prominent in the medulla. Lymphatic vessels enter the node at various points around its circumference, and efferent lymphatics leave from a depression or hilus on one side. The blood vessels to and from a lymph node also enter and leave via the hilus.

The interior of a lymph node is divided into a peripheral cortex, a central medulla and an ill-defined area between these two regions termed the paracortical zone. The cells in the cortex are predominantly B lymphocytes and are arranged in nodules. Prior to exposure to antigen these nodules are termed primary

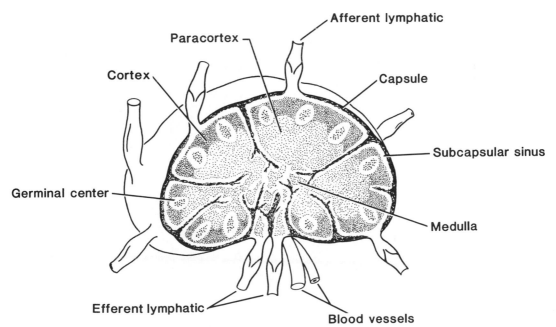

Figure 5–10. The structure of a typical lymph node.

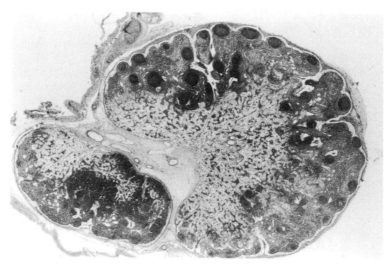

Figure 5–11. A section of bovine lymph node. × 12. (From a specimen kindly provided by Dr. W. E. Haensly.)

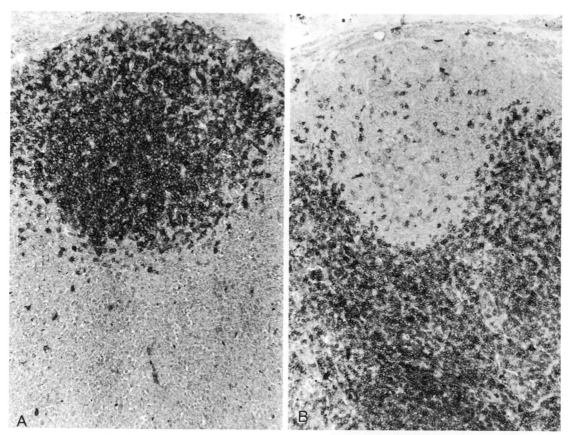

Figure 5–12. Normal bovine lymph node stained by the immunoperoxidase technique (Chapter 11) with (A) a monoclonal antibody that identifies B lymphocytes and (B) a monoclonal antibody that identifies T lymphocytes. The B cells are located in the lymph node cortex. The T cells fill the paracortical zone. (Courtesy of Drs. I. Morrison and N. MacHugh.)

follicles. In lymph nodes that have been stimulated by antigen, the cells within primary follicles expand to form characteristic structures known as germinal centers. A follicle containing a germinal center is known as a secondary follicle. Some T cells are found in the cortex, distributed in an area immediately surrounding each germinal center.

The cells in the paracortical zone are mainly T lymphocytes and are arranged in poorly defined nodules called tertiary follicles. In neonatally thymectomized or congenitally athymic animals, this area is deprived of cells and so can be considered a "thymus-dependent" area (Fig. 5–12).

The cells found in the medulla include B lymphocytes, macrophages, reticulum cells and plasma cells. These are arranged in cellular cords between the lymphatic sinuses.

Lymphocyte Circulation

Lymph flows through the calf thoracic duct at 500 ml per hour, and it contains about 1×10^8 lymphocytes per milliliter. If the thoracic duct is cannulated and the lymph removed, a calf will become severely lymphopenic within a few hours. When the lymphoid tisssues of such an animal are examined, it can be shown that T lymphocytes have disappeared from lymph node paracortical zones. Because of their rapid depletion, it is clear that thoracic duct cells must normally recirculate back to the lymphoid tissues (Fig. 5–13). In fact, the T cells that enter the vena cava from the thoracic duct spend only between two and twelve hours in blood before returning to the lymph nodes. They leave the blood stream by way of the venules of the lymph node paracortical zone. These venules possess an extremely tall endothelium (Fig. 5–14). (Except in sheep, where the endothelium in unstimulated nodes is flat, a high endothelium is induced in highly stimulated nodes where the rate of lymphocyte emigration is increased.) Circulating T cells adhere to receptors on these endothelial cells and then pass into the node by penetrating between the endothelial

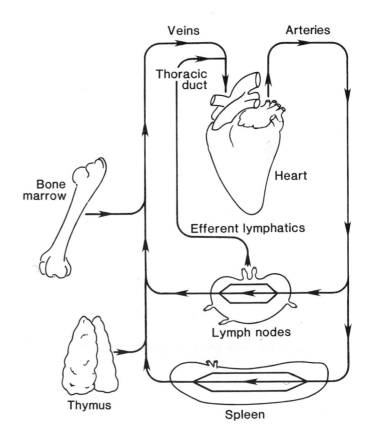

Figure 5–13. The circulation of lymphocytes. Lymphocytes found in blood may be newly formed cells passing from the bone marrow to the primary lymphoid organs or cells passing from the primary to the secondary lymphoid organs. The vast majority of these cells, however, are recirculating between the lymph nodes and the blood stream.

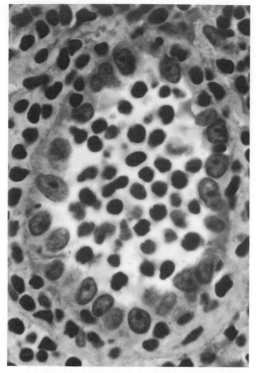

Figure 5–14. A section of human tonsil, showing a "post-capillary" venule with its high endothelium.

cells. After passing through the node, the T cells re-enter the lymphatic circulation via the efferent lymph. There is thus a continuous recirculation of T cells between lymph and blood. It is tempting to suggest that this is most appropriate for lymphocytes whose function is to survey the body for aberrant cells.

As a result of this circulation, the majority of lymphocytes found in peripheral blood are T cells (see Table 5–5). The B cells in blood are probably in transit between the bone marrow and the secondary lymphoid organs.

A small proportion of the T cells found in blood do not return to lymph nodes but leave the circulation from venules within the lymphoid tissues in the lung or intestine. These cells are specifically involved in the development of immune responses at body surfaces.

Pigs and other swine, elephants, hippopotamuses, rhinoceroses and dolphins are different! Their lymph nodes are structurally inverted so that the afferent lymphatics enter the node through the hilus and the lymph passes from the cortex at the center of the node to the medulla at the periphery before leaving through the efferent vessels (Fig. 5–15). The medulla has few sinuses but consists of a diffuse reticulum, containing cells. In addition pig lymphocytes circulate differently from other mammals. The circulating lymphocytes leave the lymph node not via the lymphatics but by way of the venules. As a result very few lymphocytes are found in pig lymph. The reasons for this difference are unknown.

Response of Lymph Nodes to Antigen

Foreign antigen deposited in tissues is carried by the flow of tissue fluid to local lymph nodes.

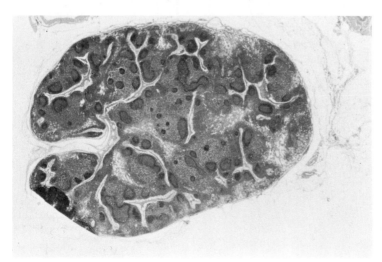

Figure 5–15. A section of a pig lymph node. Note how the germinal centers are located in the interior of the node. × 12. (From a specimen kindly provided by Dr. W. E. Haensly.)

Its fate within these nodes depends upon whether the animal has had previous exposure to the antigen. Lymph nodes possess two separate antigen-trapping systems. Macrophages in the medulla can take up antigen in the absence of antibodies. They can therefore function relatively effectively on first exposure to antigen. The other system involves dendritic cells. These cells are found within secondary follicles in the lymph node cortex. Dendritic cells have an extensive array of long cytoplasmic processes (see Fig. 2–9) and can thus form a web through which antigen must pass as it filters through the cortex. The efficiency of this web as an antigen-trapping device does depend, however, upon the presence of antibody, which is required for antigen to adhere to the dendritic cell processes.

If an animal possesses no antibodies to an injected antigen, then most of the antigen entering the node will be phagocytosed by medullary macrophages. The macrophages then migrate to the cortical follicles, and present their antigen to B and T cells. When antibody production is stimulated then the progeny of these B cells move to the medulla and begin to produce antibodies. Some of these antibody-producing cells are also released into the efferent lymph and in this way colonize other lymph nodes downstream. Several days after antibody production is first observed in the medulla, germinal centers appear in the cortex, arising as a result of proliferation of cells within primary follicles. The dividing cells are usually relatively large and pale-staining but compress the surrounding lymphocytes into a dense mantle around the germinal center (Fig. 5–16). Antigens that do not stimulate antibody production do not cause germinal center formation, and it is believed that germinal centers are required for the establishment of immunological memory.

Adherence to follicular dendritic cells is the predominant means of antigen trapping once an animal has been sensitized by previous exposure to antigen. In a secondary response the germinal centers become less obvious as the activated memory B cells migrate from the cortex to the medulla and the efferent

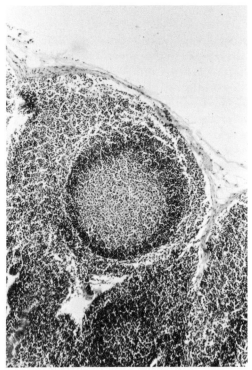

Figure 5–16. A germinal center in the cortex of a cat lymph node. Note the large, pale area in the center of the germinal center where the cells are dividing. × 120. (From a specimen kindly provided by Dr. W. E. Haensly.)

lymph. Once this stage is completed, the germinal centers then show hyperplasia and, to a limited extent, antibody production. All this movement of cells within the lymph node ensures that antibody-producing cells are kept as far away as possible from antigen-sensitive cells. As will be discussed later (Chapter 9) this prevents an immediate inhibition of the immune response through the negative feedback exerted by antibody.

When responding to antigens that stimulate a cell-mediated rather than an antibody-mediated immune response, such as, for example, skin grafts, the T cell–rich paracortical areas respond by the production of large pyroninophilic cells (pyronin is a stain for RNA; thus, a cell with pyroninophilic cytoplasm is rich in ribosomes and is probably a protein-producing cell). These large pyroninophilic cells give rise, in turn, to more small lymphocytes, which participate in the cell-mediated immune responses.

Spleen

Just as lymph nodes serve to "filter" antigen from lymph, so the spleen "filters" blood. The filtering process removes both antigenic particles and aged blood cells. In addition, the spleen stores erythrocytes and platelets and undertakes erythropoiesis in the fetus. It is therefore divided into two compartments, one for storage of erythrocytes, antigen trapping and erythropoiesis, called the red pulp; and one in which the immune response occurs, known as the white pulp (Fig. 5–17).

Structure of Splenic White Pulp

Vessels entering the spleen travel through muscular trabeculae before entering its functional areas. Immediately on leaving the trabeculae each arteriole is surrounded by a

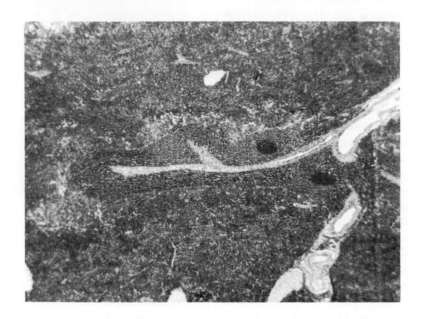

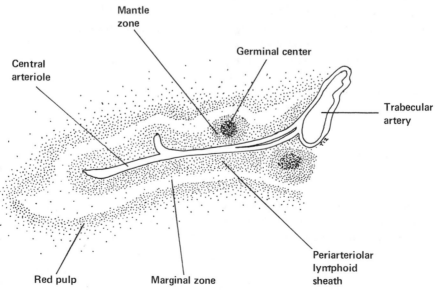

Figure 5–17. A histological section and diagram, showing the structure of the bovine spleen. × 50. (From a specimen kindly provided by Dr. J. R. Duncan.)

sheath of lymphoid tissue known, naturally enough, as the periarteriolar lymphoid sheath. The arteriole eventually leaves this sheath and branches into penicillary arterioles, which possess a characteristically thickened wall, forming a structure known as an ellipsoid. These arterioles then open, either directly or indirectly, into venous sinuses that drain into the splenic venules. The periarteriolar lymphoid sheath consists largely of T cells and is therefore depleted following neonatal thymectomy. Scattered through the sheath are primary follicles, consisting largely of B cells. On antigenic stimulation these follicles develop germinal centers and so become secondary follicles. Each follicle is surrounded by a layer of T cells, forming a mantle zone. The white pulp (that is, the periarteriolar sheath, the B cell follicles and the mantle zone) is separated from the red pulp by a marginal sinus, a reticulum sheath and a marginal zone of cells.

Response of the Spleen to Antigen

Intravenously administered antigen is trapped, in part, in the spleen, where it is taken up by macrophages located in the marginal zone and lining the sinusoids of the red pulp. These macrophages carry antigen to the primary follicles of the white pulp from which, after a few days, antibody-producing cells migrate. These antibody-producing cells colonize the marginal zone and the red pulp, and it is in these regions that antibody production is first detected. Germinal center formation also occurs in the primary follicles within a few days, although this is not directly associated with antibody production. In an animal already possessing circulating antibody, trapping by dendritic cells within the secondary follicles becomes significant. As in a primary immune response, the antibody-producing cells migrate from these follicles to the red pulp and the marginal zone where antibody production largely occurs, although some antibodies may also be produced within the hyperplastic secondary follicles.

Lymphocyte Trapping

When antigen enters the spleen or lymph nodes, it initiates lymphocyte trapping. That is, lymphocytes that normally pass freely through these organs are trapped so that they cannot leave. The mechanism of the trapping process is not clear, but the process probably occurs as a result of the interaction between antigen and macrophages, leading to the release of a factor that influences the movement of lymphocytes in some way. Trapping serves to concentrate lymphocytes in close proximity to sites of antigen accumulation and so increases the efficiency of the immune responses. Some adjuvants may also act by enhancing trapping. After about 24 hours the lymph node releases the trapped cells and shows increased cellular output for about seven days. Toward the end of this time, many of these released cells become antibody producers and memory cells.

OTHER SECONDARY LYMPHOID TISSUES AND THE SITES OF ANTIBODY PRODUCTION

Antibodies are produced in the secondary lymphoid tissues. These tissues include not only the spleen and lymph nodes but also the bone marrow, tonsils (see Fig. 12–6) and lymphoid tissues scattered throughout the body, particularly in the digestive (see Fig. 5–7), respiratory and urogenital tracts.

Although its scattered nature makes it difficult to measure, the bone marrow constitutes the largest mass of secondary lymphoid tissue in the body. Therefore, if antigen is given intravenously, it will be trapped and will stimulate antibody production not only in the spleen, but also in the bone marrow. Although the spleen produces the greatest amount of antibody in relation to its size, the bone marrow produces the greatest total amount of antibody, accounting for up to 70 per cent of the antibody produced in response to some antigens (Fig. 5–18). The lymphoid tissues of the lung may also contribute significantly to the immune response against intravenously administered antigen.

Antigen administered orally, if it can penetrate the intestinal wall without being degraded, may stimulate the intestinal lymphoid tissues. As a result, sensitized lymphocytes

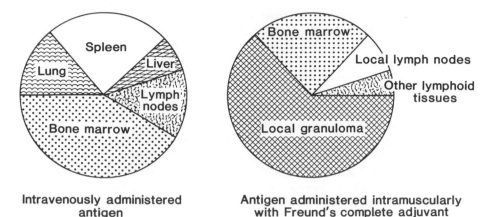

Figure 5–18. The relative contribution of different organs or tissues to antibody production following the administration of antigen either intravenously or intramuscularly with Freund's complete adjuvant.

leave the intestine, circulate in the blood stream and then colonize surfaces throughout the body. Antigenic stimulation of one part of the intestine may thus provoke antibody formation throughout the digestive tract as well as in the lung, the mammary gland, and the urogenital tract (Chapter 12). Antigen introduced directly into the nonlactating mammary gland stimulates local antibody synthesis in lymphoid nodules and in the draining lymph nodes. Antibody is therefore found in relatively high levels in milk during the subsequent lactation. Antigen administered by inhalation stimulates local antibody production in the lymphoid tissues of the respiratory tract and, if absorbed into the blood stream, will provoke a systemic immune response.

Many adjuvants, such as those containing alum or water-in-oil emulsions, act by forming an insoluble antigen-containing depot. This persistent irritation stimulates a chronic inflammatory response (Chapter 19). Antibody-forming cells develop within this chronic lesion and may contribute a significant proportion of the antibody produced when these adjuvants are used (Fig. 5–18).

ADDITIONAL SOURCES OF INFORMATION

Barclay AN. 1982. The organization of B and T lymphocytes in lymph nodes. Immunol Today *3* 330–331.

Binns RM. 1982. Organization of the lymphoreticular system and lymphocyte markers in the pig. Vet Immunol Immunopathol *3* 95–146.

Edelson RL and Fink JM. 1985. The immunologic function of skin. Sci Amer *252* 46–53.

Ekino S, Suginohara K, Urano T et al. 1985. The bursa of Fabricius: a trapping site for environmental antigens. Immunology *55* 405–410.

Firth GA. 1977. The normal lymphatic system of the domestic fowl. Vet Bull *47* 167–179.

Gershwin LJ, Lance P and Rokito AS. 1983. Comparison of analysis of bovine surface immunoglobulin bearing and peanut agglutinin binding lymphocytes by flow cytometry and fluorescence microscopy. Vet Immunol Immunopathol *5* 185–186.

Higgins DA. 1981. Markers for T and B lymphocytes and their application to animals. Vet Bull *51* 925–963.

Hopkins J and McConnell I. 1984. Immunological aspects of lymphocyte recirculation. Vet Immunol Immunopathol *6* 3–33.

Johansson C and Morein B. 1983. Evaluation of labelling methods for bovine T and B lymphocytes. Vet Immunol Immunopathol *4* 345–359.

Kajikawa O, Koyama H, Yoshikawa T et al. 1983. Use of alpha-naphthyl acetate esterase staining to identify T lymphocytes in cattle. Am J Vet Res *44* 1549–1552.

Kubai L and Auerbach R. 1983. A new source of embryonic lymphocytes in the mouse. Nature *301* 154–156.

Monroe WE and Roth JA. 1986. The thymus as part of the endocrine system. Comp Cont Ed Pract Vet *8* 24–33.

Ratcliff MJH. 1985. The ontogeny and cloning of B cells in the bursa of Fabricius. Immunol Today *6* 223–227.

Reynolds JD. 1986. Evidence of extensive lymphocyte death in sheep Peyer's patches. I. A comparison of lymphocyte production and export. J Immunol *136* 2005–2010.

Reynolds JD and Morris B. 1984. The effect of antigen on the development of Peyer's patches in sheep. Eur J Immunol *14* 1–6.

Torres-Medina A. 1981. Morphologic characteristics of the epithelial surface of aggregated lymphoid follicles (Peyer's patches) in the small intestine of newborn gnotobiotic calves and pigs. Am J Vet Res *42* 232–236.

Weiss L. 1972. Cells and Tissues of the Immune System: Structure, Functions, Interactions. Foundations of Immunology Series. Prentice-Hall, Inc, Englewood Cliffs, New Jersey.

6

The Cellular Basis of Antibody Formation

It is clear from our observation of immune responses that certain cells must be able to recognize antigens as foreign and then respond to specific epitopes on these antigens. It is also clear that the response of these antigen-sensitive cells must result either in the production of antibodies or in the production of cells that can participate in the cell-mediated immune responses. In addition, cells must be generated that can respond even more effectively to a second exposure to the same antigen—in other words, memory cells.

CLONAL SELECTION

The hypothesis that first successfully accounted for the ability of an animal to mount a specific immune response against any one of a very wide variety of antigens is known as the clonal selection theory. This theory was put forward by Nobel Prize winner Sir Macfarlane Burnet in 1959 and has now been amply confirmed. The basic postulates of Burnet's theory are as follows:

1. Lymphoid stem cells differentiate randomly to produce clones of lymphocytes, each of which is committed to respond to a single epitope.

2. Antigen binding to lymphocyte receptors triggers them to proliferate and differentiate into effector cells and memory cells.

3. The specificity of the antibodies produced by a lymphocyte is identical to that of its antigen receptors.

4. Tolerance results when a clone of antigen-binding lymphocytes is destroyed or suppressed.

It is now recognized that two populations of antigen-sensitive cells do exist: the B lymphocytes, which eventually give rise to plasma cells and produce antibody and the T lymphocytes, which mediate the cell-mediated immune responses. Antigen binding to receptors on these cells induces them to proliferate and is the initiating event in the immune responses (Fig. 6–1). The response of B cells to antigen is discussed in this chapter, the response of T cells in the next.

The Development of B Cells
(Fig. 6–2)

B cells develop from stem cells that originate in the bone marrow. These stem cells are committed to all the steps required to produce an antibody-secreting plasma cell. The first stage in the development of B cells is the appearance in their cytoplasm of heavy chains of the μ type. Next, the cell synthesizes immunoglobulin light chains, which interact with the μ heavy chains to form monomeric IgM molecules. These IgM molecules are expressed first in the B cell cytoplasm and then on its surface, where they are embedded in the cell membrane. At a slightly later stage of development the immature B cell also synthesizes cytoplasmic and membrane IgD. Thus, by the time it reaches maturity the B

cell possesses both IgM and IgD. Once these immunoglobulins appear on the B cell membrane it is able to respond to foreign antigen.

The B Cell Antigen Receptor

B cells can respond to a specific epitope because they have specific receptors for that epitope on their surface. These receptors are immunoglobulin molecules attached to the cell membrane and positioned so that their antigen-binding (Fab) sites are exposed, whereas their Fc region is buried within the cell membrane. There are about 10^4 to 10^5 of these receptor immunoglobulin molecules on the surface of each B cell. Normally, the receptors on B cells that have never encountered antigen consist of monomeric IgM and IgD. As an immune response progresses, the isotype, but not the specificity of a B cell's antigen receptors, changes. Because all the receptor immunoglobulin molecules on a single B cell are of a single specificity, an individual B cell can bind and respond only to the epitope

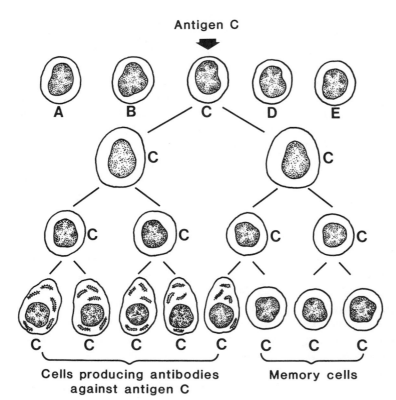

Figure 6–1. The clonal selection theory. Antigen stimulates the proliferation only of a specific clone of cells (in this case clone C). The responding clone proliferates and eventually differentiates into two populations: an antibody-producing population that releases antibody into the blood stream and a memory cell population that lives until the animal is exposed to the same antigen for a second time.

Antigen C

A   B   C   D   E

Cells producing antibodies against antigen C   Memory cells

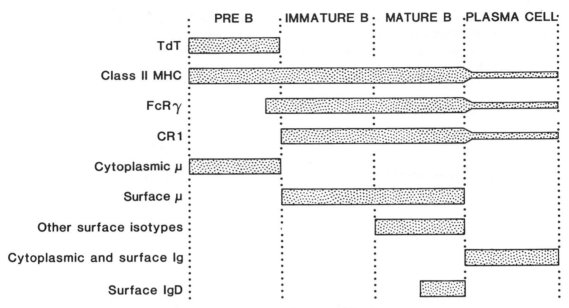

	PRE B	IMMATURE B	MATURE B	PLASMA CELL
TdT				
Class II MHC				
FcRγ				
CR1				
Cytoplasmic μ				
Surface μ				
Other surface isotypes				
Cytoplasmic and surface Ig				
Surface IgD				

Figure 6–2. The development of B cells.

against which its receptor immunoglobulins are directed.

B cells, each specific for a different epitope, are generated at random from bone marrow stem cells. It has been shown that an adult mouse spleen, for example, contains about 2×10^8 B cells capable of responding to at least 10^7 different epitopes. For some of these epitopes there may be only one or two responsive cells; for others there may be several thousand.

THE RESPONSE OF B CELLS TO ANTIGEN

The binding of antigen to a B cell-receptor immunoglobulin is not sufficient in itself to trigger an immune response. The proliferation of B cells is rigorously controlled and will normally occur only if certain critical conditions are met. These conditions are, first, that the antigen is processed by certain cells, especially macrophages, and presented to the B cell while fixed to the cell surface and, second, that certain T cells, called helper T cells, must also respond to the same antigen and secrete soluble helper factors (Fig. 6–3).

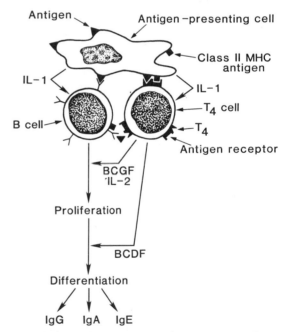

Figure 6–3. The interactions between an antigen-presenting cell, a B cell and T_4+ helper cell that lead to the development of an antibody response.

Macrophage Help

Although all macrophages phagocytose antigen, only some can process the antigen in such a way that it can stimulate an immune response. These antigen-processing macrophages are characterized by possessing proteins called class II histocompatibility antigens on their surface. (In mice these antigens are called Ia antigens. Unfortunately there is no consistent nomenclature between species. Histocompatibility antigens are discussed in detail in Chapter 8.) Class II antigen-positive macrophages permit residual foreign antigen to remain on the cell membrane, where it is up to 10 times more effective than unbound antigen in promoting an immune response. In this location the foreign antigen is physically associated with the class II antigen molecule. Although B cells can recognize the foreign antigen alone, helper T cells can only recognize a foreign antigen if it is associated with a class II antigen. As they present foreign antigen to a B cell (Fig. 6–4), macrophages also secrete a family of proteins called interleukin 1.

Interleukin 1 (IL-1) is the name given to two proteins (interleukin 1 α and interleukin 1 β) with molecular weights between 12,000 and 16,000 daltons. They are produced spontaneously by macrophages in small quantities and in much larger amounts when the macrophages are activated by such agents as endotoxin, muramyl dipeptide, bacteria, interferon-γ (IFN-γ), antigen-antibody complexes, concanavalin A or particulate antigens. IL-1 activates the helper T cells (and also B cells to a much lesser extent). Since IL-1 is also an integral component of the macrophage membrane, helper T cells may be stimulated simply by contact with macrophages.

T Cell Help

When helper T cells encounter macrophage-bound antigen linked to a class II antigen in the presence of interleukin 1, they secrete two proteins. One is called B cell growth factor (BCGF), and the other is called interleukin 2 (IL-2). BCGF consists of two molecules of 17,000 and 50,000 daltons. IL-2 is discussed in detail in the following chapter. BCGF and IL-2 act together with IL-1 to provoke B cells to respond optimally after they have been exposed to foreign antigen.

The B Cell Response

Once a B cell's receptor immunoglobulin molecules are crosslinked by foreign antigen and its BCGF and IL-2 receptors are stimulated, the B cell will go from a resting to an activated state. The activated B cell itself expresses new cell membrane class II antigens, the surface receptors become rearranged and the membrane-bound antigen becomes concentrated

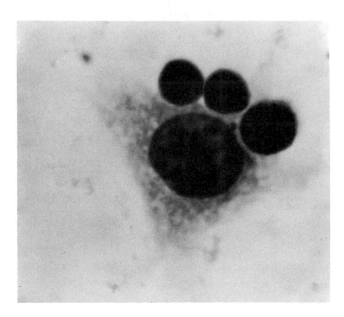

Figure 6–4. Macrophage-lymphocyte interaction. The lymphocytes are from an animal sensitized to the hapten dinitrophenol (DNP) linked to the carrier bovine serum albumin. The macrophage was coated with DNP linked to the unrelated carrier ovalbumin by means of cytophilic antibodies to ovalbumin. The three lymphocytes are therefore binding to an antigen-coated macrophage. × 1300.

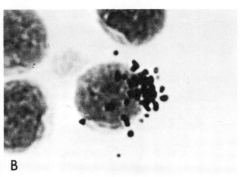

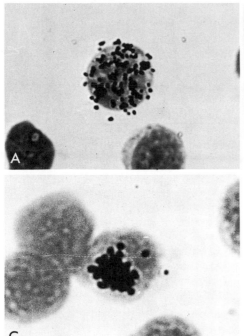

Figure 6–5. The capping phenomenon. Autoradiographs of lymph node cells from an immunized mouse incubated with bound, tritiated polymerized flagellin. A, Uniform distribution of antigen after incubation of 0°C for 30 minutes. B and C, Aggregation of antigen at a polar region after incubation at 37°C for 15 minutes. A, B, and C, × 2400. (From Diener E and Paetkan V. H. 1972. Proc. Natl. Acad. Sci. 69 2374. Used with permission. Courtesy of Dr. Diener.)

into a small region (or cap) on the B cell surface (Fig. 6–5). The antigen may then be taken into the B cell or released into the surrounding medium. The B cell then divides repeatedly. As the B cell divides it is influenced by other soluble factors secreted by T cells, called B cell differentiation factors (BCDF). After a few days, the progeny of the responding B cell gradually differentiate into two morphologically and functionally discrete cell populations. The cells in one of these populations acquire the ability to manufacture and secrete large quantities of antibody. The specificity of this antibody is identical to the specificity of the antigen receptors on the original responding B cell. These antibody-producing cells are called plasma cells. The cells in the other population remain structurally unchanged and function as memory cells (Fig. 6–6).

Plasma Cells

Because plasma cells arise by differentiation from B cells, it is possible to identify a series of stages that are morphologically intermediate between lymphocytes and plasma cells. Plasma cells are ovoid, 8 to 20 μm in diameter (Figs. 6–7 and 6–8). They are widely distributed throughout the body but are concentrated in the red pulp of the spleen, in the medulla of lymph nodes and in bone marrow. (Despite their name, they are not found in plasma.) They possess a round, eccentrically situated nucleus whose chromatin is distributed unevenly, so that the stained nucleus may resemble a clockface or cartwheel. They possess extensive cytoplasm that is strongly basophilic and pyroninophilic, as befits a cell rich in ribosomes that produce antibodies. Because these antibodies must be rapidly secreted, plasma cells also possess a large, pale-staining Golgi apparatus. Plasma cells are capable of synthesizing as many as 300 molecules of antibody per second, and on occasion this antibody may accumulate within cells to form vesicles known as Russell bodies. Normally, however, antibodies are secreted through reverse pinocytosis soon after they are formed. As pointed out before, it is important to note that the specificity of the immunoglobulin produced by these plasma cells is identical to that of the original antigen receptor on the

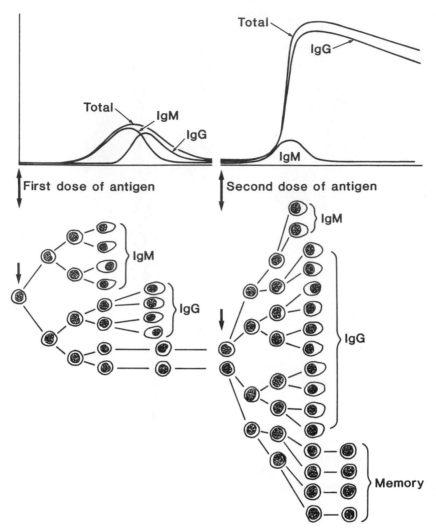

Figure 6–6. The cellular basis of the antibody response. Note how some IgG is made in the primary immune response while a little IgM is made in a secondary immune response.

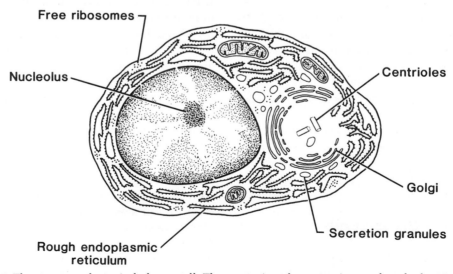

Figure 6–7. The structure of a typical plasma cell. The possession of an extensive rough endoplasmic reticulum is typical of a cell dedicated to massive protein synthesis.

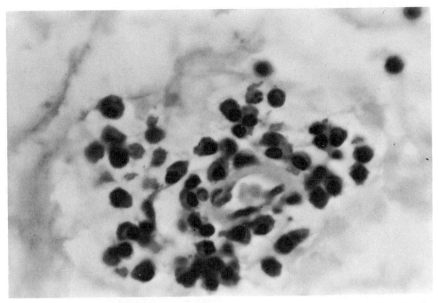

Figure 6–8. Plasma cells in the medulla of a dog lymph node. × 450. (From a specimen kindly provided by Dr. S. Yamashiro.)

parent B cell. (This is because the same genes are used to synthesize the immunoglobulin variable region.) Once fully differentiated, plasma cells die after three to six days. This is reflected in serum antibody levels as the immunoglobulins produced by these cells decline gradually through catabolism.

Plaque Assays

It is a relatively simple matter to identify individual cells producing antibody against sheep erythrocytes. The test (known as a plaque assay) can be performed by mixing a suspension of antibody-producing cells (usually spleen cells from an inoculated animal) with sheep erythrocytes and stabilizing the mixture in thin film between a slide and a coverslip. When the mixture is incubated at 37°C, antibodies released from the producing cells diffuse into the media and combine with nearby red cells. If hemolytic complement (Chapter 10) is incorporated in the media and if the antibody being produced is IgM (Chapter 4), then antibody-coated red cells will be lysed. A clear zone or plaque therefore develops around each antibody-producing cell as a result of the development of a zone of lysis (Fig. 6–9). The test may be modified to detect cells producing antibodies of other immunoglobulin isotypes by incorporating specific antiglobulins in the media. Thus anti-IgA will reveal IgA-producing cells, and so on. The test may also be employed to detect antibodies to soluble antigens if these antigens are first chemically linked to the erythrocytes.

Memory Cells

The second population of cells derived from a stimulated antigen-sensitive B cell remains morphologically indistinguishable from the parent cell. These cells possess immunoglobulin receptors of an antigen binding specificity identical to those of the parent. However, their isotype switches from IgM to IgG, IgA or IgE. These memory cells live for many months or years after the first exposure to antigen. As a result, if a second dose of antigen is given to an animal, it will encounter and stimulate many more antigen-sensitive cells than did the first dose. Consequently, a secondary immune response is quantitatively greater than a primary response, and the immunoglobulin produced is primarily of the IgG rather than the IgM isotype. The lag period is shorter in a secondary as opposed to a primary response, because more antibody is

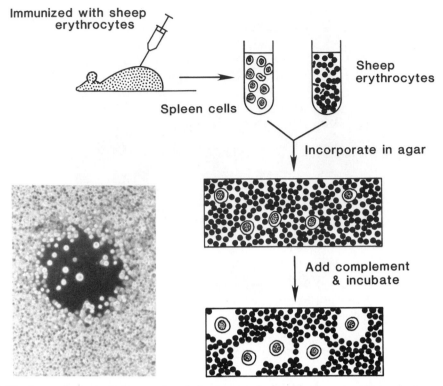

Figure 6–9. The Jerne plaque technique and a photomicrograph showing the zone of hemolysis surrounding a mouse spleen cell that is producing antibodies against sheep erythrocytes.

produced and because the lymphoid organs can process antigen much more effectively (Chapter 5). Even when circulating antibody levels have sunk to undetectable levels, there may be sufficient memory cells remaining to give an accelerated (anamnestic) response.

MYELOMAS

If control of the proliferation of B cells is lost, they may become cancerous and give rise to plasma cell tumors known as myelomas. The plasma cells in myelomas have the ability to synthesize immunoglobulins in the usual manner. Unfortunately, since plasma cells become neoplastic in an entirely random manner, the immunoglobulins that they produce are not usually directed against any antigen of practical importance. Nevertheless, myeloma cells can be grown in tissue culture, where, since they are tumor cells, they survive indefinitely.

Hybridomas

From a practical point of view it would be highly desirable to be able to set up a system to obtain large quantities of absolutely pure specific immunoglobulin directed against an antigen of interest. This can be done by fusing a normal plasma cell making the antibody of interest with a myeloma cell with the capacity for prolonged growth in tissue culture (Fig. 6–10). The resulting mixed cell is called a hybridoma.

The first stage in making a hybridoma is to generate antibody-producing plasma cells. This is simply done by immunizing a mouse against the antigen of interest and repeating the process several times to ensure that it mounts a good response. Two to four days later, its spleen is removed and broken up to form a spleen cell suspension. These spleen cells are suspended in culture medium together with a special mouse myeloma cell line.

It is usual to use myeloma cells that do not secrete immunoglobulins, since this simplifies purification later on. Polyethylene glycol is added to the mixture and induces many of the cells to fuse together. (It takes about 200,000 spleen cells on average to form a viable hybrid with one myeloma cell.) If the cell mixture is now cultured for several days, any unfused spleen cells will die. The myeloma cells would normally survive but they are eliminated by a simple trick. The myeloma cells used in the process are selected so that they lack the enzyme hypoxanthine phosphoribosyl transferase. As a result the myeloma cells cannot utilize hypoxanthine from the culture medium to manufacture purines and pyrimidines. The

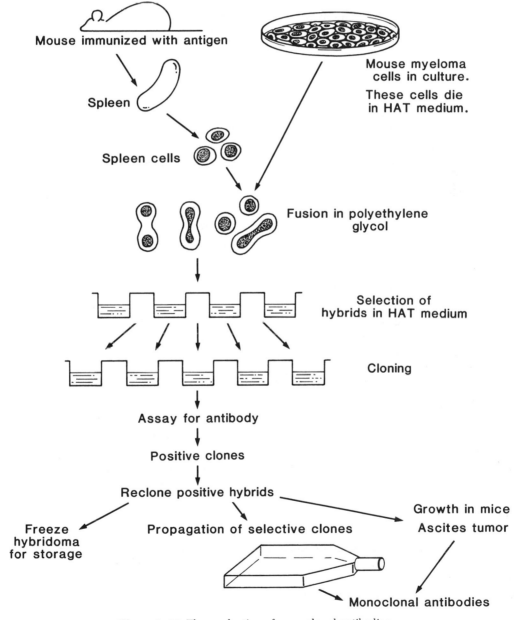

Mouse immunized with antigen

Spleen

Spleen cells

Mouse myeloma cells in culture.

These cells die in HAT medium.

Fusion in polyethylene glycol

Selection of hybrids in HAT medium

Cloning

Assay for antibody

Positive clones

Reclone positive hybrids

Freeze hybridoma for storage

Propagation of selective clones

Growth in mice Ascites tumor

Monoclonal antibodies

Figure 6–10. The production of monoclonal antibodies.

fused cell mixture is therefore grown in a culture containing three compounds; hypoxanthine, aminopterin, and thymidine (HAT medium). Aminopterin is a drug that prevents cells from making their own purines and pyrimidines. Since the myeloma cells cannot use hypoxanthine from the medium and the aminopterin stops them from making their own, then they will soon die. Hybrids made from a myeloma and a normal cell will grow because they possess the enzyme and can therefore use the hypoxanthine and thymidine in the culture medium and survive. The hybridomas divide rapidly in the HAT medium, doubling their numbers every 24 to 48 hours. On average, about 300 to 500 different hybrids can be isolated from a mouse spleen, although not all will make antibodies of interest.

If a mixture of cells from a fusion experiment is cultured in wells on a plate with about 5×10^4 myeloma cells per well, it is usual to obtain about one hybrid in every three wells. After culturing for two to four weeks, it is possible to see the growing cells, and the supernatant fluid can be screened for the presence of antibodies. It is essential to use a good sensitive assay at this time. Radioimmunoassays or ELISAs are preferred (Chapter 11). Clones that produce the desired antibody are grown in mass culture and recloned to eliminate nonantibody-producing hybrids.

Unfortunately, antibody-producing clones tend to lose this ability after being cultured for several months. Thus it is usual to make large stocks of hybridoma cells and store them frozen in small aliquots. These can then be thawed as required and grown up in bulk culture. Alternatively, the hybridoma cells can be injected intraperitoneally into mice. Since they are tumor cells, the hybridomas grow rapidly and provoke the effusion of large volumes of fluid into the mouse peritoneal cavity. This ascites fluid is rich in monoclonal antibody and can be readily harvested.

Within recent years, monoclonal antibodies have become the preferred source of antibodies for much immunological research. They are absolutely specific for individual epitopes and are available in very large quantities. Because of their purity, they can function as standard chemical reagents. They are rapidly being incorporated into clinical diagnostic techniques in which large quantities of antibody of consistent quality are required.

THE GENERATION OF ANTIBODY DIVERSITY

One immediate result of the studies on antisera to haptens described in Chapter 3 was the realization that antibodies could distinguish among epitopes differing only in minor structural configurations (see Table 3–2). This implied that an enormous number of different epitopes existed and that the number of different antibodies required to combine with these epitopes must be extremely large. It has been estimated that the immune system must therefore have the potential to produce between 10^6 and 10^8 different antibody specificities. One difficulty raised by this huge number was the assumption that an impossibly large amount of genetic material would be required to code for every potential antibody molecule.

When the structure of immunoglobulins was clarified, however, it became clear that the specificity of an antibody for its complementary epitope was due to the structure of the variable regions of the light and heavy chains, and that much of the molecule, the constant regions, had nothing to do with antigen binding. It also became clear that there must be at least two groups of genes coding for immunoglobulin peptide chains, one group of genes coding for variable regions and a separate set of genes coding for constant regions.

Immunoglobulin molecules are, in fact, coded for by three unlinked gene families. Each of these families consists of a large number of gene segments coding for variable regions (V genes) associated with one or more genes coding for constant regions (C genes). One of the families, located on chromosome 14 in man and 12 in mice, codes for immunoglobulin heavy chains. One family, on chromosome 2 in man and 6 in mice, codes for κ light chains, while the third family, on chromosome 22 in man and 16 in mice, codes for λ light chains.

The explanation of antibody diversity lies in the structure of the variable region genes.

Variable (V) Region Diversity

The variable region of an immunoglobulin light chain contains about 108 amino acids. When the first variable region genes were isolated, however, they were found to code for only the first 95 amino acids. The remaining 13 amino acids (positions 96 to 108) are coded for by one of four or five separate gene segments called joining or J segments. The formation of a complete immunoglobulin light chain gene by a B cell therefore involves recombination between one of 100 to 200 different variable gene segments and one of these four or five J gene segments (Fig. 6–11). Hence, the variable region of a light immunoglobulin chain is coded from two gene segments—V and J. The constant region of the chain is encoded by a single C gene segment located nearby on the same chromosome.

One hundred V segments and five J segments are able to be connected in 500 different ways, thus accounting for some diversity. When the gene sequences of the J segment were first determined and compared with the known amino acid sequences of the corresponding light chain region (around position 96), it was found that they commonly did not correspond. This suggested that V and J segments were capable of joining at one of several different points. The region surrounding position 96 is a hypervariable region. Recombination between V and J segments can cause the deletion of up to six nucleotides from the two segments. This deletion sometimes throws the remaining portion of the segment into a nonsense reading frame, which produces nonsense genes unable to function in the immune response. These wasted recombinants are the price paid for this additional diversity-generating mechanism. More commonly, however, the effect of this deletion is to further enhance the diversity available in the antigen-binding site.

A third source of diversity is provided by a series of mutations within the V segments. If the amino acid sequences of a large number of V regions are studied, it is possible to show a progressive departure from a basic sequence as the immune response progresses and B cells gradually differentiate into plasma cells. These differences arise as a result of changes in the nucleotide sequences within V gene segments. These changes occur as a result of mutation and selection. During the course of a B cell response to an antigen, spontaneous

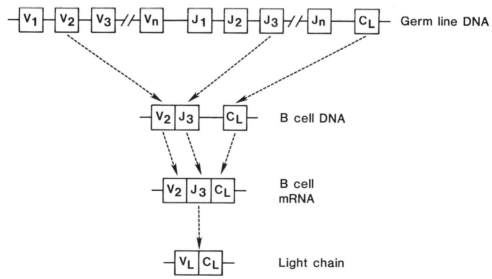

Figure 6–11. The production of an immunoglobulin light chain. One V segment, one J segment and a constant segment of DNA are joined and transcribed into mRNA. This mRNA is, in turn, translated into an intact light chain.

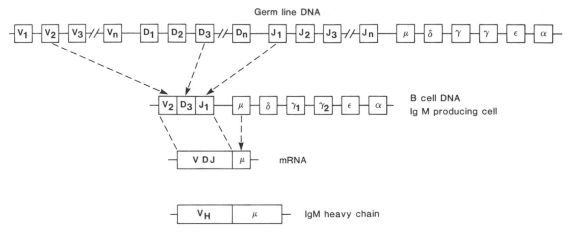

Figure 6–12. The production of an IgM heavy chain. As a B cell matures, one V, one D and one J segment are selected at random from the germ line DNA. In the immature B cell these segments are transcribed together with a μ chain gene to form mRNA. This is then translated into the complete IgM heavy chain.

mutations occur within the V gene segments. Many of these mutations will result in changes in the V region that reduce the ability of affected cells to bind antigen. As a result, these B cells will cease to be stimulated by the antigen and will die. Some of the mutations will, however, enhance antigen binding by affected cells. These B cells will therefore be selectively stimulated by the antigen and eventually predominate in that antibody response. Thus, the immunoglobulin produced during the course of an immune response becomes progressively more efficient at binding the inducing epitope.

The diversity-generating mechanisms described are very prone to error. It is not uncommon for the rearranged nucleotide sequence to code for nonsense. If this happens, the B cell has several opportunities to produce a functional antibody. A pre-B cell initially attempts to produce a functional κ chain gene. Failing this, it will switch to the other allele for a second attempt. If both κ alleles are unsuccessfully rearranged or deleted, the next attempt involves rearrangement of one of the λ alleles. The second λ allele represents the last resort. A failure here to produce a functional allele results in the development of a B cell that is incapable of binding antigen. This cell cannot therefore be stimulated by antigen and will die without participating in an immune response. (κ and λ light chains are discussed on page 40.)

The mechanisms for generating heavy chain variable regions are similar to those for light chains. The heavy chain variable region is constructed by joining not two but three distinct gene segments: a V segment, a D (diversity) segment and a J segment (Fig. 6–12). D segments code for about 10 amino acids located between the V and J segments. There are probably about 100 V segments, 50 D segments and 6 J segments. These have the potential to create 30,000 different V, D, J combinations. Since each of these combinations can also have crossover point variations, there can be thousands of different gene sequences, and thus thousands of different heavy chain variable regions created.

Isotype Selection

The immunoglobulin isotype produced by a B cell is controlled by a heavy chain switching mechanism. There is one heavy chain constant region gene for each heavy chain constant region of each immunoglobulin isotype and subisotype. (In cattle, for example, there would be six of these— —μ—δ—γ1—γ2— ε—α—.) The μ and δ heavy chain genes lie about 2 kilobases from each other. On the 3' side of these are the γ genes (the number of these depends upon the number of γ subisotypes), the ε gene and the α gene.

The first step in synthesizing a complete heavy chain is to make a complete heavy chain

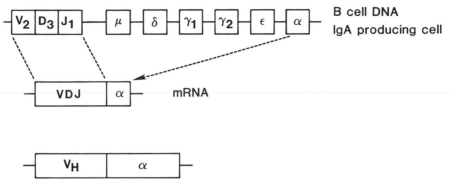

Figure 6–13. The production of an IgA heavy chain. In certain B cells, especially those located at body surfaces, the VDJ gene segment is linked directly to the α chain gene. All the intervening genes are deleted. This is transcribed into mRNA and translated into an IgA heavy chain.

gene. This is initiated by a recombination event that links a V segment with a J and D segment to the μ gene. In immature B cells both IgM and IgD are expressed simultaneously. This simultaneous expression of μ and δ genes is regulated by an RNA processing mechanism that alternately terminates the code after the μ gene, thus producing a μ chain, or splices out the μ gene, to join the V-D-J segment directly to the δ gene and so codes for a δ chain.

As it matures a B cell loses its ability to make IgD but continues to use its IgM genes. Once stimulated by antigen, the cell switches from IgM to IgG, IgE or IgA synthesis. This switch is also caused by recombination events. In this case an active V D J segment is switched from a position beside the μ gene to another site along the chromosome and results in deletion of all the intervening DNA. For example, in order to make an active IgG gene, the V-D-J sequence is moved from its position beside the μ gene and spliced into a position next to the γ gene, deleting the μ and δ genes in the process. When IgE is made, the μ, δ and γ genes are deleted.

On switching to IgA production, the μ, δ, γ and ε genes are deleted, and the variable region genes attach directly to the α gene (Fig. 6–13). It is interesting to speculate whether this switch might be triggered by specific enzymes within a tissue or organ. Thus, it is possible that antibody production could be regulated at body surfaces by an enzyme that deletes the intervening μ and γ

genes and thus permit B cells in those tissues to synthesize only IgA or IgE.

ADDITIONAL SOURCES OF INFORMATION

Baltimore D. 1981. Somatic mutation gains its place among the generators of diversity. Cell 26 295–296.

Boss MA. 1983. Enhancer elements in immunoglobulin genes. Nature 303 281–282.

Cerruti-Sola S, Kristensen F, Vandevelde M and de Weck AL. 1984. Interleukin 1- and 2-like activities in the dog. Vet. Immunol. Immunopathol. 6 261–272.

Early P and Hood L. 1981. Allelic exclusion and nonproductive immunoglobulin gene rearrangements. Cell 24 1–3.

Gearhart PJ and Bogenhagen DF. 1983. Clusters of point mutations are found exclusively around rearranged antibody variable genes. Proc. Natl. Acad. Sci. 80 3439–3443.

Leder P. 1983. Genetic control of immunoglobulin production. Hospital Practice 18 73–82.

Marcin KB and Cooper MD. 1982. New views of the immunoglobulin heavy-chain switch. Nature 298 327–328.

Marx JL. 1983. Immunoglobulin genes have enhancers. Science 221 735–737.

Miedema F and Melief CJM. 1983. T-cell regulation of human B-cell activation. Immunol. Today 6 258–259.

Robertson M. 1983. Control of antibody production. Nature 301 114.

Robertson M and Hobart M. 1981. Antibodies, Introns and Biosynthetic Versatility. Nature 290 543–554.

Saklatvala J, Sarsfield SJ and Townsend Y. 1985. Pig interleukin 1. Purification of two immunologically different leukocyte proteins that cause cartilage resorption, lymphocyte activation and fever. J Exp Med 162 1208–1222.

Tonegawa S. 1983. Somatic generation of antibody diversity. Nature 302 575–581.

Unanue ER. 1980. Cooperation between mononuclear phagocytes and lymphocytes in immunity. N. Engl. J. Med. 303 977–985.

7

The Cellular Basis of Cell-Mediated Immunity

In contrast to B cells, T cells serve many different functions. T cells are essential for protection against intracellular bacteria, against viruses and virus-infected cells, against foreign tissue grafts and against some tumor cells. They also mediate the characteristic inflammatory response known as delayed hypersensitivity. Some T cells act as effectors in the cell-mediated immune response by producing biologically active glycoproteins called lymphokines, and others are capable of destroying foreign or abnormal cells directly. Some T cells act to enhance the response of other T or B cells to antigen and are therefore known as helper cells. Others function as suppressor cells and inhibit the responses of other T and B cells. Even within these subgroups there are subdivisions. For example, some helper cells are non-antigen specific, whereas others help the response to a specific antigen only.

Notwithstanding this complexity, all T cells possess the common property of having been processed in the thymic environment during their maturation process.

Note: Our detailed knowledge of the T cell response is based upon studies in man and mice. Unfortunately, there is little logic in the terminology used to describe the lymphocyte membrane antigens in mice, Thy 1, Lyt 1, Ia and so forth. In humans, the system is more rational. The human T cell antigens have been labeled T1, T2, T3 and so forth. However, a suggestion has recently been made to modify this simple system by changing the T prefix to CD (Cluster of Differentiation). Recently, investigators working on lymphocyte antigens of domestic animals have tended to use the T prefix with a species initial, e.g., PT1, PT2 for pigs, BoT4, BoT8 for cattle. For the sake of clarity, therefore, the following description uses the terminology for T cell surface antigens used in man.

THE DEVELOPMENT OF T CELLS

The progressive development of T cells may be followed from a prethymic stage, through the thymus and out into the secondary lymphoid organs (Fig 7–1). It can be shown that T

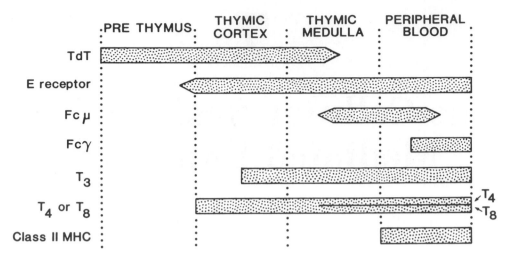

Figure 7–1. The development of T cells.

cell surface receptors and cell membrane antigens develop at specific stages in the development process. For example, the enzyme terminal deoxynucleotidyl transferase (TdT) is found in prethymic cells and in cells in the thymic cortex but is lost as the cells mature and migrate into the thymic medulla and is absent from mature T cells in peripheral blood. The sheep erythrocyte receptor (T11), in contrast, only appears on T cells as they mature in the thymus and is therefore found on mature cells in peripheral blood. The class II histocompatibility antigen is absent from all immature T cells and only develops on activated mature T cells. Immature thymocytes initially possess both T4 and T8 antigens but lose one of these as they leave the thymus.

T Cell Heterogeneity

Each T cell subpopulation can be characterized by its cell-surface antigens and by its receptors (Fig. 7–2). Thus, all mature T cells possess T3 antigens on their surface. About two thirds of the T lymphocytes in blood

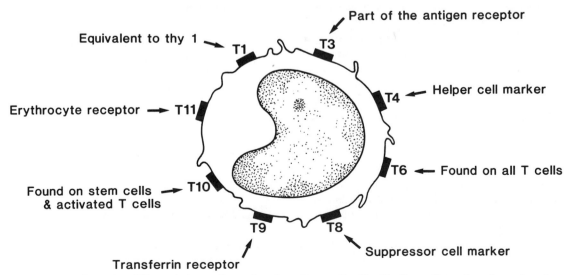

Figure 7–2. The major differentiation antigens found on human T cells. Similar antigens have been found on the T cells of domestic animals.

possess a surface antigen called T4 and function as helper cells. The remaining one third of circulating cells possess another antigen called T8 and function either as suppressor cells or as cytotoxic cells. These suppressor T cells possess Fc receptors for IgG, whereas the helper T cells have Fc receptors for IgM.

THE T CELL ANTIGEN RECEPTOR

Although B cells can bind and respond to an antigen if it is on a cell membrane or in solution, T cells will only respond to a foreign antigen when it is closely associated with a class I or class II histocompatibility antigen on another cell. Both the T cell and its target cell must have identical histocompatibility antigens. Thus cytotoxic (T8$^+$) T cells can only kill targets that share class I histocompatibility antigens with them. In contrast, helper (T4$^+$) T cells will only promote an immune response if the antigen is presented to them on cell membranes that share common class II antigens with them. Thus the T cell antigen receptor must be able to recognize not only the foreign antigen but also a histocompatibility antigen. For this reason, these receptors are composed of several different proteins.

Because T lymphocytes can recognize specific antigen they must possess specific cell-membrane receptors for that antigen. In man this receptor molecule is called Ti. Ti is a 90,000 dalton protein consisting of two peptide chains (α and β). Each chain is composed of four domains, two extracellular domains, a hydrophobic transmembrane domain and a C-terminal cytoplasmic tail. The β chain shows marked variability in the amino acid sequence of its N-terminal domain and probably plays a major role in antigen binding. The α chain, on the other hand, has relatively little sequence variability and is probably less important in antigen binding than the β chain. A third chain associated with the T cell receptor is called the γ chain. The function of this chain is unknown. Studies on the genes coding for the β chain show that there are two genes for the constant regions (Cβ), a cluster of genes

for a J region and a D region (Jβ. and Dβ.), and less than 30 variable region (Vβ) genes. The antigen binding site on the β chain derives its structure from variable amino acid sequences in the N-terminal domain. The variability in these sequences seems to be entirely due to recombinant diversity between multiple V, D and J genes and not to somatic mutation. The α chain is also coded for by multiple linked genes including Cα, Jα, and Vα gene segments. The α and β subunits have significant sequence homology with immunoglobulins and therefore belong to the immunoglobulin superfamily.

The Ti receptor molecule is also linked to the T cell by a T3 molecule. T3 consists of three peptide chains, γ, δ, and ϵ and has a total molecular weight of 66,000 daltons. Tiβ is directly linked to T3γ.

The T cell antigen receptor therefore consists of a Ti molecule associated with a T3 molecule. However, T cells must also be able to recognize class I and class II antigens in very close proximity to the foreign antigen. It has been suggested that a T4 or T8 molecule, depending upon the subset of the T cell, is closely linked to the Ti molecule and serves this purpose. For example, antibodies against the T4 antigen will block the helper effect of T4$^+$ cells. Antibodies against the T8 antigen block the cytotoxicity of T8$^+$ cells. Antibodies to T3 block both of these effects. Thus T3, T4 and T8 antigens must all be involved in recognition of target cells. It is suggested therefore that a cell with Ti linked to T4 can recognize a foreign antigen linked to a class II histocompatibility antigen on the surface of an antigen-presenting cell and trigger the events that result in helper cell function (Fig 7–3). A T cell possessing Ti linked to T8 can recognize antigen (for example, a virus protein) linked to a class I histocompatibility antigen on the surface of an infected cell and trigger the events that lead to cytotoxicity. Although an attractive theory, the precise functions of T4 and T8 and their relation, if any, to the Ti molecule are still unclear.

We know very little about the antigen binding abilities of suppressor cells. It has been suggested that T$_s$ cells use the α chain primarily for antigen recognition.

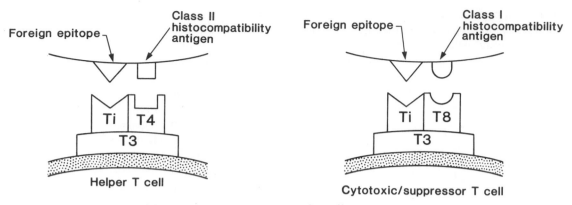

Figure 7–3. The structure of the T cell antigen receptor on helper/effector cells (T4⁺) and on suppressor/cytotoxic cells (T8⁺).

THE RESPONSE OF T CELLS TO ANTIGEN (Fig. 7–4)

Three interacting cells are required in order for a T cell to respond optimally to antigen—an antigen-presenting cell, an effector T cell (T8⁺) (the cell that will actually mediate the response), and a helper T cell (T4⁺).

An effector T cell can only recognize the foreign epitope if it is located on the surface of an antigen-presenting cell such as a macrophage, a B cell or a dendritic cell. The epitope must also be closely associated with, perhaps even physically linked to, a class I histocompatibility antigen. The effector cell binds both the foreign epitope and the class I antigen through its Ti/T8/T3 receptor complex. As a result of this interaction the effector cell begins to express interleukin 2 receptors.

The helper T cell also recognizes a foreign epitope on the surface of an antigen-presenting cell. However, in this case, the epitope must be associated with a class II histocompatibility antigen. The helper cell binds both the foreign epitope and the class II antigen through its Ti/T4/T3 receptor complex. (The epitopes recognized by the effector cell and the helper cell need not be identical.)

During this recognition process, the antigen-presenting cell secretes IL-1. The combined stimulus of foreign epitope, class II antigen and IL-1 induces the helper T cell to secrete a protein called interleukin 2 (IL-2).

The interleukin 2 released by the helper cell binds to the interleukin 2 receptors on the effector cell. As a result, the effector cell is stimulated to undertake DNA synthesis and division. Once the effector cell is activated, the continued presence of IL-2 is sufficient to maintain its clonal expansion.

The presence of antigen and interleukin 1 also stimulates the helper cell to make more interleukin 2 receptors. The interleukin 2 then

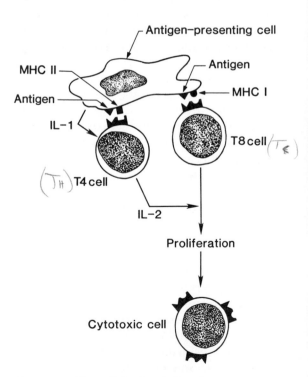

Figure 7–4. The cellular interactions between an antigen-presenting cell, a T8⁺ cytotoxic cell and a T4⁺ helper cell.

binds to these receptors and so stimulates additional IL-2 release, thus accelerating the entire process.

Antigen-sensitive T8$^+$ effector cells respond to antigen and interleukin 2 by dividing and eventually generating both memory cell and effector cell populations. The responding cells are somewhat larger than unstimulated lymphocytes, and their cytoplasm is pyroninophilic, reflecting their ability to make proteins. These cells are capable of performing a number of different functions; for example, they can synthesize and secrete numerous glycoproteins known as lymphokines and they can participate in direct cytotoxic reactions on contact with foreign or altered cells.

Antigen-Presenting Cells

Although macrophages have traditionally been considered to be the most important antigen-presenting cells, it is now clear that many other cell types also have this ability. These include B cells, endothelial cells and dendritic cells. B cells bind native antigen by means of their immunoglobulin receptors, then ingest and process it and present the antigen, in association with class II histocompatibility antigens, to T cells. The importance of B cells as antigen-presenting cells can be demon- strated by showing that T cell responses are seriously impaired in B cell–deprived animals.

Vascular endothelial cells can also take up antigen, synthesize IL-1 and, under the influence of interferon, express class II histocompatibility antigens. They can therefore act as effective antigen-presenting cells. Even skin keratinocytes can produce factors similar to IL-1, express class II histocompatibility antigens and present antigen to T cells.

Dendritic cells have large amounts of class II histocompatibility antigens on their surface and are therefore potent antigen-presenting cells. Langerhans cells are the most important antigen-presenting cells in the skin; they play an important role in the development of skin allergies, delayed hypersensitivity and allergic contact dermatitis (Chapter 23).

LYMPHOKINES

Lymphokines are proteins with molecular weights between 25,000 and 75,000 daltons. They are released mainly from activated T cells, but B cells may produce them in response to nonspecific stimulants such as bacterial lipopolysaccharides or PPD tuberculin. Lymphokines possess a wide range of biological activities (Table 7–1), and at least 90 different lymphokine-mediated activities have

Table 7–1 SOME IMPORTANT LYMPHOKINES

Regulatory Factors	Actions
Interleukin 2	Initiates and maintains T cell proliferation
Interleukin 3	Promotes T cell and mast cell development
γ Interferon	Modulates lymphocyte function
B cell growth factor	Promotes B cell responses
B cell differentiation factor	Promotes B cell differentiation
Antigen-specific helper and suppressor factors	Regulate T and B cell function
Inflammatory Mediators	
Skin-reactive factors	Increase vascular permeability
Macrophage Activity Modulators	
Migration inhibitory factors	Inhibit macrophage movement
Leukocyte inhibitory factors	Inhibit neutrophil movement
γ Interferon	Activates macrophages
Macrophage fusion factor	Induces giant cell formation
Macrophage chemotactic factor	Chemotactic for macrophages
Cytotoxic Effects	
Lymphotoxins	Kill nearby cells
Tumor necrosis factor	Kills tumor cells
Perforins	Kill target cells
Other Activities	
Fibroblast stimulation factor	Increases collagen production

been recognized. Unfortunately, these activities are a reflection of the many different methods used to assay them rather than of true heterogeneity. In general, lymphokines are neither antigen-binding nor antigen-specific. Lymphokines act on many different types of cells to induce functional changes. The interleukins are probably the most important of the lymphokines.

Interleukins

Four interleukins are known. Interleukin 1 is derived from macrophages and thus is a monokine, not a lymphokine. Its role is to promote interleukin 2 (IL-2) production by T cells. Interleukin 2 (IL-2), originally called "T cell replacing factor" (TCRF), is a family of glycoproteins. The molecular weights of the IL-2 proteins vary between species; rat, human and pig IL-2 have a molecular weight of around 15,000 daltons; sheep and bovine IL-2 is about 17,200 daltons; and canine and mouse IL-2 have a molecular weight of around 30,000 daltons. There may be several different forms of IL-2 in a single species of animal but this is probably due to a variable carbohydrate component. All forms of IL-2 appear to have identical biological activities. They are produced by helper T cells and are required to stimulate a response by antigen primed effector T cells and B cells (to a lesser extent). IL-2 induces the production of γ interferon in spleen cell cultures, and can render some T cells cytotoxic. It also stimulates the production of BCGF. IL-2 has a very short half-life (3.7 minutes) in the blood stream. Like the interferons, IL-2 is somewhat toxic, causing fever, chills and malaise after injection into animals. The inability of newborn rodents to mount an immune response may be due in part to a deficiency of IL-2.

Interleukin 3 is also derived from T cells. It serves to stimulate the maturation of immature T cells and to promote the differentiation of certain mast cell populations (Chapter 20).

A lymphokine that has a function similar to that of IL-2 is B cell growth factor (BCGF). BCGF is released by helper T cells and acts on B cells, promoting their response to antigen. There are two of these factors, BCGF I and BCGF II, each with slightly different biological activities.

Two different groups of investigators have described interleukin 4. Unfortunately, they described two different molecules! Students are advised to avoid this subject at present.

Interferons (Table 7–2)

Interferons are a family of glycoproteins synthesized by cells in response to virus infection, immune stimulation or a variety of chemical stimulators. They all have the ability to inhibit virus replication by interfering with viral RNA and protein synthesis. Three major classes of interferon are recognized: interferon alpha (IFN-α), a family of at least sixteen different molecules derived from virus-infected leukocytes; interferon beta (IFN-β), a single protein derived from virus-infected fibroblasts; and interferon gamma (IFN-γ), a lymphokine derived from T cells and NK cells after exposure to IL-2. (Interestingly, T cells can also produce IFN-α if they are infected by a virus.) The molecular weights of interferons vary according to the method used to induce them but

Table 7–2 INTERFERONS

Type	Number	Source	Molecular Weight (daltons)	Stability at pH 2	Inducers
IFN-α	>16	Leukocytes	16,000–20,000	Stable	Viruses Polynucleotides
IFN-β	1	Fibroblasts	20,000	Stable	Viruses Polynucleotides
IFN-γ	1	Lymphocytes	20,000–25,000	Labile	Mitogens Antigens

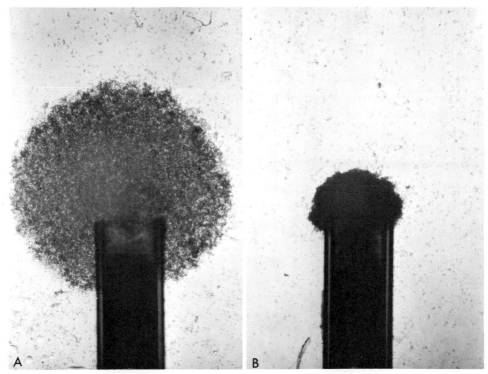

Figure 7–5. The macrophage migration inhibition test. Guinea pig peritoneal macrophages will normally migrate out of a glass capillary tube (A). In the presence of a supernatant derived from antigen-treated bovine lymphocytes (MIF), macrophage migration is inhibited (B). (Courtesy of Dr. B. N. Wilkie.)

they generally lie between 16,000 and 25,000 daltons. IFN-γ occurs in two forms, with molecular weights of 20,000 and 25,000 daltons. IFN-α and IFN-β are stable at pH 2, whereas IFN-γ is labile at low pH. All are heat stable and only weakly antigenic.

Interferon and Cell Functions

Interferons have both enhancing and inhibitory effects on cell functions. Their most important inhibitory effect is a slowing of the growth of normal and neoplastic cells. Gamma interferon will prevent the migration of macrophages out of a capillary tube in a culture chamber. This involves incubation of a mixture of macrophages and lymphocytes in a capillary tube resting on the flat bottom of a tissue culture chamber. In the presence of antigen the lymphocytes produce interferon. The interferon prevents the spontaneous migration of the macrophages out of the tube (Fig. 7–5). This activity used to be ascribed to a specific lymphokine called migration inhibi-

tory factor (MIF). It is assumed to be of benefit to an animal by ensuring that macrophages remain in the vicinity of antigen invasion.

Gamma interferon enhances the ability of macrophages to kill invading bacteria or protozoa by causing macrophage "activation." This activation is essential for the development of resistance to certain pathogenic microorganisms. For example, certain bacteria, notably *Mycobacterium tuberculosis, Rhodococcus equi, Corynebacterium pseudotuberculosis, Brucella abortus, Listeria monocytogenes* and the Salmonellae, as well as the protozoan parasite *Toxoplasma gondii*, are normally able to live and grow inside macrophages (Fig. 7–6). Because of their intracellular growth, antibodies cannot confer protection against these organisms. However, during the course of infections by these agents, a cell-mediated immune response is stimulated, in which T cells release IFN-γ. This interferon causes the macrophages to increase in size, mobility and metabolic activity (Table 7–3 and Fig. 7–7). The number of their Fc receptors

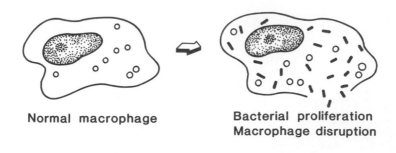

Normal macrophage   Bacterial proliferation
                                      Macrophage disruption

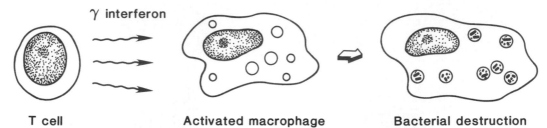

γ interferon

T cell   Activated macrophage   Bacterial destruction

Figure 7–6. Normal macrophages are not able to destroy bacteria such as *Listeria monocytogenes*. However, if activated by IFN-γ released by T cells, the macrophages become activated and acquire the ability to destroy the bacteria.

increases so that phagocytosis is enhanced. The lysosomes in these macrophages enlarge and contain increased amounts of hydrolytic enzymes, while they also secrete increased quantities of IL-1. As a result, destruction of the intracellular organisms occurs (Fig. 7–8).

Gamma interferon has either enhancing or suppressor effects on B cell function, depending on the timing of the treatment. If given late in the immune response, interferon enhances antibody production. If given prior to antigen administration, interferon is suppressive.

The interferons also have a complex effect on cell-mediated immune responses. Thus

Table 7–3 FEATURES OF ACTIVATED MACROPHAGES

Increased
   Size
   Spreading
   Pinocytosis
   Phagocytosis
   Secretion of lysosomal enzymes
   Membrane ruffling
   Oxidative metabolism
   Microbicidal activity
   Tumoricidal activity

they can depress the mixed lymphocyte reaction but also enhance graft rejection. They can, depending on dose and timing, enhance or suppress the delayed hypersensitivity reaction. Interferons enhance the activities of cytotoxic T cells by inducing T cells to produce both the interleukin 2 receptor and interleukin 2. On the other hand, they also enhance suppressor cell activity by stimulating the synthesis of prostaglandins, ACTH and endorphins. Thus, paradoxically, interferons may be immunosuppressive at the same time as they increase host resistance to tumors and to viruses.

The interferons induce the appearance of differentiation markers on cells. They act on myeloid cells, macrophages and B cells to enhance the expression of receptors for IgG (FcγR). All three interferons enhance the expression of class I histocompatibility antigens. Gamma interferon induces the appearance of class II antigens on endothelial cells, myeloid cells, dendritic cells and fibroblasts as well as on macrophages. When T cells release interferon during the course of graft rejection, it induces the appearance of class II antigens on endothelial cells of the graft as

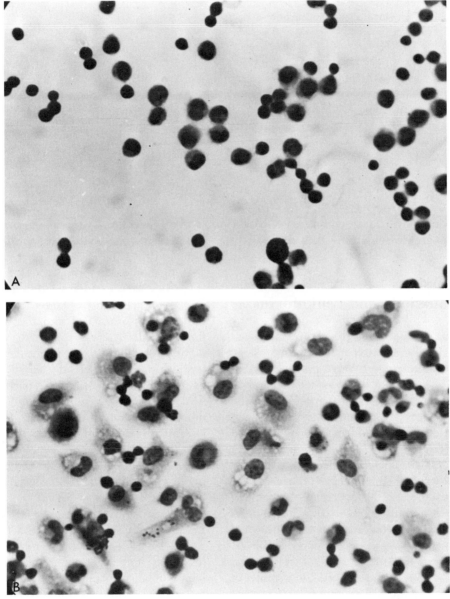

Figure 7–7. Monolayers of mouse peritoneal macrophages. *A*, From a normal mouse. *B*, From a mouse that had recovered from infection with *Listeria monocytogenes*. These macrophages are "activated." × 450.

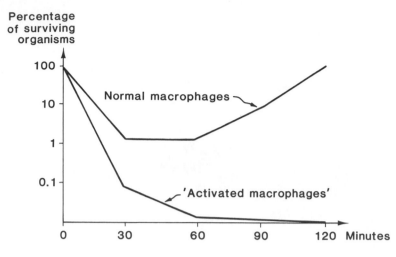

Figure 7–8. The destruction of *Listeria monocytogenes* when grown in the presence of normal macrophages or "activated" macrophages from *Listeria*-infected mice.

well as on the host's macrophages (Chapter 18). This greatly enhances the intensity of graft rejection.

Cytotoxicity and Leukotoxins

Some T8$^+$ cells develop the ability to bind to foreign or altered tissue cells and destroy them. This can be a very rapid process. Within seconds after contact between a T cell and its target, the organelles and the nucleus of the target cell disrupt simultaneously. The T cell can then disengage itself and move on to find another target. The mechanisms involved in this process are unclear. It is known that the T8$^+$ cell must first recognize both a foreign antigen and a class I histocompatibility antigen on the target cell surface. The T cell then attaches to the target and secretes either cytotoxic proteins known as perforins or soluble proteins called lymphotoxins. Perforins are normally stored in the cytoplasmic granules of T cells. After the T cell comes into contact with its target and the appropriate signal is given, the T cell's Golgi apparatus and microtubules align themselves so that the granules are released at the region of cell contact. Once the granules contact the target, the perforin molecules polymerize in a calcium-dependent reaction to form tubular structures called polyperforins (see Fig. 18–7). The polyperforins insert themselves into the target membranes

so that they form transmembrane channels. As a result, the target cell is disrupted by osmotic lysis (Fig. 7–9).

Under some circumstances, IL-2-stimulated cytotoxic lymphocytes need not come into direct contact with the target, releasing soluble lymphotoxins (LT) into the surrounding fluid instead. There is some debate about the number of different LT molecules. Some investigators claim that only one LT molecule exists with a molecular weight of about 60,000, while others suggest that there are several different LT molecules. In mice, for example, at least six different lymphotoxin molecules have been described with molecular weights ranging from 200,000 to 12,000 daltons. Lymphotoxins appear to be especially toxic for neoplastic cells. They disrupt cell membranes and permit endonucleases in tissue fluid to reach the cell's DNA. LT can act synergistically with IFN-γ since the interferon seems to prime the target for LT killing. Soluble lymphotoxins are much less efficient at cytotoxicity than are perforins. They also suffer from nonspecificity. Any cell, including the cytotoxic lymphocyte, that is in the neighborhood when the free lymphotoxin is released may be destroyed at the same time.

Under some circumstances, macrophages may be able to bind and destroy target cells without ingesting them. This may be either a slow, antibody-independent process or a rapid, antibody-dependent process (ADCC,

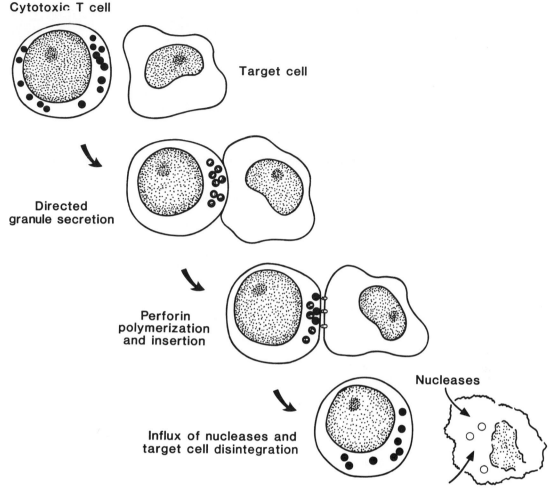

Figure 7–9. The destruction of a target cell by perforins released by a cytotoxic T cell. The polymerized perforins insert themselves into the target cell membrane and permit nucleases to gain access to the cell interior. Electron micrographs of polyperforins are seen in Figure 18–7.

see subsequent section). Macrophages that have been activated by mediators such as IFN-γ can act by either process. Irrespective of the mechanism of attachment, target cell destruction probably occurs as a result of the secretion of cytotoxic factors from macrophages. The macrophage "toxins" have not been firmly identified but could include proteases, lysozyme, interferon, hydrogen peroxide, arginase or tumor necrosis factor.

The tumor necrosis factors (TNF) are two related proteins. TNF-α, or cachexin, is released from macrophages by exposure to stimulants such as endotoxin, BCG or IL-2, but is distinct from IL-1. TNF-β is a T cell–derived lymphotoxin. As their name suggests the TNFs can cause destruction of some tumor cells. They also have a physiological role in regulating the growth of normal cells.

Other Mechanisms of Cytotoxicity
(Fig. 7–10)

Two other mechanisms of cell-mediated toxicity, although not mediated by T cells, may be mentioned here for comparison. Cells that possess receptors for the Fc region of immunoglobulins may bind to foreign target cells or bacteria by means of specific antibody and then become cytotoxic. Cells capable of this include monocytes, eosinophils, neutrophils and a population of small non-T, non-B small lymphocytes, which may be called killer (K) or null cells and which are probably identical

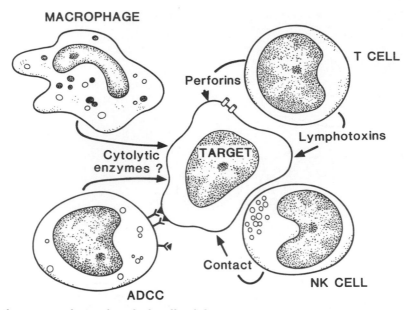

Figure 7–10. The major pathways by which cells of the immune system can cause destruction of nucleated target cells. These targets would normally be tumor cells or virus-infected cells.

to NK cells (see page 259). The mechanism of this antibody-dependent cell-mediated cytotoxicity (ADCC) is unknown. However, neutrophils and eosinophils probably act through a respiratory burst mechanism (Chapter 2), which causes destruction of target-cell membranes. ADCC is slower and less efficient than direct T cell–mediated cytotoxicity.

Finally, normal animals possess a population of natural killer (NK) cells, which have the ability to destroy virus-infected or tumor cells in the absence of previous sensitization. NK cells are not T cells, but they may be related to them. Their mode of action is unknown, but their activity is greatly enhanced by interferons. NK cells are discussed at length in Chapter 19.

Other Lymphokines

Other lymphocyte-derived glycoproteins that modify macrophage behavior include a macrophage chemotactic factor, which attracts these cells to sites of antigen-T cell interaction, and a factor that stimulates macrophage migration. It is not surprising therefore that intradermal inoculation of some lymphokine preparations into an animal leads to the de-

velopment of an inflammatory reaction characterized by mononuclear cell infiltration and resembles delayed hypersensitivity (Chapter 23). Another form of lymphocyte-mediated skin reaction that may be induced by the intradermal inoculation of certain antigens is known as cutaneous basophil hypersensitivity, because the reaction site is extensively infiltrated with basophils (Chapter 23). This reaction is due, in some cases, to the release of a basophil-chemotactic lymphokine from sensitized T cells. A lymphokine called interleukin 3 is necessary for the development of some mast cell populations (Chapter 20). Similarly, in certain systemic helminth infestations such as trichinosis, it has been suggested that the massive eosinophilia so characteristic of this condition may be mediated, at least in part, by an eosinophil-mobilizing lymphokine.

ADDITIONAL SOURCES OF INFORMATION

Acuto O and Reinherz EL. 1985. The human T-cell receptor: structure and function. N. Engl. J. Med. *312* 1100–1111.
Cummins JM and Rosenquist BD. 1982. Partial protection of calves against parainfluenza-3 virus infection by nasal

secretion interferon induced by infectious bovine rhino-tracheitis virus. Am. J. Vet. Res. *43* 1334–1338.

Daemen AJJM, Buurman WA, Linden CJ, Groenewagen G and Kootstra G. 1984. Canine IL-2: Characterization and optimal conditions for production. Vet. Immunol. Immunopathol. *5* 247–258.

Deeg HJ, Wulff JC, DeRose S et al. 1982. Unusual distribution of Ia-like antigens on canine lymphocytes. Immunogenetics *16* 445–457.

Gasbarre LC, Urban JF and Romanowski RD. 1983. Porcine interleukin 2: parameters of production and biochemical characterization. Vet. Immunol. Immunopathol. *5* 221–236.

Imboden JB, Weiss A and Stobo JD. 1985. Transmembrane signaling by the T3–antigen receptor complex. Immunol. Today *6* 328–331.

Katz EH, Hansburg D and Schwartz RH. 1983. The Ia molecule of the antigen presenting cell plays a critical role in immune response gene regulation of T cell activation. J. Mol. Cell Immunol. *1* 3–14.

Kronenberg M, Malissen B and Eisen HN. 1985. Genes, structures and function of T lymphocyte antigen receptors. Immunol. Today *16* 281–286.

MacKay R, Maddox JF, Gogdin-Ewens KJ and Brandon MR. 1985. Characterization of two sheep lymphocyte differentiation antigens, SBU-T1 and SBU-T6. Immunology *55* 729–737.

Marrack P and Kappler J. 1986. The T cell and its receptor. Sci. Am. *254* 36–45.

Miller-Edge M and Splitter GA. 1984. Bovine interleukin 2 (IL-2) production and activity on bovine and murine cell lines. Vet. Immol. Immunopathol. *7* 119–130.

Podack ER. 1985. The molecular mechanism of lymphocyte-mediated tumor cell lysis. Immunol. Today *6* 21–27.

Robb RJ. 1984. Interleukin 2: the molecule and its function. Immunol. Today *5* 203–209.

Robertson M. 1984. Receptor gene rearrangement and ontogeny of T lymphocytes. Nature *311* 305–306.

Ruddle NH. 1985. Lymphotoxin redux. Immunol. Today *6* 156–159.

Torti FM, Dieckmann B, Buetler B et al. 1985. A macrophage factor inhibits adipocyte gene expression: an in vitro model of cachexia. Science *229* 867–869.

Toy JL. 1983. The interferons. Clin. Exp. Immunol. *54* 1–13.

8

Histocompatibility Antigens

T cells have three major functions: cytotoxicity for abnormal or foreign cells, helper activity that promotes the immune response, and suppressor activity that suppresses the immune response.

Since cytotoxic T cells may be called upon to destroy abnormal cells in any part of the body, their activities are regulated by proteins found on the surface of all potential targets. These proteins are called class I histocompatibility antigens.

Since helper T cells must interact with B cells and antigen-presenting cells in order to promote an immune response, their activities are regulated by proteins found on the surface of these cells. These proteins, restricted to B cells, activated T cells (but not resting T cells) and antigen-presenting cells such as macrophages, dendritic cells and Langerhans cells, are called class II histocompatibility antigens (Table 8–1).

The histocompatibility antigens of both classes are coded for by genes located close together on one chromosome. Together, these genes form a gene complex known as the major histocompatibility complex. Because histocompatibility antigens are detected most easily on blood leukocytes they are denoted by the initials of the species followed by LA (leukocyte antigen). Thus HLA denotes the major histocompatibility antigens in humans; DLA denotes those in dogs; BoLA, those in bovines;

Table 8–1 COMPARISON OF CLASS I AND CLASS II MHC ANTIGENS

Property	Class I	Class II
Detection	Serological	Mixed lymphocyte culture
Distribution	All nucleated cells	B cells, macrophages and other antigen-presenting cells
Function	Regulation of T cell recognition	Regulation of the immune response

SLA, those in swine and so forth. In mice and chickens the major histocompatibility antigens are known as H2 and B respectively, since they were first recognized as blood-group antigens.

TERMINOLOGY

The following definitions are offered as an aid to those who may have forgotten any genetics they once knew.

Genes are units of DNA that code for the amino acid sequence of a polypeptide chain. Genes can exist in two or more alternative forms known as alleles. Alleles are located on chromosomes at sites called loci. In the case of histocompatibility antigens, as many as 30 different alleles can be coded for at one locus, but in any individual animal a single locus can contain only one gene. Because chromosomes are paired, one being inherited from each parent, alleles are also inherited in pairs. Since there may be three or more class I loci and no more than two alleles inherited at each locus in any individual animal, the number of possible allelic combinations is very large. A gene complex is a cluster of related genes, occupying a restricted area of a chromosome. The term haplotype is used to describe the complete set of alleles at all loci within a gene complex on a single chromosome.

CLASS I HISTOCOMPATIBILITY ANTIGENS

When the class I histocompatibility antigens of different individuals of a species are compared, tremendous antigenic diversity is en-

countered. This diversity, or polymorphism, occurs because at each class I locus there may be 30 to 60 different alleles. The number of class I loci also varies between species. In mice, for example, there are eight different loci. In humans, six loci have been identified, but in most of the domestic species only one or two class I loci are known. The class I gene loci are arranged in a consistent pattern along the chromosome within the MHC (Fig. 8–1).

The Structure of Class I Antigens

All class I antigens indentified so far have been found to be membrane-bound glycoproteins of 45,000 daltons, consisting of a single peptide linked to a molecule of β2 -microglobulin (Fig. 8–2). The peptide chain is divided into three domains each of about 100 amino acids bound together by intrachain disulfide bonds that fold the molecule into three globular subunits. The chain is attached to the cell at its carboxy-terminus by a peptide that penetrates the cell membrane and extends for a short distance into the cytoplasm.

The polymorphism of class I molecules occurs as a result of variations in the amino acid sequence in the amino-terminal domain of each molecule. The carboxy-terminal domains have a constant sequence and, because they are related in structure to the domains of immunoglobulins, they are members of the immunoglobulin superfamily (Chapter 4).

The β2–microglobulin molecule found associated with the class I antigen is not coded for by genes in the MHC but is synthesized

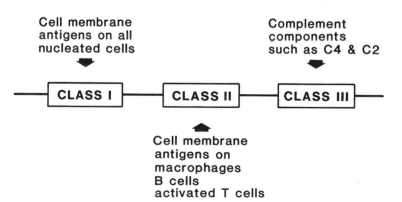

Figure 8–1. The three classes of major histocompatibility complex-coded antigens.

CLASS I

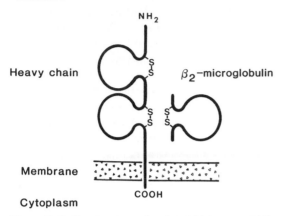

Figure 8–2. The structure of a class I histocompatibility antigen.

elsewhere in the cell and attaches to the class I antigens on the rough endoplasmic reticulum before they are expressed on the cell surface.

The Function of Class I Antigens

One function of the T cell–mediated immune system is the identification and destruction of virus-infected cells. In order to do this, the T cells must clearly recognize the presence of virus antigen on the cell membrane. It is also essential, however, that the cytotoxic T cells recognize the class I antigens of the target cell at the same time. This is readily demonstrated experimentally by showing that cytotoxic T cells will destroy virus-infected target cells only if the T cells and their targets possess identical class I antigens. The T8 protein on the surface of cytotoxic T cells may be the molecule that recognizes the class I antigen on target cells. This requirement for identity of the class I antigens is known as MHC restriction, and it plays a major role in regulating the activity of cytotoxic T cells (Fig. 8–3).

CLASS II HISTOCOMPATIBILITY ANTIGENS

Class II histocompatibility antigens are coded for by genes located within the MHC. In the species studied so far, up to three different class II loci have been described and each locus contains between 12 and 40 alleles.

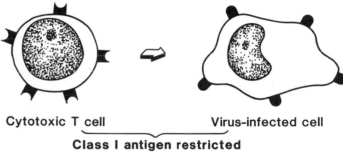

Cytotoxic T cell   Virus-infected cell

Class I antigen restricted

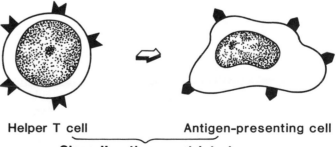

Helper T cell   Antigen-presenting cell

Class II antigen restricted

Figure 8–3. The phenomenon of MHC restriction. A cytotoxic T cell will only destroy a target with identical class I antigens. A helper T cell will only recognize antigen from a presenting cell with identical class II antigens.

The Structure of Class II Antigens

The class II antigens are glycoproteins, each consisting of two non-covalently linked polypeptide chains (Fig. 8–4). One chain, the α or heavy chain has a molecular weight of 34,000 daltons, while the other, the β or light chain, is between 26,000 and 28,000 daltons. Class II molecules do not contain β2-microglobulin. Like class I molecules, class II molecules show polymorphism as a result of variations in the amino acid sequence of the amino-terminal domain of their β chain. The α chain has a constant structure. The amount of class II antigens on the cell surface is enhanced in rapidly dividing cells.

> Class II structures also contain a third chain called the γ chain. This is an invariant intracellular chain that seems to be involved in cellular protein transport. Its immunological function is unknown.

The Function of Class II Antigens

Class II antigens regulate the interactions between regulatory T cells, B cells and antigen-presenting cells. These antigen-presenting cells include some macrophages, dendritic cells, endothelial cells and epithelial cells. If the interactions between helper T cells and macrophages or B cells are investigated, it can be readily shown that cell cooperation will

CLASS II

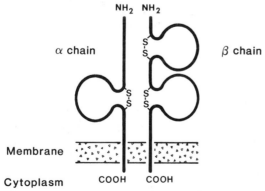

Figure 8–4. The structure of a class II histocompatibility antigen.

only occur if the helper T cell and the cells it interacts with have identical class II antigens on their surfaces (Fig. 8–3). Helper T cells can therefore recognize class II molecules on the surface of antigen-presenting cells. Indeed, these helper T cells only recognize foreign antigen if it is presented to them in close physical association with a class II antigen. It is believed that the T4 molecule on the helper T cell surface may function as a receptor for class II antigens.

Class II antigens are also able to regulate whether or not an animal will mount an immune response to a specific epitope. For example, the synthetic antigen TGAL is a branched-chain peptide consisting of a lysine backbone with alanine side chains to which tyrosine and glutamic acid residues are attached. If TGAL is injected into inbred strains of mice, one strain, called CBA, does not mount an immune response, while another strain, called C57Bl, responds by making a high level of antibodies. If mice of these two strains are crossed, the F1 animals are found to mount a strong response to TGAL. Further studies show that the ability to mount an immune response to TGAL is controlled by a single gene. When a large number of different mouse strains are tested for the presence of this immune response gene, it is obvious that the gene is closely associated with certain histocompatibility antigens. Careful genetic studies have shown that immune response genes code for specific class II antigens on the surface of lymphocytes. Indeed, it is possible to use antisera directed against specific class II antigens to block the immune response to a specific foreign antigen in responder animals.

The control exercised by class II antigens on the immune responses only becomes readily apparent if the response to single simple foreign epitopes is investigated. It is much more difficult to demonstrate genetic control of the response to a complex protein. When the immune system encounters such a molecule, it mounts a set of responses against each individual epitope on the molecule. The net result is therefore the sum of several different immune responses.

Interferon and MHC Antigens

Interferon enhances the expression of class I and class II antigens on cells either by inducing the synthesis of new MHC antigens or by promoting the production of increased quantities of antigen. Since interferon is produced by T cells attacking foreign tissue grafts, it can increase the expression of class II antigens on the grafted cells and so enhance graft rejection.

The I-J Antigens

The class II histocompatibility antigens of the mouse are coded for by genes located in a segment known as the I region. Studies have shown that mouse suppressor T cells possess a characteristic cell membrane protein called I-J, whose genes appear to be located in the I region. Unfortunately, when the I region is mapped there is no room for I-J genes. This paradox is unresolved, although it has been suggested that I-J is coded for by a gene located on chromosome four, whose expression is controlled by the class II histocompatibility genes.

CLASS III HISTOCOMPATIBILITY ANTIGENS

Gene loci that regulate the synthesis and level of some components of the complement system are also located within the MHC and are known as class III genes. In mice, one region, known as S, contains the genes that code for C1, C4 and C2 as well as for the C3 receptor. In man the class III genes code for variants of the C4 molecule as well as for factor B of the alternate complement pathway (Chapter 10). Class III gene loci have been identified within the MHC of horses and swine.

HISTOCOMPATIBILITY ANTIGENS AND DISEASE

Since the function of the products of the major histocompatibility complex is to regulate immune function, it is logical to assume that their genes also influence susceptibility to diseases in which immune responses play a significant role. Thus, preliminary evidence in cattle suggests that links exist between possession of certain BoLA antigens and resistance to bovine leukosis, squamous cell eye carcinoma, trypanosomiasis and susceptibility to the tick *Boophilus microplus*. Possession of BoLA w16 is linked to susceptibility to mastitis. BoLA w6 and BoLA w16 have been shown to be associated with high, and BoLA w2 with low antibody responses to human serum albumin. (The w prefix indicates that the allele has been tentatively accepted by an international workshop.) In chickens, possession of the haplotypes, B2, B6, B14 and B21 is associated with resistance to Marek's disease. Possession of haplotypes B1, B3, B5, B15 and B19 is associated with susceptibility to this condition. Chickens homozygous for B1 generally have high adult mortality, are highly susceptible to Marek's disease and respond poorly to such antigens as *Salmonella pullorum* or human serum albumin. In the OS strain of chickens, homozygous B1 or B4 birds are much more susceptible to autoimmune thyroiditis than are B3 birds. Similar associations have been observed in humans.

Selection for specific histocompatibility antigens has great potential for use in the genetic selection of disease-resistant strains of domestic animals.

THE MHC OF DOMESTIC ANIMALS

Every mammal studied in sufficient detail has been shown to possess a complex containing genes coding for class I and class II histocompatibility antigens as well as for complement components (class III). The precise arrangement and number of loci do, however, vary between species (Fig. 8–5). While not all loci have yet been described for each domestic species, this is undoubtedly a result of a lack of investigation rather than of their absence.

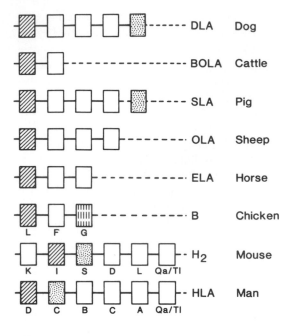

Key:

☐ Class I loci

▨ Class II loci

▦ Class III loci

▥ Class IV locus

Figure 8–5. The general arrangement of the major histocompatibility complex in the domestic animals and man.

The BoLA System

Class I (44,000 dalton) proteins and class II (33,000 and 29,000 dalton) proteins are present on bovine lymphocyte membranes. DNA probes for HLA class I and class II genes can hybridize with bovine DNA, and monoclonal antibodies against human and mouse class II antigens can bind to their bovine homologs. At the present time only one class I BoLA locus is internationally accepted on the basis of serological testing, although claims have been made for a second class I and several class II loci. The class I locus (A) has 17 well-defined alleles and at least four more putative alleles. These class I alleles can be detected by tests using cell-mediated lympholysis. MHC-restricted cytotoxicity has been shown to occur in the destruction of cells infected

with the parasites *Theileria parva* and *T. annulata* (Chapter 17). The bovine blood group antigen M' is closely linked to the allele BoLA w16 and to resistance to mastitis (M'+ animals are resistant to mastitis). The genes for C4 (the fourth component of complement) are probably located within the BoLA MHC.

The ELA System

There are 10 accepted alleles (ELA w1 to ELA w10) at one locus and a single specificity ELY-2 at another locus in the horse. Horses also possess a lymphocyte alloantigen called ELY-1 that is inherited independently of the ELA antigens. Susceptibility to sweet itch, an allergic condition associated with insect bites, is linked to the presence of ELA w7.

The SLA System

Both class I and class II antigens have been identified biochemically on the surface of swine lymphocytes. By means of specific typing antisera it has been possible to show that there are probably three class I loci containing at least 26 alleles. These three loci have been labeled SLA-A SLA-B, and SLA-C. There is also good evidence from MLR (page 102) and biochemical studies that a class II locus is present in swine. Swine class I antigens consist of two peptide chains one of which is β2–microglobulin. Class I antigens have been detected on lymphocytes, platelets, granulocytes, hepatocytes, kidney cells and sperm. Soluble class I antigens have been detected in the serum. Two families of class II antigens have been found on B cells and on a subpopulation of T cells. They are also present on boar sperm in low concentrations. Pigs have a class III locus located within the SLA complex that codes for C4.

Preliminary studies have shown that low growth performance in large white pigs is associated with possession of SLA 4, SLA 5 and SLA 20. High carcass fatness in Landrace pigs is associated with SLA 1, SLA 15 and SLA 18.

The OLA and GLA Systems

At least thirteen class I alleles controlled by three loci (OLA-A, OLA-B, and OLA-C) have been identified in sheep, and resistance to scrapie and to caseous lymphadenitis appears to be associated with possession of certain of these. Claims have been made for the presence of 13 class I alleles at two linked loci, and for three class II alleles at a single locus in the goat.

The DLA System

Dogs are known to possess three DLA class I loci. Ten specificities are recognized at the first locus DLA-A and six at the second locus DLA-B. A third class I locus with three distinct specificities is known as DLA-C. It is believed that these class I antigens have a similar distribution to those in other species. Preliminary experiments have also shown that they are composed of two peptide chains, one of which is probably $\beta2$–microglobulin.

By use of the MLR assay it has been possible to show that dogs probably have a single class II locus with at least three different alleles. Monoclonal antibodies against human class II antigens will react with antigens on canine tissues, and the proteins so recognized contain two peptide chains. A class III locus coding for C4 has been identified in the dog.

Avian Lymphocyte Antigens

Since chickens have nucleated red cells, they possess histocompatibility antigens on their erythrocytes. Three different loci are recognized. BF antigens are class I antigens found on all nucleated cells. BL antigens are class II antigens found on B cells and monocytes. BG antigens are found on red cells only and have been classified as class IV histocompatibility antigens by some investigators. The expression of the BL antigens on B cells is controlled by a non-MHC gene called Bu1. The antigenic molecules themselves are similar in structure to those found in mammals.

HISTOCOMPATIBILITY ANTIGENS AND GRAFT REJECTION

The surgical transplantation of tissues between genetically different individuals has no natural counterpart. Sperm are the only cells naturally transplanted. Surgical transplantation is therefore entirely artifactual and the mechanisms of graft rejection must be interpreted in this light.

In general, when a tissue or organ is transplanted into a genetically dissimilar recipient, the recipient will mount an immune response against the histocompatibility antigens present on the grafted cells. The class I antigens in the graft stimulate an antibody response. The class II antigens, on the other hand, stimulate a cell-mediated response from the host. Grafts that differ minimally from the recipient will generally be much more successful than grafts that are highly incompatible.

When dogs are given kidney grafts from donors incompatible at both the class I and the class II loci, they survive for about 10 days (see Table 18–1). If, on the other hand, they are compatible at both loci, graft survival is prolonged to about 40 days. A more impressive result is obtained with canine liver grafts, which survive for about 8 days in unrelated animals and for 200 to 300 days in DLA-identical recipients. (The failure of DLA-compatible grafts to survive indefinitely is due to the cumulative effects of a large number of minor histocompatibility differences.) If animals are given grafts compatible at the class I loci but incompatible at the class II loci, or vice versa, then graft survival is intermediate between complete compatibility and complete incompatibility.

The class I antigens, being present on all the nucleated cells of the graft, can readily provoke an antibody response from the recipient. The class II antigens are, however, found only on a few cells in the grafted tissue, B cells and macrophages, for example. Nevertheless, it is clear that the intensity of graft rejection is directly related to the number of lymphocytes and other class II positive cells present within the graft. Removal of these cells by careful flushing or by pretreatment of the donor with cytotoxic drugs greatly reduces the intensity of the rejection process.

Tissue Typing

Because class I antigens provoke a strong antibody response they can be identified and "typed" by specific antisera. For this reason, they are sometimes known as serologically defined (SD) antigens. It is possible to obtain specific antisera against each individual class I allele and to determine which of these antisera will kill an animal's leukocytes in the presence of complement. By using a set of these antisera it is possible to identify, or "type," all the class I antigens present on the cells of an individual.

Class II antigens are detected by measuring their ability to stimulate incompatible lymphocytes to divide. They are therefore also called lymphocyte-defined (LD) antigens. Class II antigens may be detected by culturing a mixture of lymphocytes from donor and recipient *in vitro*. If incompatible, both cell populations are stimulated to divide by the presence of foreign class II antigens. This division may be quantitated by measuring the uptake of tritium (^{3}H)-labeled thymidine by the cells, since thymidine is used only by dividing cells that are actively synthesizing DNA. This technique is known as the mixed lymphocyte reaction (MLR). If one of the cell populations is prevented from reacting by pretreatment with an immunosuppressive drug (Chapter 27), then the inactivated cells act as "targets" and it is possible to type the class II antigens on the inactivated cells.

A simple and rapid test for histocompatibility is to take lymphocytes from a potential graft recipient and inject them into the skin of a potential donor. If the injected cells are not compatible with the recipient, then both injected lymphocytes and the recipient's lymphocytes will attack and destroy the nearest foreign tissue and so provoke an inflammatory skin reaction. This reaction is known as the normal lymphocyte transfer test. It mainly measures compatibility at the class II loci; the intensity of the inflammatory response provides an indication of the degree of incompatibility between donor and recipient.

HY ANTIGENS

Skin grafts from male donors placed on histocompatible females are usually rejected; however, the reverse is not the case. This occurs because male cells carry a histocompatibility antigen coded for by genes on the Y chromosome and called the HY antigen. The HY antigen is the inducer of the testes in male fetuses. Thus in twin cattle with fused placental blood vessels, HY antigen released by a male calf can be carried to its female twin and cause masculinization. Such a female calf will be infertile and is known as a freemartin (Chapter 21). Antibodies directed against the HY antigen will kill cells carrying the HY antigen in the presence of complement. It is possible, therefore, to treat a sperm suspension with anti-HY and selectively kill the sperm carrying HY—the male sperm. This has been successfully accomplished in mice where, for example, in one experiment the sex ratio was changed to obtain 95.8 per cent females and only 4.2 per cent males.

An alternative approach to manipulating sex ratios is to selectively destroy male embryos by treating them with anti-HY and complement. In one mouse experiment, 86 per cent of the embryos surviving after treatment were female. By using fluorescent labeled anti-HY it is also possible to determine the sex of isolated embryos. In field trials it has proved possible, by using this technique, to correctly identify the sex of six out of seven bovine embryos.

There is no doubt that some or all of these techniques will eventually find a use in influencing the sex ratio in domestic animals. This will have a very significant effect on the dairy industry especially, where the tendency for the sex ratio to be 1:1 has been very inconvenient.

ADDITIONAL SOURCES OF INFORMATION

Bailey E, Antczak DF, Bernoco D, et al. 1984. Joint report of the second international workshop on lymphocyte alloantigens of the horse. Animal Bld. Gps. Biochem. Gen. *15* 123–132.

Benacerraf B. 1981. Role of MHC gene products in immune regulation. Science *212* 1229–1238.

Hood L, Steinmetz M and Goodenow R. 1982. Genes of the major histocompatibility complex. Cell *28* 685–687.

Kirszenbaum M, Renard C, Geffrotin C, et al. 1985. Evidence for mapping pig C4 gene(s) within the pig major histocompatibility complex (SLA). Animal Bld. Gps. Biochem. Gen. *16* 65–68.

Larsen B, Jensen NE, Madsen P, et al. 1985. Association of the M blood group system with bovine mastitis. Animal Bld. Gps. Biochem. Gen. *16* 165–173.

Lee J and Trowsdale J. 1983. Molecular biology of the major histocompatibility complex. Nature *304* 214–215.

Lew AM, Lillehoj EP, Cowan EP, et al. 1986. Class I genes and molecules: an update. Immunology *57* 3–18.

Marx JL. 1982. Cloning the genes of the MHC. Science *216* 400–402.

Matzinger P and Zamoyska R. 1982. A beginner's guide to major histocompatibility complex function. Nature *297* 628.

McDevitt HO. 1985. The HLA system and its relation to disease. Hospital Practice *20* 57–72.

Newman MJ and Antczak DF. 1983. Histocompatibility polymorphisms of domestic animals. Adv. Vet. Sci. Comp. Med. *27* 2–76.

Nixon DF, Ting JP and Frelinger JA. 1982. Ia antigens on non-lymphoid tissues: their origins and functions. Immunol. Today *3* 339–342.

Preston PM, Brown GCD and Spooner RL. 1983. Cell-mediated cytotoxicity in *Theileria annulata* infection of cattle with evidence for BoLA restriction. Clin. Exp. Immunol. *53* 88–100.

Rosa F and Fellous M. 1984. The effect of gamma-interferon on MHC antigens. Immunol. Today *5* 261–262.

Skoskiewicz MJ, Colvin RB, Schneeberger EE and Russell PS. 1985. Widespread and selective induction of major histocompatibility complex-determined antigens *in vivo* by γ-interferon. J. Exp. Med. *162* 1645–1664.

Spooner RL. 1985. The bovine MHC. Bola Newsletter *1* 3–9.

9

Regulation of the Immune Responses

The interactions between T cells, B cells and macrophages form a complex network, and our understanding of this network is in a state of dynamic change. As a result, students studying this area for the first time may find its complexity discouraging. If you go slowly, however, and make sure that you understand each section you should have little difficulty. Remember that all physiological processes are subject to careful and rigorous controls. It is certain that the immune system is not unique in its complexity and that the patterns of cellular interaction that immunologists have discovered are only a reflection of the superb sophistication of all biological processes.

WHY REGULATE?

The immune responses, both cell- and antibody-mediated, although essential for the protection of the body, may cause severe damage if permitted to act in an unregulated fashion (Fig. 9–1). Failure to control the specificity of an immune response may permit the production of autoantibodies and so result in autoimmune disease. Failure to mount an adequate immune response may result in immunodeficiency and increased susceptibility to infection. In contrast, excessive antibody formation may cause a disease such as amyloidosis. Failure to control the lymphocyte proliferation

Depressed immune reactivity	Excessive immune reactivity
⇧ Susceptibility to infection	⇧ Autoantibodies
⇧ Spontaneous tumors	⇧ Amyloidosis
	⇧ Lymphoid tumors
	⇧ Allergies

Figure 9–1. The consequences of either depressed or excessive immune reactivity.

105

Depressed cellular activity	Enhanced cellular activity
⇧ cAMP	⇩ cAMP
⇩ cGMP	⇧ cGMP
⇧ PGE1	⇧ Insulin

Figure 9–2. The effects of changes in the levels of cyclic nucleotides, prostaglandin E1 and insulin on cellular activities.

that occurs in immune responses may lead to the development of lymphoid tumors. Failure to control the mother's immune response to the fetus may lead to abortion. It is obvious, therefore, that the immune responses must be carefully regulated to ensure that the only responses permitted to occur are appropriate in both quality and quantity. As might be anticipated, many different control mechanisms exist in order to accomplish this task.

PHYSIOLOGICAL CONTROL OF CELLULAR ACTIVITY

Many of the activities of cells, such as secretion or division, are regulated by alterations in the ratio of two intracellular molecules, cyclic AMP (cyclic adenosine-3′,5′-monophosphate) and cyclic GMP (cyclic guanosine-3,′5′-monophosphate). If the relative level of cyclic AMP in a cell is raised or the level of cyclic GMP lowered, then cellular functions tend to be inhibited. In contrast, if cyclic GMP is raised or cyclic AMP lowered, then cellular activities are enhanced (Fig. 9–2). Many, perhaps all, of the mechanisms that regulate

immune responses do so by altering the cyclic AMP/cyclic GMP ratio within cells (Table 9–1).

A second physiological regulator of cellular activity is the hormone insulin. Activated T and B cells possess receptors for insulin. When insulin binds to these cells, it stimulates their metabolic activities.

Prostaglandins also regulate cellular activity. The prostaglandins are a family of complex fatty acids some of which are produced by macrophages and bind to receptors on T cells. These prostaglandins raise cyclic AMP levels in lymphocytes. As a result they inhibit the production of interleukin 2 and therefore cause immunosuppression. They may be responsible for some cases of tolerance, since prostaglandin inhibitors such as indomethacin may permit tolerant B cells to respond to antigen. Prostaglandins of the E group are probably the most important in suppressing immune reactivity.

Leukotrienes, another family of specialized fatty acids, are also immunoregulatory. Leukotriene B_4, for example, enhances suppressor T cell activity, IFN-γ production, T cell and NK cell cytotoxicity as well as IL-1 and IL-2 production.

Table 9–1 ROLE OF CYCLIC AMP IN SOME IMMUNOLOGICAL PHENOMENA*

Cell	Stimulus That Elevates Cyclic AMP	Effect of Elevated Cyclic AMP
Lymphocyte	Antibodies Immune complexes Suppressor cells Prostaglandins	Inhibition of antigen-stimulated differentiation and division
Macrophage	Some ingested bacteria and protozoa	Inhibition of lysosome-phagosome fusion
Mast cells	E prostaglandins Histamine	Inhibition of antigen-induced histamine release

*Cyclic AMP generally acts to inhibit cellular activities, although the overall effect is modulated by the cyclic AMP/cyclic GMP ratio.

GENETIC CONTROL OF THE IMMUNE SYSTEM

The cell interactions that are so important in generating immune responses are rigorously regulated by class II histocompatibility antigens on the surfaces of interacting cells. It is not clear, however, just how these antigens function. As pointed out in the previous chapter, it is possible to show that animals may be either responders or nonresponders to specific epitopes. It is also clear that the ability to respond to a specific epitope is regulated by immune response genes and that these genes code for class II antigens. Two mechanisms have been proposed to account for this phenomenon. One hypothesis suggests that the class II molecules influence the development of the T cell repertoire during embryonic development. As a result, clones of T cells capable of recognizing that specific epitope in association with the nonresponder class II molecule fail to develop. The second hypothesis suggests that the presence of the nonresponder class II molecule prevents T cells from responding to the epitope. However, experiments show that T cells derived from another animal may respond normally to an epitope linked to a nonresponder class II molecule. This suggests that there is nothing intrinsically wrong with the epitope-nonresponder molecule complex. It has also been shown that in some cases a specific class II molecule can prevent the response to one epitope while at the same time permitting the response to a related epitope. This suggests that the class II molecule does regulate the ability of T cells to recognize a specific epitope.

REGULATION BY ANTIGEN

The immune responses are antigen driven. Once antigen is eliminated, then the stimulus for lymphocyte proliferation (but not immunoglobulin synthesis) is removed and the immune response ceases. If antigen persists, then the stimulus persists, lymphocytes continue to proliferate and the immune response is prolonged. This type of prolonged response is observed after immunization with poorly metabolized antigens, such as some bacterial polysaccharides, or with antigen incorporated in water-in-oil emulsions or insoluble adjuvants.

Antigen-sensitive lymphocytes can respond to antigen by producing antibodies or effector T cells only if that antigen is presented to them in an appropriate dose and manner. If the amount of antigen encountered by an antigen-sensitive cell is excessive, then instead of responding to antigen by division and differentiation, lymphocytes may become unreactive or even be eliminated and a state of tolerance will result. If the amount of antigen is insufficient or if it is presented to T cells in an inappropriate fashion, then suppressor T cells will be preferentially stimulated and tolerance will also result (Fig. 9–3).

Tolerance is a state in which an animal becomes unresponsive to a specific antigen. The most obvious example of tolerance is seen in the failure of animals to make antibodies against normal body components. Burnet and Fenner suggested in 1948 that the development of this self-tolerance depended upon the state of maturation of the antigen-sensitive cells at the time they first encounter antigen.

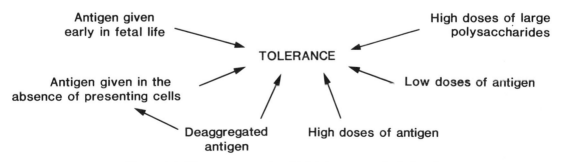

Figure 9–3. The many ways in which tolerance can be induced.

They suggested that antigen-sensitive cells became specifically unresponsive if exposed to an antigen during fetal life but that after birth these cells responded to new antigens by mounting a conventional immune response. As evidence for this suggestion they pointed to the existence of chimeric calves. In about 90 per cent of dizygotic twin calves, the placental blood vessels fuse and the blood of the two calves mixes freely. Circulating hematopoietic stem cells are therefore free to intermingle in each calf. Consequently, when these calves are born they possess two populations of erythrocytes, some originating from one animal and some from its twin. In spite of being genetically and antigenically dissimilar, the calves are fully tolerant of each other's blood cells.

A variation on this "natural" experiment can be performed in the laboratory if cells from one inbred strain of mice are inoculated into the fetuses of a second inbred strain. When the inoculated mice are born they are completely tolerant to cells of the donor strain, so they can, for instance, accept skin grafts indefinitely from that strain. This experiment confirmed (at least in mice) Burnet and Fenner's suggestion that antigen given *in utero* provokes tolerance rather than immunity. The switch from tolerance induction to normal immune responses occurs soon after birth in laboratory rodents, at the time when the newborn rodent acquires the ability to make interleukin 2. If a T cell encounters antigen in the absence of IL-2, then tolerance will develop. If IL-2 is present, then a normal immune response will result. Thus, if IL-2 is given to newborn mice, it will permit them to respond to injected antigens. In domestic mammals, the young are born at a much more mature stage of immunological development than in rodents. As a result the ability to mount an immune response develops at a much earlier stage of fetal life (Chapter 13). The ability to cause experimental tolerance in the fetus demonstrates how self-tolerance can occur. Most self-antigens are present in the fetus and thus can induce tolerance long before an animal is able to mount an immune response to extrinsic antigens.

Tolerance may also be induced in adult animals. As pointed out earlier, the conditions under which a T cell or a B cell will respond to an antigen are highly restrictive, and antigen must be presented to these cells in an appropriate dose and manner. If antigen is administered to animals in doses ranging from very low to very high, it is found that very low and very high doses are tolerogenic, whereas medium doses provoke an immune response. Very low doses of antigen induce tolerance only in T cells, whereas very high doses render both B cells and T cells unresponsive. Because helper T cells are needed for a B cell response to occur, tolerance of either type will block antibody production.

Protein solutions normally contain a mixture of aggregated and single molecules. Aggregated protein molecules are rapidly phagocytosed by macrophages and are thus highly immunogenic. If a protein solution is ultracentrifuged so that these aggregates are removed, the antigen solution becomes highly tolerogenic. It is believed that this is because the single antigen molecules can reach antigen-sensitive T cells directly without having undergone macrophage processing.

A different type of tolerance is provoked by high doses of polysaccharide antigens. These antigens can bind irreversibly to B cell antigen receptors and thus block the further response of these cells to antigens.

The Mechanisms of Tolerance

Although tolerance may be induced in many different ways, the precise mechanisms involved at the cellular level remain unclear. In self-tolerance induced in fetal animals, responsive T cells are not completely eliminated, since some self-reactive cells can be detected in adult animals if very sensitive techniques are used. In tolerance induced by very low doses of antigen or by ultracentrifuged antigens, suppressor cells are preferentially stimulated. In contrast, very high doses of antigen probably cause deletion of reactive T cells.

All these forms of tolerance gradually wane as antigen is eliminated. If the antigen persists in the body, as occurs in self-tolerance, then the tolerant condition may be maintained indefinitely. Once the antigen is eliminated,

B cells regain their reactivity rapidly, whereas T cells take considerably longer to recover.

REGULATION BY ANTIBODY

Antibody or immune complexes usually exert a negative feedback on immune responses. For example, IgG antibody to a specific antigen can depress the production of IgM or IgG to the same antigen, and high levels of IgM depress the further synthesis of IgM. This feedback process ensures that immunoglobulin levels in normal animals remain relatively constant regardless of the degree of antigenic stimulation to which they are subjected. It was once considered that this negative feedback was mediated by antibody that combined with antigen to mask its epitopes and so removed the stimulus for cell proliferation. It is likely, however, that this is a minor mechanism, since negative feedback requires the presence of intact Fc regions on the inhibitory immunoglobulin molecules and $F(ab)'_2$ fragments are unable to block an antibody response. B cells possess Fc receptors, and the binding of antibodies or immune complexes to these receptors causes these cells to turn off by increasing intracellular levels of cyclic AMP. Suppressor T cells also possess Fc receptors, and antibody or immune complexes may act through these to stimulate suppressor cell activities.

When serum immunoglobulin levels are abnormally elevated, as occurs in plasma cell tumors (myelomas) (Chapter 26), these feedback mechanisms can depress normal immunoglobulin synthesis. As a result, animals with myelomas are immunosuppressed and are thus very susceptible to secondary infection. A similar phenomenon occurs in newborn animals that acquire immunoglobulins passively from their mother. The presence of maternal antibody, while conferring temporary immunity, prevents the successful vaccination of these newborn animals, since it effectively inhibits immunoglobulin production.

It is also of interest to note that antibody-producing cells migrate away from the lymph node cortex and the lymph follicles of the spleen, where the antigen-sensitive cells react with antigen (Chapter 5). Presumably, if this movement did not take place, then the presence of high concentrations of immunoglobulin in close proximity to antigen-sensitive cells might cause the immune response to switch off prematurely.

The isotype as well as the quantity of immunoglobulin produced during an immune response is also carefully regulated. Most unstimulated B lymphocytes have both IgD and IgM on their cell membrane. During the course of an immune response, these cells switch to the production of IgG, IgA or IgE, and this switch is regulated by T cells through the release of B cell differentiation factors. In the absence of T cells the switch in inefficient, and IgM production persists at a relatively low level. Antigens such as bacterial lipopolysaccharides, polymerized flagellin and pneumococcal polysaccharide that do not stimulate T cells readily but can induce B cells to respond in the absence of T cells, generate a persistent IgM response with no switch to IgG production. As might be anticipated, neonatal thymectomy does not depress the responses to these antigens. They may therefore be considered to be thymus independent antigens. Neonatal bursectomy may also result in a failure of the IgM-to-IgG switch, suggesting that the bursa is responsible for this process in birds.

Immunological Networks

When an antibody response occurs, large amounts of immunoglobulin are produced. The idiotypes found on the variable regions of these immunoglobulins function as epitopes and will provoke the production of autoantibodies against themselves. These anti-idiotype autoantibodies also possess idiotypes. As a result they, in their turn, function as epitopes and provoke anti–anti-idiotype antibodies (Fig. 9–4). This process could, theoretically, proceed indefinitely. This concept has been developed into a hypothesis that a network of interacting idiotype–anti-idiotype reactions are provoked in any antibody response and that these reactions serve to regulate antibody formation. Thus antibody formation is nor-

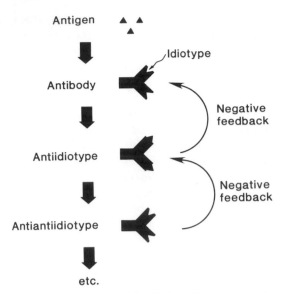

Figure 9–4. The principle of the idiotype network. Each immunoglobulin induces the production of antibodies directed against its own idiotypes. These antiidiotype antibodies exert a negative feedback on antibody production.

mally suppressed by the anti-idiotype response, the anti-idiotype response is suppressed by the anti–anti-idiotype response and so forth. The net effect of this will be to cause rapid termination of the antibody response. The concept is more complex than this, however, since, under some circumstances, antiidiotypes may enhance an antibody response.

REGULATION BY REGULATORY CELLS

It has already been described how helper T cells are required in order for B or T lymphocytes to respond to antigen. There also exist T lymphocytes whose function is to inhibit the immune response. These are known as suppressor T cells. Helper and suppressor T lymphocytes can be identified by analysis of the surface antigens found on peripheral blood lymphocytes. Helper cells possess the T4 antigen, whereas suppressor cells possess T8. Changes in the ratio of T4 and T8 cells in blood are reflected in different levels of immune reactivity. Thus elevated T8 or lowered T4 numbers are associated with a state of

immunosuppression (AIDS, for example), whereas raised T4 or depressed T8 numbers are characteristic of some autoimmune diseases. Suppressor cells suppress immune responses by releasing soluble suppressor factors, at least fifteen of which have been described. Some of these factors act directly on antigen-sensitive B or T cells; others act on helper T cells. Some of these factors are antigen-specific and others are nonspecific. At least three different types of antigen-specific suppressor factors have been described. These include a single chain polypeptide, a two chain polypeptide carrying antigen-specific and class II MHC determinants and a two chain protein that suppresses the antibody response by binding to idiotypes on B cells.

Epitopes differ in their ability to stimulate the immune system. Some are weak and stimulate a poor response, others stimulate a strong response. Some stimulate suppressor cell activity, others stimulate helper cell activity. Some stimulate T cells; others stimulate B cells. The immune response provoked by any individual antigenic molecule will represent the sum of all the responses against all the epitopes on that molecule. Epitopes may therefore be classified according to the cell type they stimulate, i.e., B cell, helper T cell or suppressor T cell.

It has proved difficult to identify the important differences between these three types of epitope. The epitopes that stimulate antibody formation must be presented to B cells in an undistorted fashion. (We know this because antibodies are directed against the intact, native molecule.) The ability of a determinant to stimulate a B cell is critically dependent on its conformation. If the antigen is treated so that the shape of its epitopes change, then its ability to stimulate a specific B cell response is impaired. If the epitopes that stimulate helper T cell activity are analyzed, it is apparent that their conformation is much less important than in the epitopes that stimulate B cells. Indeed it appears that helper T cells recognize new epitopes that arise as a result of processing by antigen presenting cells. Helper T cells also appear to recognize sequences of amino acids rather than their three dimensional conformation.

It is still not clear what features of an epitope are preferentially recognized by suppressor T cells. These suppressor epitopes have been identified on proteins and can be isolated. They vary in their suppressive potency. Some suppressor epitopes are so potent that they can prevent an animal responding to the intact antigen. Others only function after being revealed by treatment of the antigen with proteolytic enzymes. The differences between helper and suppressor epitopes may be caused by the manner in which the antigen is presented by macrophages or other cells.

Suppressor cells also function as part of a network. Thus it has been demonstrated in mice that one population of suppressor T cells may induce differentiation of a second population of suppressor T cells. This second population induces differentiation of a third population of suppressor cells. The characteristics and specificity of each of these three suppressor cell populations differ. Thus they act at different times during an immune response, recognize different epitopes and produce different suppressor factors.

The plant lectin concanavalin A has the ability to stimulate suppressor cell activity nonspecifically. Thus if a lymphocyte culture is taken from an animal and exposed to concanavalin A, the cells acquire the ability to suppress other *in vitro* immune reactions. The supernatant fluid from a concanavalin A–treated lymphocyte culture is rich in soluble suppressive factors and can suppress the response of other lymphocytes to antigen.

Suppressor cells function throughout an animal's life. Thus, the poor ability of newborn animals to mount an immune response is due in part to suppressor cell activity, as is the decline in immune competence seen in old animals. The unreactivity of pregnant animals toward their fetuses is ascribed in part to suppressor cells, as is the normal decline following the primary immune response. Tolerance may be caused, in some cases, by suppressor cell activity. Thus, tolerance to self-antigens is largely suppressor cell–mediated. Loss of suppressor cells can therefore result in the development of autoimmune responses. The immune suppression seen in some viral diseases, in cancer and following

trauma or burns has been shown to be due, at least in part, to suppressor cell activity. Some allergic individuals, such as those who suffer from type I hypersensitivity reactions, appear to have depressed suppressor cell function. The administration of desensitizing shots to these individuals can lead to clinical improvement by promoting suppressor cell function. There is, indeed, no doubt that suppressor T cells function as major regulators of immune reactivity.

Suppressor Macrophages

Macrophages may also function as suppressor cells by releasing PGE_2. This inhibits lymphocyte proliferation and differentiation and blocks the production of IL-2, MIF, MAF and other lymphokines. Treatment of B cell tolerant animals with cyclooxygenase inhibitors such as indomethacin may lead to restoration of their immune responsiveness, suggesting that B cell tolerance may also be caused by prostaglandins.

OTHER REGULATORY FACTORS

In recent years it has been possible to show that many normal body constituents may have the ability to regulate immune reactivity. In some cases subsequent investigation has shown that this regulation is due to an ability to influence suppressor cell populations. For example, α fetoprotein, a protein synthesized in large quantities by the fetal liver, is potently immunosuppressive and may therefore contribute to the immunological acceptance of the fetus by the mother. α Fetoprotein has been shown to be a potent stimulator of suppressor T cell activity and it also inhibits class II antigen expression by macrophages, thus blocking antigen presentation.

Another immunosuppressive factor is C-reactive protein (CRP). This is an acute phase protein, found normally in low concentrations in serum, whose level increases rapidly within hours of infection, inflammation or tissue damage (Chapter 19). In addition to being immunosuppressive, CRP can promote phagocyto-

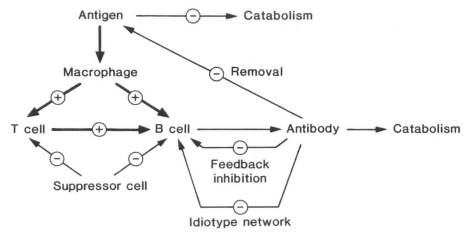

Figure 9–5. Some of the major interactions that regulate the immune response. As can readily be seen, the enhancing effects generally stem from the presence of antigen. Suppressive effects, in contrast, are caused by the antibody itself or by suppressor cells.

sis, inhibit platelet function and activate complement. Its function is unknown, but it has been suggested that CRP prevents the occurrence of autoimmunity to intracellular antigens released from damaged tissue.

The nervous system hormones known as endorphins and encephalins also influence immune reactivity and provide a rational basis for the obvious effects of the nervous system on immune reactivity. For example, α-endorphin is immunosuppressive but encephalins are immunostimulating; some lymphocytes can synthesize and release endorphins.

Histamine, another ubiquitous, pharmacologically active agent, can bind to T cells through specific H2 receptors. In doing so, it raises the cyclic AMP level within these cells and depresses their activity. Conversely, if the histamine binds to lymphocyte H1 receptors, it enhances their activity. If histamine binds to the H2 receptors of suppressor cells, it stimulates their activity. It may therefore serve to regulate T cell activity in general.

Immune Regulation

It should be clear to the reader that there exists a complex system of interacting factors that control immune reactivity (Fig 9–5). A moment's consideration should reveal that this is an inevitable and consistent feature not only

of the immune system but also of all body systems.

In order for any complex multicellular organism to survive and function, it is essential that an efficient yet flexible control system exist. In this respect, the immune system is not unique. It happens to be the first of the body's systems to have been analyzed in detail, but it may be predicted that other body systems will be found to be equally complex.

ADDITIONAL SOURCES OF INFORMATION

Bankert RB, Bloor AG and Jou Y-H. 1982. Idiotypes: their presence on B- and T-lymphocytes and their role in the regulation of the immune response. Vet Immunol. Immunopathol. *3* 147–184.

Bielefeldt-Ohmann H, Filion LG and Babiuk LA. 1983. Bovine monocytes and macrophages: an accessory role in suppressor-cell generation by Con A and in Lectin-induced proliferation. Immunology *50* 189–197.

Chang TW. 1985. Regulation of immune response by antibodies: the importance of antibody and monocyte Fc receptor interaction in T-cell activation. Immunol. Today *6* 245–249.

Ellis JA and Demartin JC. 1985. Ovine concanavalin A-induced suppressor cells: generation, assay, age-related effects and reevaluation of mechanism of suppression. Immunology *54* 353–362.

Geha RS. 1981. Regulation of the immune response by idiotypic-antiidiotypic interactions. N. Engl. J. Med. *305* 25–28.

Gilbert KM and Hoffmann MK. 1983. Suppressor B lymphocytes. Immunol. Today *4* 253–255.

Hadden JW and Coffey RG. 1982. Cyclic nucleotides in

mitogen-induced lymphocyte proliferation. Immunol. Today 3 299–304.

Heron I, Cahill R and Trnka Z. 1982. The appearance of specific helper cells in lymph of immunized sheep. Int. Arch. Allergy Appl. Immunol. 68 157–163.

Kapp JA, Pierce CW and Sorensen CM. 1984. Antigen-specific suppressor T-cell factors. Hospital Pract. 11 85–98.

Marx JL. 1983. Chemical signals in the immune system. Science 221 1362–1364.

Ninnemann JL. 1984. Prostaglandins and immunity. Immunol. Today 5 170–178.

Pleszcynski MR. 1985. Immunoregulation by leukotrienes and other lipoxygenase metabolites. Immunol. Today 6 302–307.

Rosenthal AS. 1980. Regulation of the immune response—role of the macrophage. N. Engl. J. Med. 303 1153–1156.

Taylor RB. 1984. Mechanism of T-cell tolerance. Nature 307 317.

10

Antigen-Antibody Interaction and the Complement System

Up to this point, the immune responses have been considered part of an isolated system concerned only with the elimination of antigen from the body. However, body systems rarely, if ever, act in total isolation, and the immune system is no exception, since it acts in conjunction with many other systems to produce a wide variety of different effects. Although most of these consequences may be considered to be physiological when operating normally, it is not uncommon for them, when operating in apparent excess of the normal body requirements, to produce lesions that are considered to be pathological. It should, however, be pointed out that in declaring a reaction to be pathological, we must consider not only the immediate discomfort of an animal but also the influence of this reaction on the animal's long-term survival and therefore on the survival of the species as a whole. For example, antigen-antibody interactions commonly lead to the development of acute inflammatory reactions. If these reactions involve critical locations such as the walls of blood vessels or the upper respiratory tract, they may be extremely uncomfortable or even life-threatening. Nevertheless, they do serve to hasten the elimination of antigen and this may greatly outweigh the risks incurred by not eliminating it.

ANTIGEN-ANTIBODY INTERACTION AS AN INITIATING EVENT IN PHYSIOLOGICAL PROCESSES

The properties of antibody molecules complexed with antigen are very different from those of free antibody (Fig. 10–1). For example, when antibody molecules bind antigen they acquire the ability to bind to receptors on phagocytic cells and thus function as opsonins. New epitopes also appear on this antigen-bound antibody. These epitopes are regarded by the immune system as foreign and provoke the formation of autoantibodies known as rheumatoid factors (Chapter 25). The new epitopes and new biological activities are associated with changes in the immunoglobulin Fc region. Normally, the Fc region is partially masked by the Fab regions. When the antibody binds antigen through the Fab regions the shape of the molecule changes. The active sites on the Fc region are exposed and are then able to exert their biological functions.

A second mechanism by which immunoglobulins exert their biological activity is through a dose effect. One active site on a single immunoglobulin molecule may be, by itself, insufficient to initiate many reactions. When several antibody molecules bind closely together on the surface of an antigen, however, the combined stimulus may be sufficient to initiate subsequent reactions.

THE COMPLEMENT SYSTEM

There are several physiological processes that, if activated in the absence of effective controls, may lead to disastrous consequences. Examples of these include the clotting system, the fibrinolytic system, and the kinin system. Uncontrolled activation of these systems can lead to uncontrollable hemorrhage, to extensive intravascular thrombosis or to increases in vascular permeability, respectively. Therefore, in order to ensure that uncontrolled activation does not occur, all of these systems are regulated by mechanisms that involve a series of interlinked enzyme reactions. The general principle of these interlinked reactions is that the products of one reaction catalyze a second reaction whose products can catalyze a third reaction and so on (Fig. 10–2). Since many of these intermediate products either are present in limiting quantities, have a very short half-life or are easily inhibited, it is possible to ensure that the reactions do not proceed to completion in an uncontrolled fashion. Chain reactions of this type are known as cascade reactions and usually require some form of trigger to initiate the reaction chain.

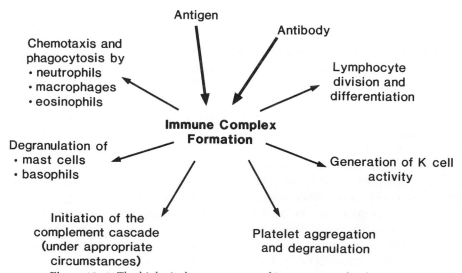

Figure 10–1. The biological consequences of immune-complex formation.

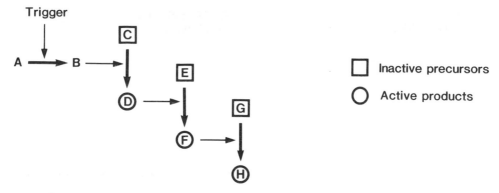

Figure 10–2. The principle of cascade reactions. A "trigger" initiates the conversion of an inactive proenzyme A to an active enzyme B. Enzyme B then acts to convert a proenzyme C to an active enzyme D. Enzyme D in turn converts proenzyme E to enzyme F, and so forth.

In the case of the blood clotting cascade, for example, activation of Hageman factor by altered surfaces serves as the initiating event that sets the cascade in motion.

In addition to the three systems mentioned previously, there exists another system whose activation may result in the disruption of cell membranes and, as a result of this disruption, cause the destruction of either cells or organisms. This system is termed the complement system (because it complements the antibody system). The complement system must be carefully regulated, since uncontrolled generation of the products of the system may lead to massive cellular destruction and tissue damage.

The complement system may be considered to consist of three distinct reaction pathways. Two of these pathways represent alternative procedures for the activation of the third component of the cascade. The third, or terminal, pathway is not a true cascade reaction but a series of aggregations by which a membrane-damaging complex is generated from the activated third component. Complement components are either labeled numerically with the prefix C, i.e., C1, C2, C3 and so forth, or designated by letters of the alphabet, i.e., B, D, P, etc. There are at least 15 of these components; they are all serum proteins and together they make up about 10 per cent of the globulin fraction of serum. The molecular weights of the complement components vary between 80,000 daltons for C9 to 400,000 daltons for C1q. Their serum concentrations

in humans vary between 3mg/100 ml of C2 to 130 mg/100 ml of C3. Complement components are synthesized at various sites throughout the body. For example, the C1 subcomponents are synthesized in macrophages and fibroblasts; C2, C5, C3, H, P, D, B and C4 in macrophages; and C3, C6 and C9 in the liver. The levels of C1, C4 and C2 in serum are controlled by class III genes in the major histocompatibility complex (Chapter 8).

Classical Pathway for Activation of C3 (Fig. 10–3)

The classical pathway of complement activation, so called because it has been known for many more years than the alternate pathway, is initiated by antigen-antibody interaction on surfaces such as cell membranes. The process may be initiated by combination of an antigen with either a single molecule of IgM or two, closely spaced, IgG molecules. The active sites on the Fc region of the immunoglobulin molecules exposed by combination with antigen can bind and activate the first component of complement (C1). C1 is a trimolecular complex containing three subcomponents (C1q, C1r and C1s) held together as a single unit by a calcium ion. The binding of C1q to an immunoglobulin molecule results in activation of C1r. The activated C1r then cleaves a fragment off C1s so that the C1s develops proteolytic activity. C1q may also be activated by bacteria such as *Staphylococcus aureus* and

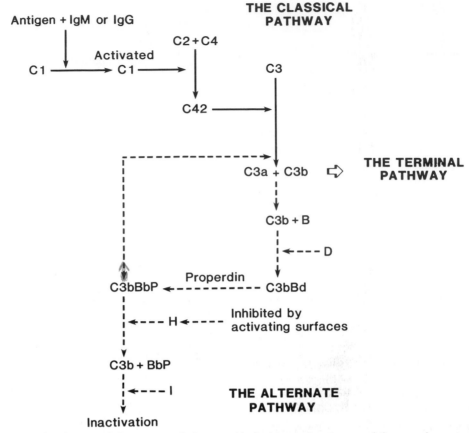

Figure 10–3. The classic (solid arrows) and alternate (dashed arrows) pathways of the complement cascade.

some strains of *Escherichia coli*. The natural substrates of activated C1s are the complement components C4 and C2. C1s acts on both of these molecules to generate a new enzyme called C42. C42 is a protease that binds to cell surfaces, and acts on the next component, C3, to split it into two fragments, known as C3a and C3b. One molecule of C42 (also known as C3 convertase) may act on several hundred molecules of C3 in this way, resulting in a relatively large quantity of C3b being deposited on the antigen surface.

Alternate Pathway for Activation of C3

The alternate pathway (whose factors are denoted by letters of the alphabet B, D, P, etc.) provides a mechanism by which C3 convertase activity may be generated in the absence of

antibody. In normal plasma C3 slowly, continuously and spontaneously breaks down to C3a and C3b (Fig. 10–3). The C3b thus formed adheres to cell surfaces where it binds to factor B. This C3bB complex is then split by an enzyme D to form C3bBb. The C3bBb can act as a C3 convertase, but it is extremely unstable and must therefore be stabilized by binding factor P, also known as properdin, to form C3bBbP. However, there are two inhibitors in normal serum called factors H and I. Factor H splits the C3bBbP complex into C3b and BbP. Factor I can then inactivate the C3b. Thus, the C3 convertase of the alternate pathway is normally destroyed as soon as it is formed. Factor H is strongly inhibited, however, by the presence of surfaces that do not contain sialic acid. These include bacterial and fungal cell walls, helminth cuticles, some tumor cell membranes and aggregated immunoglobulins. Consequently, if any of these

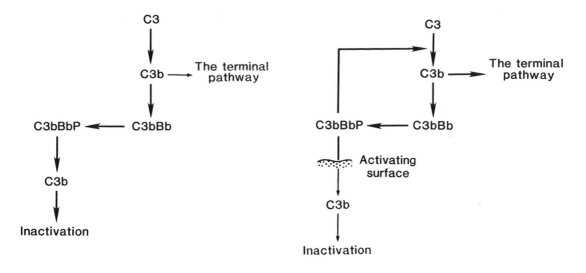

In normal serum   **In the presence of an activating surface**

Figure 10–4. The activation of the alternate pathway in the presence of activating surfaces results in the generation of large amounts of C3 convertase, which would otherwise be destroyed.

surfaces are present, factor H will be inactivated, and C3bBbP will not be destroyed but will remain able to act on native C3 to generate C3a and C3b (Fig. 10–4). Because of this positive feedback loop, very large quantities of C3b can be rapidly generated in the presence of activating surfaces. Thus, the alternate pathway provides a route by which potential invaders—bacteria, fungi or helminths—can activate complement despite the absence of antibody.

Terminal Complement Pathway
(Fig. 10–5)

The final stage of the complement pathway differs from the processes involved in the production of the two C3 convertases in that it is not a cascade reaction in the strict sense. Apart from the enzymatic activation of C5, the terminal pathway involves the aggregation of complement components out of solution and into a large macromolecular complex bound

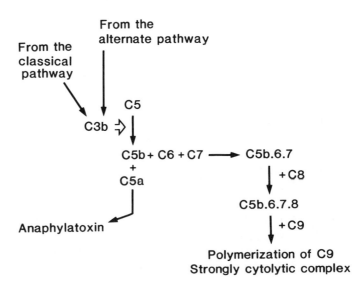

Figure 10–5. The terminal complement pathway.

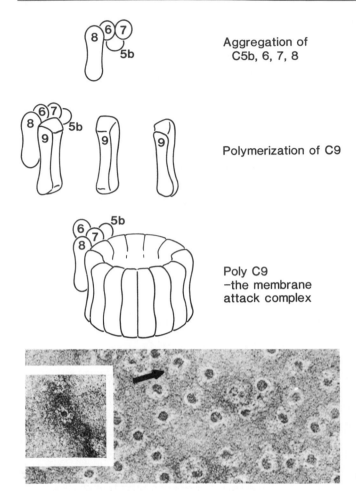

Aggregation of
C5b, 6, 7, 8

Polymerization of C9

Poly C9
−the membrane
attack complex

Figure 10–6. The formation of poly C9 by the terminal complement pathway and an electron micrograph of human poly C9-complement lesions on an erythrocyte membrane. The insert shows a mouse complement lesion. The arrow points to a possible C5b678 complex. Compare these lesions to the NK cell polyperforins in Figure 18–7. (From Podack ER and Dennert G. 1983. Nature *307* 442. Used with permission.)

to the cell surface. Thus, C3b acts on C5 to split it into C5a and C5b. A stable complex, C5b67, is then formed from the aggregation of C5b, C6 and C7. Then C8 can bind to this complex to form a structure with some membrane-damaging properties (it possibly activates cell membrane phospholipases). The C5b678 complex also provides the stimulus for polymerization of C9. When this happens, 12 to 15 C9 molecules bind together to form a tubular structure (Fig. 10–6). This tubular poly C9 can insert itself into cell membranes. It is believed that cell lysis occurs as a result of the escape of the cell contents through the central channel of poly C9. (It is also known, however, that small C9 polymers that do not form tubes are also lytic, so the mechanism of lysis remains unclear.) C9 is a member of a class of proteins known as perforins. Similar

perforins are probably involved in the destruction of target cells by cytolytic T cells and NK cells (see Fig. 18–7). These tubular polymerized complexes are called polyperforins.

Inhibitors of the Complement System (Table 10–1)

As might be expected, there exist a number of naturally occurring inhibitors of the complement pathways. One of the most important of these is the inactivator of C1. Normally, when C1 acts on C2 it splits off a small polypeptide with kinin-like activity. The amount of C2 kinin produced is controlled by the C1 inactivator. In individuals with a congenital deficiency of this inactivator (a condition known as hereditary angioedema), exces-

Table 10–1 COMPLEMENT REGULATORY
PROTEINS

Component	Action
Factor H	Splits C3bBb to C3b and Bb
Factor I	Splits C3b to inactive fragments
C4 binding protein	Accelerates decay of C42
C1 inactivator	Prevents production of C2 kinin
S protein	Enhances the attachment of C5b67 to membranes

sive amounts of C2 kinin are produced. The C2 kinin increases vascular permeability, and affected individuals therefore suffer from attacks of widespread edema. If this edema involves the larynx, it may close off the airway and cause the victim to suffocate.

Several different proteins act to regulate the activities of C42 and C3b. These include factor H and factor I, which normally ensure that the alternate pathway is regulated, and the C3 convertase of the classical pathway, C42, is regulated by a C4 binding protein. A protein called S enhances the attachment of C5b67 to membranes and thus reduces the possibility of nearby cells being damaged by free complexes. Several cell membrane proteins also block complement activity. It is assumed that this is a safety feature to protect cells against inappropriate lysis.

Genetics of the Complement System

C2 and C4 as well as factor B are coded for by class III genes in the MHC. Some of these proteins show allotypic variation. Thus, canine C4 is encoded at a single locus with at least five codominant alleles. The genes for the complement controlling proteins, factor H, C4 binding protein and the major cell membrane receptor for complement, CR1, are also linked in a gene cluster outside the MHC. The gene for C3 is on the same chromosome as the MHC but is not part of the complex.

BIOLOGICAL CONSEQUENCES OF COMPLEMENT ACTIVATION
(Fig. 10–7)

Cell Adherence

Many cells possess receptors for complement components. These receptors are called CR1, CR2 and so forth; the most important of these is CR1. CR1 is found on neutrophils, macrophages, platelets (not in primates) and B cells where it can bind C3b strongly and C4b weakly. Particles coated with C3b can there-

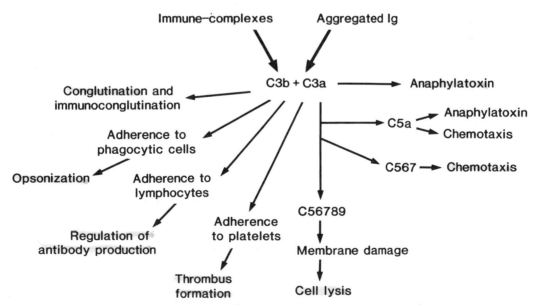

Figure 10–7. The biological consequences of complement activation.

fore bind to these cells in a process called immune adherence. The CR2 receptors are found on some B cells and neutrophils. They bind the breakdown products of C3. Monocytes, B cells, neutrophils and some null cells have a receptor for C1q, while B cells also have a receptor for factor H.

Opsonization

Because phagocytic cells possess both Fc and C3 receptors, they bind both antibody and complement-coated particles. If, for some reason, the particles cannot be ingested, then neutrophils may be induced to secrete their lysosomal enzymes into the surrounding tissues. These enzymes then cause tissue damage and activate C3 and C5. If complement coated particles bind to platelets, the platelets are induced to secrete the vasoactive amines, histamine and serotonin.

Immune Regulation

B cells but not T cells possess CR1 receptors. It is probable that these are involved in regulation of the immune response. Thus complement depletion can delay antibody responses, prevent the switch from IgG to IgM production and impair the development of germinal centers and immunological memory. Notwithstanding this, the actions of complement are complex since C3a is immunosuppressive, blocking the activities of helper T cells and cytotoxic T cells. In contrast, C5a stimulates the secretion of IL-1 and therefore enhances B cell and T cell proliferation as well as cytotoxic T cell activity.

Complement-Mediated Chemotaxis

When the complement cascades are activated, several potent chemotactic agents are generated. These include C5a, C5b67 and Bb. They do not have identical properties. Thus C5b67 is chemotactic only for neutrophils and eosinophils but C5a attracts these cells and macrophages and basophils as well. C5a rapidly loses

a terminal arginine *in vivo* to form C5a des arg (Chapter 19).

Complement and Blood Clotting

The complement system is closely linked to the clotting system (Fig. 10–8). For example, not only do complement-lysed cells activate the clotting cascade through Hageman factor, but C3b directly promotes thrombus formation by causing platelet aggregation. Because of this, extensive cell lysis or immune complex formation that occurs within the blood stream may provoke intravascular coagulation. This is commonly observed in acute graft rejection, in which destruction of graft vascular endothelium by complement can cause intravascular thrombosis and graft destruction. In hemolytic disease of newborn calves (Chapter 21), massive complement-mediated destruction of erythrocytes can provoke disseminated intravascular coagulation and death.

Complement-Mediated Inflammation

The major contribution of the complement system to the inflammatory process is attracting leukocytes to sites of complement activation. However, proteolytic enzymes such as plasminogen that are released from neutrophils or macrophages as they ingest particles can also activate C1 or C3 and thus enhance the process significantly. The anaphylatoxins C3a and C5a enhance inflammation by promoting the release of mast cell and platelet vasoactive factors. C3b-induced platelet aggregation also provides a source of inflammatory mediators.

Complement-Mediated Cell Clumping

When C3 is split into C3a and C3b, this exposes an epitope on the C3b that is not normally recognized as self by the body. The generation of C3b therefore results in the formation of autoantibodies against this newly

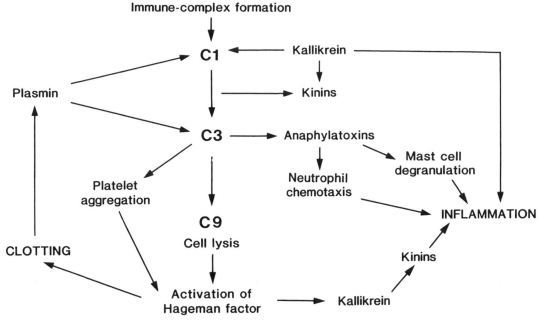

Figure 10–8. Some of the interactions between the complement, clotting, and inflammatory systems. In some ways they can be considered to be different manifestations of a single system.

formed epitope. These autoantibodies are known as immunoconglutinins (Chapter 24). Immunoconglutinins will clump any particles with fixed C3 on their surface and probably enhance their opsonization. In bovidae (i.e., cattle, buffalo, etc.) there also exists a serum protein known as conglutinin, which binds to one of the breakdown products of C3. Conglutinin can cause C3b-coated particles to clump (strictly speaking, conglutinate). The biological significance of conglutinin is not known.

COMPLEMENT DEFICIENCIES
(Table 10–2)

The effects of a congenital deficiency in individual complement components varies greatly. Thus, a deficiency in a component of the classical pathway may have little visible effect as a result of a compensatory increase in the activity of the alternate pathway and vice versa.

The most severe consequences occur in humans or animals deficient in C3. This is for two reasons. First, C3 is a vitally important opsonin and, second, because C3 is essential to the functioning of both the classical and alternate pathways. Brittany spaniels have been reported to have a congenital deficiency of C3 that is inherited as an autosomal recessive condition. Dogs that are homozygous for this deficiency have no detectable C3 (Fig. 10–9), whereas heterozygous animals have C3 levels that are approximately half of normal. The homozygous animals suffered from recurrent sepsis, pneumonia and local bacterial infections. The organisms involved included Clostridia, *E. coli*, and Klebsiella. Some af-

Table 10–2 SOME CONDITIONS IN WHICH COMPLEMENT LEVELS ARE REDUCED

Disease	Mechanism
Immune complex diseases (type III hypersensitivity)	Complexes bind complement
Gram-negative septicemia	Bacteria activate the alternative pathway
Congenital deficiencies	Failure of complement synthesis

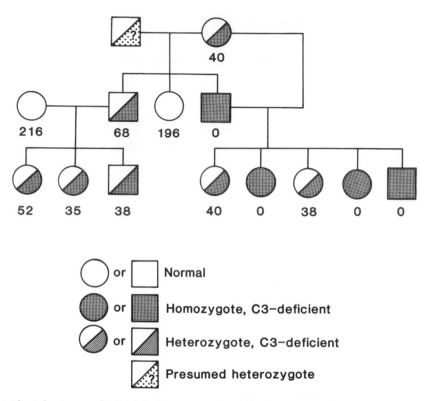

Figure 10–9. The inheritance of a C3 deficiency in a colony of Brittany spaniels. The number below each circle or square represents the animal's C3 level as a percentage of a standard reference serum. The mean level in healthy spaniels was 126. (From Winkelstein JA, Cork LC, Griffin DE, et al. 1981. Science *212* 1169–1170. Used with permission.)

fected dogs developed amyloidosis or glomerulonephritis. Heterozygous animals are clinically normal.

Some Finnish-Landrace lambs have a very low serum C3 level associated with the presence of a glomerulonephritis (Chapter 22). However, hybrids between this breed and Dorsets may also have low serum C3 and yet be quite healthy.

ANTIGEN-ANTIBODY INTERACTION AND MODULATION OF CELLULAR BEHAVIOR (Fig. 10–10, Table 10–3)

Many cells possess surface receptors specific for C3b or for immunoglobulin Fc regions (see Table 6–2). These receptors presumably function as a means of transmitting some form of signal to the cell. Thus, immune complexes binding to macrophages or neutrophils initiate changes in cellular activity, leading to phagocytosis of the inducing immune complexes. The precise mechanisms involved in the phagocytic process are not clear, but it appears that the immune complexes stimulate cell membrane activity. This increased activity may lead to complete enclosure of the complexes within the cell or, if the amount of cell-bound immune complex is small, serve to move the cell toward the complexes in a form of chemotaxis.

A second type of response seen following antigen-antibody–cell membrane interaction is degranulation, such as occurs in mast cells, platelets and, occasionally, neutrophils. For example, if antigen binds and "bridges" two mast cell–fixed IgE molecules, then intracellular enzymes are activated and cause the cell to release the contents of its granules into the extracellular fluid (Chapter 20). Platelets bound to immune complexes release not only

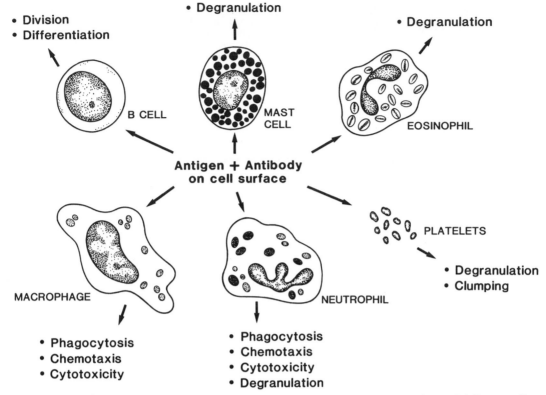

Figure 10–10. The results of the combination of antigen and antibody on the surfaces of different cells.

vasoactive factors but also procoagulants and adenosine diphosphate, which potentiates the reaction. On occasion, neutrophils respond to immune complexes by releasing the contents of their lysosomes into extracellular fluid.

A third form of response to antigen-antibody interaction is the generation of cytotoxic activity (Chapter 7). Cells that can participate in this process (ADCC) and destroy foreign (allogeneic) cells include macrophages, neutrophils and null lymphocytes. All these cells may exert their cytotoxicity regardless of whether they first bind to antibody-coated target cells or if they bind antibody first and then bind to antigens on target cell surfaces (see Table 6–5). A similar toxic effect may be mediated by eosinophils that bind to helminths, destroying them through IgG bound to the helminth surface (Chapter 17).

Most serum immunoglobulins cannot bind to cell Fc receptors unless they are first complexed with antigen. Nevertheless, some antibodies, known as cytophilic or cytotropic antibodies, may bind to Fc receptors even when uncomplexed. Examples of cytophilic antibodies include IgE antibodies, which are cytophilic for mast cells, and sheep IgG2, which is cytophilic for neutrophils and appears to act as a cell-bound opsonin, since it enhances the phagocytic ability of these cells.

Table 10–3 SOME OF THE CONSEQUENCES OF ANTIGEN-ANTIBODY INTERACTION ON CELL SURFACES

Cell Type	Consequence
Macrophage	Phagocytosis, chemotaxis, cytotoxicity
Neutrophil	Phagocytosis, chemotaxis, cytotoxicity, degranulation
Eosinophil	Degranulation, helminthicidal activity
Platelet	Degranulation, clumping
Mast cell	Degranulation
B lymphocyte	Differentiation and division
Null lymphocyte	Cytotoxicity

ADDITIONAL SOURCES OF INFORMATION

Chan AC, Karp DR, Shreffler DC and Atkinson JP. 1984. The 20 faces of the fourth component of complement. Immunol. Today *5* 200–203.

Colton HR. 1983. The complement genes. Immunol. Today *4* 151–153.

Day MJ, Kay PM, Clark WT, et al. 1985. Complement C4 allotype association with and serum C4 concentration in an autoimmune disease in a dog. Clin. Immunol. Immunopathol. *35* 85–91.

Fearon DT. 1984. Cellular receptors for fragments of the third component of complement. Immunol. Today *5* 105–110.

Fearon DT, and Austen KF. 1980. Current concepts in immunology. The alternative pathway of complement— A system for host resistance to microbial infection. N. Engl. J. Med. *303* 259–263.

Holers VM, Cole JL, Lublin DM, Seya T and Atkinson JP. 1985. Human C3b- and C4b- regulatory proteins: a new multi-gene family. Immunol. Today *6* 188–192.

Leid RW, Coley SC, Blanchard DP and Perryman LE. 1985. Equine alternative pathway activation by unsensitized rabbit red blood cells. Vet. Immunol. Immunopathol. *9* 71–85.

Menger M and Aston WP. 1985. Isolation and characterization of the third component of bovine complement. Vet. Immunol. Immunopathol. *10* 317–331.

Mueller R, Boothby JT, Carroll EJ and Panico L. 1983. Changes in complement values in calves during the first month of life. Am. J. Vet. Res. *44* 747–750.

Osler AG. 1976. Complement Mechanisms and Functions. Foundations of Immunology Series. Prentice-Hall, Inc., Englewood Cliffs, N.J.

Pangburn MK, Schrieber RD and Muller-Eberhard HJ. 1981. Formation of the initial C3 convertase of the alternative complement pathway. J. Exp. Med. *154* 856–867.

Podack ER, Esser AF, Biesecker G and Muller-Eberhard HJ. 1980. Membrane attack complex of complement. A. Structural analysis. J. Exp. Med. *151* 301–313.

Polley MJ and Nachman R. 1978. The human complement system in thrombin-mediated platelet function. J. Exp. Med. *147* 1713–1721.

Porter RR and Reid KBM. 1978. The biochemistry of complement. Nature *275* 699–704.

Winkelstein JA, Cork LC, Griffith DE, et al. 1981. Genetically determined deficiency of the third component of complement in the dog. Science *212* 1169–1170.

Winkelstein JA, Johnson JP, Swift AJ, et al. 1982. Genetically determined deficiency of the third component of complement of the dog: *in vitro* studies on the complement system and complement-mediated serum activities. J. Immunol. *129* 2598–2602.

II
SEROLOGY

11

Serology: The Detection and Measurement of Antibodies

The science of detection of specific antibodies in body fluids is known as serology. Serologic techniques fall into three broad categories (Table 11–1). The tests that are most sensitive in terms of the quantity of antibody detectable are the primary binding tests, which directly measure the binding of antigen to antibody. In contrast, secondary binding tests measure the results of antigen-antibody interaction *in vitro*. Theoretically, therefore, these tests are less sensitive than the primary binding tests, but they are usually simpler to perform. The results of antigen-antibody interactions include precipitation of soluble antigens, agglutination of particulate antigens and activation of the complement cascade. Tertiary binding tests measure the protective effect of antibodies in an animal. They, therefore, are indicative not only of the binding of antigen to antibody but also of the opsonizing ability of

Table 11–1 THE SMALLEST AMOUNT OF ANTIBODY PROTEIN DETECTABLE BY CERTAIN SELECTED IMMUNOLOGICAL TESTS

Tests	μg Protein/ml
Primary Binding Tests	
ELISA	0.0005
Competitive radioimmunoassay	0.00005
Secondary Binding Tests	
Ring test	18
Gel precipitation	30
Bacterial agglutination	0.05
Passive hemagglutination	0.01
Hemagglutination inhibition	0.005
Complement fixation test	0.05
Virus neutralization	0.00005
Bactericidal activity	0.00005
Antitoxin neutralization	0.06
Tertiary (In Vivo) Tests	
Passive cutaneous anaphylaxis	0.02

these complexes as well as the phagocytic and destructive abilities of the cells of the mono-nuclear-phagocytic system.

REAGENTS EMPLOYED IN SEROLOGIC TESTS

Serum

The most common source of antibody is serum obtained by allowing a blood sample to clot and the clot to retract. Serum may be stored frozen and used when desired. If necessary, the serum can be depleted of complement activity by heating to 56° C for 30 minutes.

Complement

Complement is a normal constituent of all fresh serum, but the complement in fresh, unheated guinea pig serum is the most efficient in hemolytic tests. Serum used as a source of complement for serologic applications should be stored frozen in small volumes and, once thawed, it should be used promptly. It should not be repeatedly frozen and thawed.

Antiglobulins

As described in Chapter 4, because immuno-globulins are complex proteins, they can function as antigens when injected into an animal

of a different species. For example, purified dog immunoglobulins can be injected into rabbits. The recipient animals respond by making specific antibodies known as antiglob-ulins. Depending on the purity of the injected immunoglobulin, it is possible to make non-specific antiglobulins against immunoglobulins of all isotypes or very specific antiglobulins directed against single isotypes (or even against specific allotypes or idiotypes) (Chapter 4). Antiglobulins are essential reagents in many immunological tests.

Monoclonal Antibodies

It is possible to fuse myeloma cells with normal plasma cells that are actively producing specific antibody. The resulting hybridomas can be selected so that they will combine the most desirable qualities of both parent cells and produce very large quantities of homogeneous, specific antibody when cultured. (For details see Chapter 6.) These hybridoma-derived monoclonal antibodies are pure and specific, can be used as standard chemical reagents and can be obtained in almost unlimited amounts. Monoclonal antibodies derived from hybridomas are frequently used to replace conventional antiserum in immunodiagnostic tests.

PRIMARY BINDING TESTS

Primary binding tests are performed by allowing antigen and antibody to combine and then measuring the amount of immune complex formed. It is usual to use radioisotope, fluorescent dye or enzyme labeling in order to identify one of the reactants. After allowing the reaction to proceed to equilibrium, the immune complexes are separated from the uncombined material, and the amount of label in the immune complexes is then determined.

Radioimmunoassays

Radioimmunoassays for Antibody

One widely employed primary binding test for antibody is called the RAST (Radioallergosorbent Test) (Fig 11–1). In this technique,

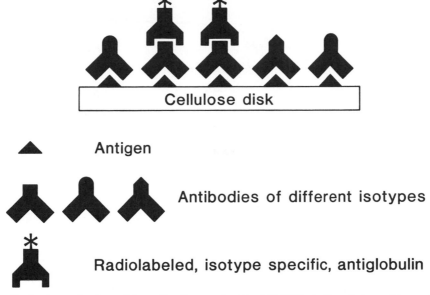

Figure 11–1. The basic mechanism of the radioallergosorbent test (RAST). Antigen is bound to a cellulose disk. When incubated in serum, antibodies to the antigen bind to the disk. These antibodies can be detected after incubation in a radiolabeled antiglobulin solution and washing.

antigen-impregnated cellulose discs are immersed in test serum so that specific antibody binds to the antigen. After washing, the disc is immersed in a solution containing radiolabeled antiglobulin.

The antiglobulin binds to the disc only if antibodies have first bound to the antigen. By determining the radioactivity associated with the disc it is possible to measure the level of antibody activity in the serum. If antiglobulins specific for a single immunoglobulin isotype are used, it is possible to determine the activity of antibodies of that isotype in a serum. The RAST is most commonly used to measure levels of specific IgE in allergic animals.

Radioimmunoassays for Antigen

Competitive immunoassays are widely employed to detect antigen. These are based on the principle that unlabeled antigen may displace radiolabeled antigen from immune complexes. The amount of labeled antigen displaced is directly related to the amount of unlabeled antigen added. Several different assays of this type have been developed. They differ in the way in which the antigen is labeled and measured. The most commonly used of these is the competitive radioimmunoassay in which antigen is labeled with an isotope such as tritium, carbon 14 or iodine 125. When radiolabeled antigen is mixed with its specific antibody, they combine to form immune complexes that may be precipitated out of solution with ammonium sulfate. The radioactivity of the supernatant fluid provides a measure of the amount of unbound antigen. If unlabeled antigen is added to the mixture of labeled antigen and unbound antibody, it will compete with the labeled antigen for antibody-binding sites. As a result, some labeled antigen will be unable to bind antibody, and the amount of radioactivity in the supernatant will be increased. If a standard curve is first constructed by using known amounts of unlabeled antigen, then the amount of antigen in a test sample may be measured by reference to this standard curve (Fig. 11–2).

This type of test is extremely sensitive and is commonly used for detecting trace amounts of drugs. For example, morphine may be measured in urine at concentrations of 10^{-8} to 10^{-10} M by means of a competitive radioimmunoassay.

Immunofluorescence Assays

Fluorescent dyes are also commonly employed as labels in primary binding tests; the most

Free radioactivity

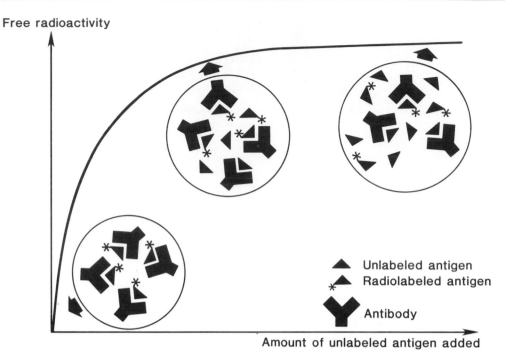

Amount of unlabeled antigen added

Figure 11–2. The principle of competitive radioimmunoassay. Unlabeled antigen will displace labeled antigen from immune complexes. The amount of labeled antigen released is proportional to the amount of unlabeled antigen added.

important is fluorescein isothiocyanate (FITC). FITC is a yellow compound that is readily conjugated to immunoglobulins without affecting their reactivity. When irradiated with invisible ultraviolet or blue light at 290 and 145 μm, it re-emits visible green light at about 525 μm. FITC-labeled immunoglobulins may be employed in a number of techniques, the most important of which are the direct and indirect fluorescent antibody tests (Table 11–2).

Direct Fluorescent Antibody Test
(Fig. 11–3)

The direct fluorescent antibody test is used to identify the presence of antigen. Antibody directed against a specific antigen such as a bacterium or virus may be labeled with FITC. A tissue or smear containing this organism may be fixed to a glass slide and incubated with a labeled antiserum and then washed to remove unbound antibody. If examined by

Table 11–2 COMPARISON OF TECHNIQUES INVOLVED IN DIRECT AND INDIRECT FLUORESCENT ANTIBODY TESTS

Test	Direct Fluorescent Antibody Test	Indirect Fluorescent Antibody Test
Requirements	Antigen? Fluorescent-labeled antibody	Antigen Fluorescent-labeled antiglobulin Antibody?
Method	1. Put FITC-labeled antibody onto suspected antigen preparation 2. Wash and examine	1. Put suspected antiserum onto known antigen preparation 2. Wash, then cover with FITC-labeled antiglobulin 3. Wash and examine
Detects	Fluorescence indicates presence of antigen	Fluorescence indicates presence of antibodies in serum

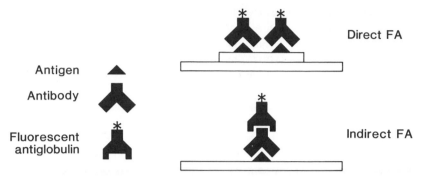

Figure 11–3. The direct and indirect fluorescent antibody assays. The direct test is used to detect antigen by means of FITC-labeled antibody. The indirect fluorescent antibody test may be used to detect either antigen or antibody. The antigen, in a section, smear or culture, will bind antibody from serum. After washing, this antibody may be detected by binding to FITC-labeled antiglobulin.

dark field illumination under a microscope with an ultraviolet light source, the antigenic particles that have bound the labeled antibody are seen to fluoresce brightly. This direct test can be used to identify bacteria when their numbers are very low. For example, it can be used when examining the feces of animals suspected of shedding *Mycobacterium paratuberculosis* or when examining smears from lesions for the presence of *Fusobacterium necrophorum*, *Listeria monocytogenes* or the clostridial organisms (Fig. 11–4). It may also be employed to detect viruses growing in tissue culture or in tissues from infected animals. It is thus possible to detect rabies virus in the brains of infected animals and antigens of the feline leukemia virus on the surface of infected cells by means of this technique (see Fig. 16–8).

Indirect Fluorescent Antibody Test (IFA)
(see Fig. 11–3)

The indirect fluorescent antibody test may be used for the detection of antibodies in serum or for the demonstration and identification of antigens in tissues or cell cultures. When testing for antibody, antigen is employed as a

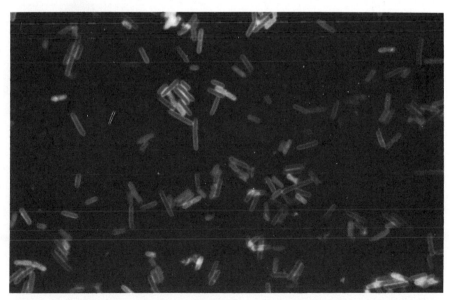

Figure 11–4. Direct immunofluorescence of a smear of *Clostridium chauveoi*. (Courtesy of Dr. C. L. Gyles.) (See also Figs. 16–8 and 25–6.)

tissue smear, section or cell culture on a slide or coverslip. This is incubated in a serum suspected of containing antibodies to that antigen, and the serum is then washed off, leaving only specific antibodies bound to the antigen.

These bound antibodies may be visualized after incubating the smear in FITC-labeled antiglobulin serum. When the antiglobulin is removed by washing and the slide examined, fluorescence indicates that antibody was present in the test serum. The quantity of antibody in the test serum may be estimated by examining increasing dilutions of serum on a number of different antigen preparations.

The indirect fluorescent antibody test has a number of advantages over the direct technique. Since each antibody molecule binding to antigen will itself bind several labeled antiglobulin molecules, fluorescence will be considerably brighter than in the direct test. Similarly, by using antiglobulin sera specific for each immunoglobulin isotype, the isotype of the specific antibody present in the serum may also be determined. All tests of this nature must be accompanied by the use of appropriate controls.

Immunoenzyme Assays

The most important of these techniques are the enzyme-linked immunosorbent assays (ELISAs). As with other primary binding tests they may be used to detect and quantitate either antibody or antigen.

ELISA Tests

In the indirect ELISA for antibody, wells in polystyrene plates are first filled with the antigen solution. Protein antigens bind firmly to polystyrene so after unbound antigen is removed by vigorous washing, the wells remain coated with antigen. The coated plates can be stored until required. The serum being tested is added to the wells so that specific antibodies in the serum may bind to the antigen on the well wall (Fig. 11–5). After incubation and washing to remove unbound

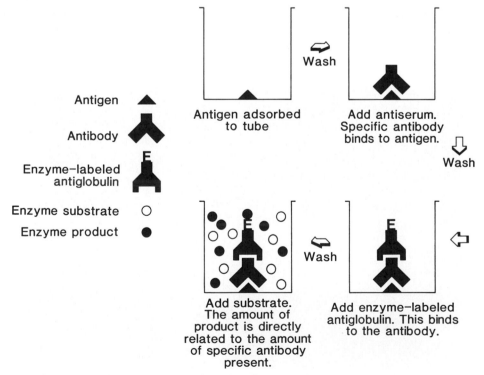

figure 11–5. The ELISA technique. Antigen is bound to the walls of a polystyrene tube or wells in polystyrene plates. The presence of bound antibody is detected by means of an enzyme-labeled antiglobulin.

antibody, the presence of bound antibodies is detected by addition of an antiglobulin chemically linked to an enzyme. This complex binds to the antibody and, following incubation and washing, may be detected and measured by addition of the enzyme substrate. The enzyme and substrate are selected so that a colored product develops in each well. The intensity of the color that develops is proportional to the amount of enzyme-linked antiglobulin that is bound, which, in turn, is proportional to the amount of antibody present in the serum being tested. The color intensity may be estimated visually or, preferably, determined spectrophotometrically.

A modification of this technique that is used to detect antigen involves first coating polystyrene wells with specific antibody. The antigen solution is then added, followed, after washing, by specific antibody, enzyme-labeled antiglobulin and substrate, as described for the indirect technique. In this test, the intensity of the color reaction is related directly to the amount of bound antigen. Tests of this type are used to detect circulating virus in cats with feline leukemia.

Because of its simplicity, the indirect ELISA has been widely used for the immunodiagnosis of many bacterial, viral and parasitic infections.

Immunoperoxidase Techniques

Enzymes conjugated to immunoglobulins or antiglobulins may also be used to identify specific antigens in tissue sections. Horseradish peroxidase is the most widely employed label. The tests are performed in a manner similar to that for the immunofluorescence tests. Thus, in the direct immunoperoxidase test, the tissue section is treated with the

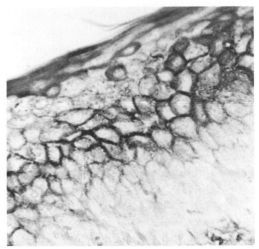

Figure 11–6. A section of dog skin stained by the immunoperoxidase technique. The dog suffered from an autoimmune disease called pemphigus foliaceus in which antibodies bind to the skin intercellular cement. The immunoperoxidase reveals these antibodies as a dark deposit between the cells. (Courtesy of Dr. G. Elissalde.) Compare this with Figure 25–6, which shows a similar lesion stained by immunofluorescence.

enzyme-labeled antibody. After washing, the tissue is then incubated in the appropriate enzyme substrate. Bound antibody is detected by the presence of a brown deposit at the site of antibody binding (Fig. 11–6). In the indirect test, bound antibody is detected by means of a labeled antiglobulin. This technique has very significant advantages over the immunofluorescence techniques in that the tissue can be examined by conventional light microscopy and the tissue can be stained so that structural relationships are easier to see.

A very successful variant is the peroxidase antiperoxidase technique (Fig. 11–7). This is a three-step method. First, the tissue sections are coated with a rabbit antibody to the tissue antigen. Second, they are treated with an

Figure 11–7. The peroxidase-antiperoxidase technique. Bound antibody is detected by the binding of peroxidase-antiperoxidase immune complexes through an antiglobulin.

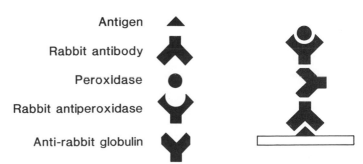

Antigen

Rabbit antibody

Peroxidase

Rabbit antiperoxidase

Anti-rabbit globulin

antigen. Second, they are treated with an antirabbit globulin. Finally, they are treated with an immune complex consisting of rabbit antiperoxidase bound to peroxidase. These immune complexes bind to free binding sites on the antiglobulin and can then be detected using the appropriate substrate.

Enzyme Labels. Although about 20 different enzymes have been used in enzyme immunoassays, the most popular choices include alkaline phosphatase, horseradish peroxidase and β-galactosidase. These enzymes are inexpensive and readily assayed. Recently, it has been demonstrated that enzyme assays involving the production of luminescent or fluorescent products, for example luciferase, may be many times more sensitive than conventional enzyme assays. The disadvantage of labels of this type is that they require sophisticated instruments to detect and measure the luminescence produced.

Western Blotting

One solution to the problem of identifying protein antigens in a complex mixture is to use a technique known as western blotting (Fig. 11–8). This is a three-stage primary binding test. Stage 1 involves electrophoresis of the protein mixture on gels so that each component is resolved into a single band. Stage 2 is the blotting or transfer of this protein from the gel to an immobilizing paper. This is accomplished by placing a nitrocellulose membrane on top of the gel and sandwiching the two between sponges saturated with buffer. The sandwich is supported between rigid plastic sheets placed in a buffer reservoir, and an electrical current is passed between the sponges. The protein bands are rapidly transferred from the gel to the nitrocellulose membrane without loss of resolution.

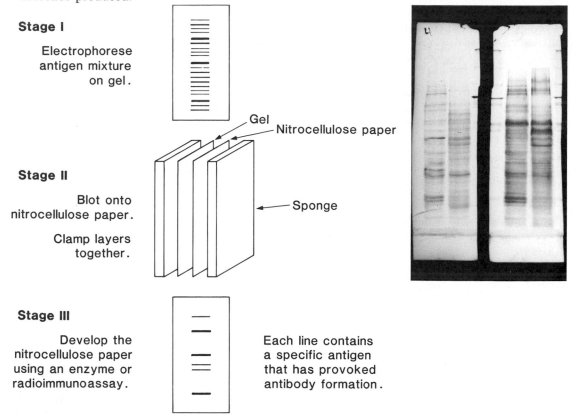

Stage I

Electrophorese antigen mixture on gel.

Gel
Nitrocellulose paper

Stage II

Blot onto nitrocellulose paper.

Clamp layers together.

Sponge

Stage III

Develop the nitrocellulose paper using an enzyme or radioimmunoassay.

Each line contains a specific antigen that has provoked antibody formation.

Figure 11–8. The Western blotting technique. Serum is separated by electrophoresis on gel, blotted onto nitrocellulose paper and the antigen bands are revealed by use of specific antibody and an enzyme- or isotope-labeled antiglobulin. The blotting stage may be a passive transfer or, alternatively, an electric potential may be used to accelerate the process. The photograph shows the results of electrophoresing two extracts of the liver fluke (*Fasciola hepatica*). The blot was then exposed to normal (left) and hyperimmune (right) bovine serum. Each dark band represents an antigen recognized by the bovine serum. (Courtesy of Dr. C. Hicks.)

SEROLOGY: THE DETECTION AND MEASUREMENT OF ANTIBODIES **137**

The third stage involves visualization of transferred antigens by means of an enzyme immunoassay or radioimmunoassay. When an enzyme immunoassay is employed, the membrane is first incubated in specific antiserum. After washing, an enzyme-labeled antiglobulin solution is added. When this is removed by washing, substrate is added, and color develops in the bands in which antibody is bound to antigen. When isotope-labeled antiglobulin is used, an autoradiograph must be made and the labeled band identified by darkening of a photographic emulsion.

Avidin-Biotin Immunoassay

Although radioisotopes and enzymes have commonly been used as labels for primary binding tests, each possesses certain disadvantages. For example, isotopes may have a short half-life, are potentially hazardous and may require expensive detection devices. Enzymes, although stable and relatively cheap, are large molecules that may inhibit antibody activity or lose enzymic activity in the process of conjugating them to antiglobulin.

One alternative to the use of enzymes and radioisotopes as labels is to use the small molecule biotin and its specific binding protein, avidin. Biotin has a molecular weight of only 244 daltons and can be very easily and gently bound to proteins without affecting their biological activity. Avidin is a small protein found in egg white that binds very strongly and specifically to biotin. Avidin may be conjugated with an enzyme such as horseradish peroxidase. This avidin-peroxidase complex will rapidly and specifically bind to biotin-labeled proteins and thus form a very effective and sensitive label.

Other Labels Used in Primary Binding Tests

Several other labels have been used as alternatives to radioisotopes, enzymes or fluorescent dyes in primary binding tests. For example, reagents linked to the iron-containing protein ferritin may be used to identify the location of antigens on cell surfaces examined by electron microscopy. The ferritin molecule

is a protein of 700,000 daltons, containing 23 per cent iron as ferric hydroxide or phosphate. The iron is concentrated within the molecule, and on electron microscopy can be detected as a characteristic electron-dense spot. Therefore, if ferritin is linked to an immunoglobulin, the location of antigen may be readily observed on electron micrographs.

SECONDARY BINDING TESTS

Secondary binding tests are two-stage processes. The first stage is the interaction between antigen and antibody, a reaction that is associated with the development of noncovalent bonds. As a result it may be reversed in solutions of high ionic strength or low pH. The second stage is determined by the physical state of the antigen. Thus, if antibodies combine with soluble antigens in solution under appropriate conditions, the complexes precipitate. If the antigens are particulate (e.g., bacteria or erythrocytes), then they agglutinate (clump). Under other circumstances, the combination of antigen and antibody may lead to activation of the complement system, which can also be detected and measured.

Precipitation

If a suitable amount of a clear solution of soluble antigen is mixed with antiserum and incubated at 37° C, the mixture becomes cloudy within a few minutes, then flocculent and finally a precipitate settles to the bottom of the tube within an hour or so. If increasing amounts of soluble antigen are mixed with a constant amount of antibody, the amount of precipitate that results is determined by the relative proportions of the reactants. No obvious precipitate is formed at low antigen concentrations. As the amount of antigen increases, larger quantities of precipitate result, until the amount is maximal. With the addition of more antigen, the amount of precipitate gradually diminishes, until none is observed in tubes containing a large excess of antigen (Fig. 11–9). Horse antibodies behave in a somewhat different fashion in precipitin tests,

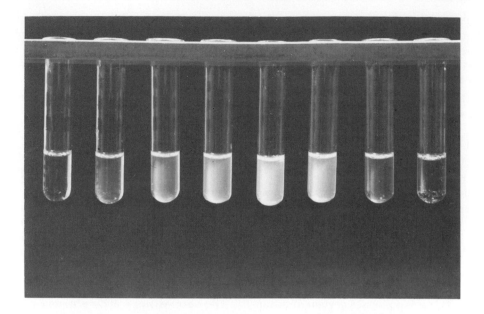

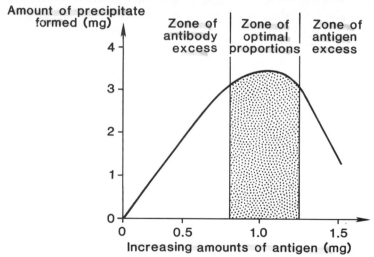

Figure 11–9. The effect of mixing increasing amounts of antigen (bovine serum) with a constant amount of antibody (rabbit antiserum). The tube with the greatest amount of precipitate is the one in which the ratio of antigen to antibody is in optimal proportions. A quantitative precipitation curve of the test shows this effect graphically.

producing a distinct flocculation over a very narrow range of antigen concentrations. This is a particular property of the IgG(T) subisotype (Fig. 11–10).

In the first stage of these reactions, only a little antigen is complexed to antibody, and little precipitate is deposited. Since antibody is in excess, free antibody may be found in the supernatant fluid. In the tubes in which the most precipitation occurs, both antigen and antibody are completely complexed and

neither can be detected in the supernatant fluid. This is known as the equivalence zone, and the ratio of antibody to antigen is here said to be in optimal proportions. When antigen is added to excess, then little precipitate is formed, although soluble immune complexes are present and free antigen may be detected in the supernatant fluid.

These results may be explained by the fact that antibodies are usually bivalent and are, therefore, able to cross-link only two epitopes

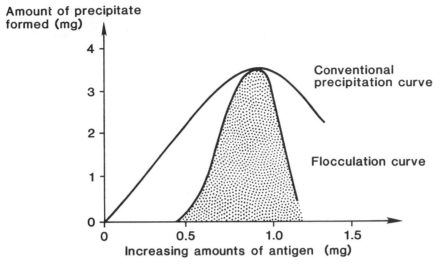

Figure 11–10. A quantitative precipitation curve of the type obtained when horse serum is used as a source of antibody. Flocculation occurs only over a narrow range of antigen-antibody mixtures.

at a time, but complex antigens are generally multivalent, possessing a relatively large number of epitopes. In the mixtures containing excess antibody, each antigen molecule is covered with antibody, preventing cross-linkage and thus precipitation. When the reactants are in optimal proportions, the ratio of antigen to antibody is such that extensive cross-linking and lattice formation occur. As this lattice grows in size it becomes insoluble and eventually precipitates (Fig. 11–11). In mixtures in which antigen is in excess, each antibody molecule is bound to a pair of antigen molecules. Further cross-linkage is impossible in this case, and since these complexes are small and soluble, no precipitation occurs. The cells of the mononuclear-phagocytic system are most efficient at binding and removing complexes formed at optimal proportions and in antibody excess. Small immune complexes formed in antigen excess are poorly removed by phagocytic cells but are deposited within vessel walls and in glomeruli, where they contribute to an acute inflammatory response classified as a type III hypersensitivity reaction (Chapter 22).

Laser Nephelometry. Nephelometry is the measurement of light scattering by particles in suspension. If optically clear solutions of antigen and antibody are mixed, the resulting precipitate will make the mixture appear cloudy. By shining the beam of a helium-neon laser through the solution, the quantity of immune complexes formed can be accurately measured. This method can be used in diagnostic tests for the very rapid assay of antibodies.

Immunodiffusion

If antigen and antibody solutions are layered one on top of the other in a tube without mixing, the components will diffuse into each other. Where the ratio of the reagents is in optimal proportions, a band of precipitate forms. A technique such as this, sometimes called an Ascoli test or a "ring" test, has been used to detect anthrax bacilli in hides. Antiserum against *Bacillus anthracis* is allowed to react in a capillary tube with an extract of hide suspected of being derived from an infected animal. A line of precipitate at the interface of the two fluids constitutes a positive reaction. Unfortunately, this technique requires a certain steadiness of hand, and the result is easily obscured if the two solutions are inadvertently mixed. The reaction, however, can be stabilized by conducting the test in gels.

A simple precipitation technique is to cut round wells 5 mm in diameter and about 1 cm apart in a layer of agar in a Petri dish. One well is then filled with soluble antigen, the

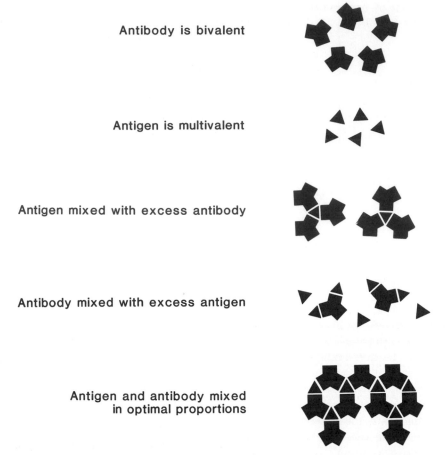

Antibody is bivalent

Antigen is multivalent

Antigen mixed with excess antibody

Antibody mixed with excess antigen

Antigen and antibody mixed
in optimal proportions

Figure 11–11. The mechanism of precipitation. In both antigen- and antibody-excess small, soluble immune complexes are produced. At optimal proportions, however, large insoluble complexes are generated.

other with antiserum; the reactants will diffuse radially. A circular concentration gradient is therefore established for each reactant, and these eventually overlap. Thus, optimal proportions for the occurrence of precipitation will occur in one zone of the superimposed gradients, and an opaque white line of precip-

itate will appear in this region (Fig. 11–12). This technique is known as the double diffusion test or the Ouchterlony technique after its inventor.

If the solutions used contain several different antigens and antibodies, each component is unlikely to reach optimal proportions in

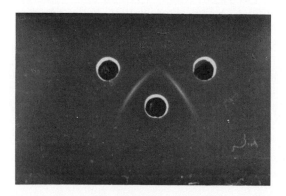

Figure 11–12. Precipitation in agar gel. Antigen and antibody, diffusing from their respective wells, precipitate in a region where optimal proportions are achieved. In this example the bottom well contains antibody. The antigen is identical in both of the top wells and, as a result, the precipitation lines fuse to show complete identity.

exactly the same position. Consequently, a separate line of precipitate is produced for each interacting set of antigens and antibodies present. This test may also be used to determine the relationship between antigens. If two antigen wells and one antibody well are set up as shown in Figures 11–12 and 11–13, then lines will form between each antigen well and the antibody well. If these two lines are confluent, then the two antigens are considered to be identical. If the lines cross over, then the two antigens are different, whereas if the lines merge with spur formation, then a partial identity exists, indicating that one antigen possesses epitopes not present in the other. The double diffusion technique may be used to identify the presence of either soluble antigen or antibodies in body fluids; for example, the Coggin's test is a double diffusion method for detecting the presence of antibodies against equine infectious anemia virus in horses. In this test an extract of infected horse spleen or a cell culture antigen is reacted with the serum of the horse being tested in agar gel, and the occurrence of a line of precipitate constitutes a positive reaction. A similar test may be employed to identify cattle infected with bovine leukemia virus. The antigen in this case is semipurified viral glycoprotein.

Radial Immunodiffusion (Fig. 11–14). If antigen is allowed to diffuse into agar in which specific antiserum is incorporated, then a ring of precipitate indicating the zone of optimal proportions will form around the well. The area of this ring is directly related to the amount of antigen added to the well. If the technique is first standardized using known amounts of antigen, then a standard curve may be constructed and unknown solutions of antigen accurately assayed. This technique is used to measure immunoglobulin levels in serum. A reversed radial immunodiffusion test employing antigen-impregnated agar has been used with success for the measurement of antibodies to *Mycoplasma mycoides* and some other organisms.

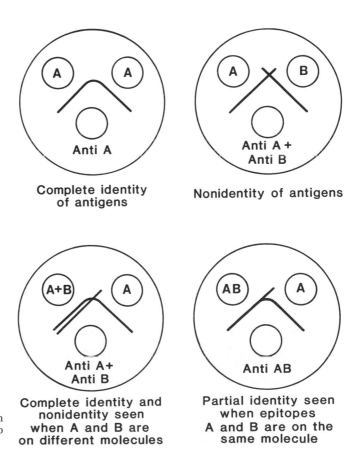

Figure 11–13. The use of the gel-diffusion technique in determining the relationship between two antigens.

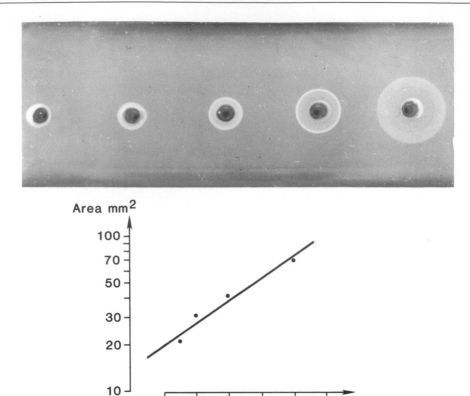

Figure 11–14. Radial immunodiffusion. In this case antiserum to bovine IgA is incorporated in the agar and is used to measure bovine serum IgA levels.

Immunoelectrophoresis and Related Techniques

Although double diffusion techniques give a separate precipitation line for each antigen-antibody system in a mixture, it is often difficult to resolve all the components in a complex mixture. One technique that may be used to improve the resolution of the system is to separate the antigen mixture by electrophoresis prior to undertaking immunodiffusion. This technique is known as immunoelectrophoresis and is commonly employed to identify proteins in body fluids. Immunoelectrophoresis involves the electrophoresis of the antigen mixture in agar gel in one direction. A trough is then cut in the agar just to one side and parallel to this line of separated proteins. Antiserum is placed in this trough and allowed to diffuse laterally. When the diffusing antibodies encounter antigen, curved lines of precipitate are formed. One arc of precipitation forms for each of the constituents

in the antigen mixture (Fig. 11–15). This technique can be used to resolve the proteins of normal serum into between 25 and 40 distinct precipitation bands. The exact number depends upon the strength and specificity of the antiserum employed (Fig. 11–16). By means of this technique it is possible to detect the absence of a normal serum protein such as occurs in animals with a congenital deficiency of some complement components. It is also possible to detect the presence of excessive amounts of an individual component, as is found in animals with a myeloma (Chapter 26).

If instead of permitting antigen to diffuse into agar-containing antiserum as in the radial immunodiffusion technique, the antigen is driven into the antiserum agar by electrophoresis, then the ring of precipitate around each well becomes deformed into a rocket shape. The length of each rocket is proportional to the amount of antigen placed in each well. This technique, known as electroimmunodif-

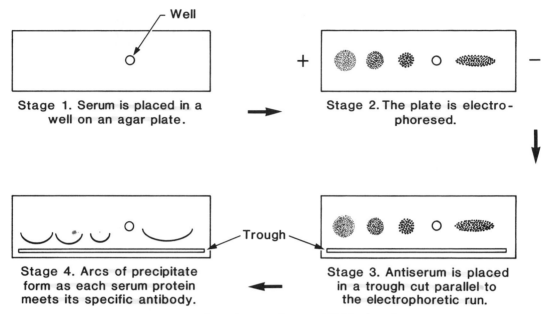

Stage 1. Serum is placed in a well on an agar plate.

Stage 2. The plate is electrophoresed.

Stage 4. Arcs of precipitate form as each serum protein meets its specific antibody.

Stage 3. Antiserum is placed in a trough cut parallel to the electrophoretic run.

Figure 11–15. The technique of immunoelectrophoresis.

fusion or rocket electrophoresis, may be employed to quantitate antigen (Fig. 11–17).

When electrophoresed in agar gel, some antibodies move toward the cathode because of a flow of buffer through the agar in that direction. This phenomenon is called electroendosmosis. If an antigen is strongly negatively charged so that it moves toward the anode in spite of this flow, then it is possible to drive antigen and antibody together by electrophoresis by suitably arranging the wells in an agar plate. A line of precipitate may be produced in this way within a few minutes. This technique is known as counter immunoelectrophoresis and may be used for the rapid identification of bacteria and mycoplasma and for the diagnosis of viral diseases such as

Aleutian disease of mink (Fig. 11–18). In this case, solutions containing the Aleutian disease agent and antibody are electrophoresed in such a way that they are driven together. The development of a line of precipitate within 30 to 40 minutes indicates the presence of antibodies in the test serum and suggests that the mink is infected. By using large sheets of agar it is possible to test large numbers of sera within a few minutes.

TITRATION OF ANTIBODIES

Although the detection of antibodies or antigen is sufficient for many tests, it is usually desirable to arrive at some estimate of the

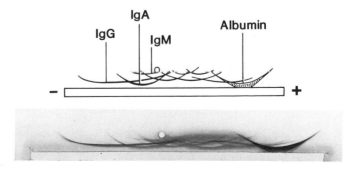

Figure 11–16. Immunoelectrophoresis of pig serum, showing the lines of precipitation produced by some of the major serum proteins. (See also Fig. 26–7.)

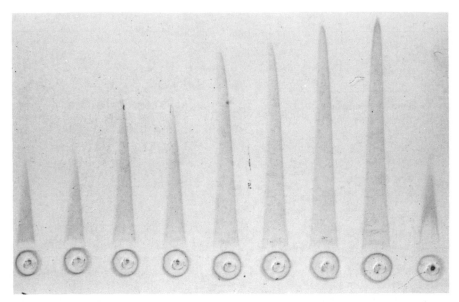

Figure 11–17. Electroimmunodiffusion. In this example, lactoferrin from bovine milk is measured. The height of each "rocket" is proportional to the amount of antigen placed in the wells at the bottom. (Courtesy of Dr. R. Harmon.)

amount of reactants present. In the case of tests designed to detect the presence of specific antibody, this estimation is often accomplished by titration. Titration is a procedure in which the serum being tested is diluted in a series of decreasing concentrations in a set of tubes (Fig. 11–19). The solution in each tube is then tested for activity in the test system. The reciprocal of the highest dilution giving a positive reaction is known as the titer,

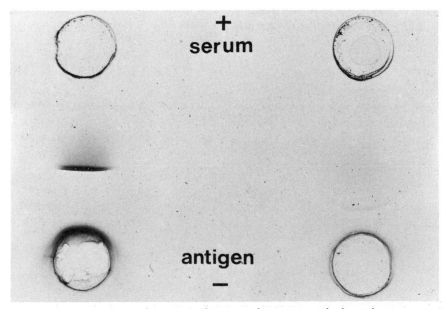

Figure 11–18. Counter-immunoelectrophoresis. In this example, serum antibody to the Aleutian disease virus is detected by its reaction with a preparation of viral antigen. *Left*, a positive reaction; *right*, a negative reaction. (Courtesy of Dr. S. H. An.)

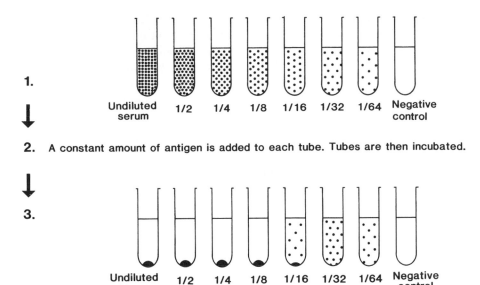

Figure 11–19. The principle of antibody titration. Serum is first diluted in a series of tubes. A constant amount of antigen is then added to each tube, and the tubes are incubated. At the end of the incubation period, the last tube in which a reaction has occurred is identified. In this example, agglutination has occurred in all tubes up to a serum dilution of 1/16. The agglutination titer of the serum is said to be 1/16.

or titre (depending on geographical location), and provides an estimate of the amount of antibody in that serum.

Agglutination

Antibodies can cross-link particulate antigens, resulting in their clumping or agglutination. Agglutination may be produced by mixing a suspension of antigenic particles, such as bacteria, with antiserum. Antibody combines rapidly with the particles—the primary interaction—but agglutination is a much slower process, since adherence between particles occurs only when they touch each other. Normally, these suspensions are stable, their particles prevented from clumping by a negative charge or "zeta potential" on their surface. However, immunoglobulins are positively charged and, on coating the particles, they neutralize this zeta potential. As a result, the particles can approach closely and agglutination may occur.

Antibodies differ in their ability to promote agglutination. IgM antibodies are considerably more efficient agglutinators than IgG antibodies (Table 11–3). If excessive antibody is added to a suspension of antigenic particles, then, just as in the precipitation reaction, it is pos-

Table 11–3 ROLE OF SPECIFIC IMMUNOGLOBULINS IN DIAGNOSTIC TESTS

Property*	IgG	IgM	IgA	IgG(T)
Agglutinating	+	+ + +	+	−
Complement-fixing (heterologous guinea pig complement)	+	+ + +	−	−
Precipitating	+ + +	+	±	±
Neutralizing	+	+ +	+	+
Time of appearance after exposure to antigen	3–7 days	2–5 days	3–7 days	3–7 days
Time to reach peak liter	7–21 days	5–14 days	7–21 days	7–21 days

*The properties listed may vary somewhat between species.

sible for each particle to be so coated by antibody that agglutination is inhibited. This lack of reactivity seen at high concentrations of antibody is termed a prozone. Another cause of prozone formation is the presence of antibodies that do not cause agglutination even when bound to the particles. These nonagglutinating antibodies are known as incomplete antibodies. The reason for their lack of agglutinating activity is not completely understood; one possible reason is that the epitopes with which they react lie deep within the surface coat of the particle, so deep that cross-linking cannot occur. An alternative suggestion is that they are capable of only restricted movement in their hinge region (Chapter 4), causing them to be functionally monovalent.

Antiglobulin Tests

If it is necessary to test for the presence of incomplete antibodies on the surface of particles such as bacteria or erythrocytes, a direct antiglobulin test may be used (Fig. 11–20). The washed particles are mixed with an antiglobulin serum, and if incomplete antibodies are present, agglutination will occur. In order to test for the presence of incomplete antibodies in a serum, an indirect antiglobulin test is used. In this technique, the serum being tested is first incubated with antigen particles

that bind the incomplete antibodies. After washing to remove unbound antibody, the coated particles are mixed with an antiglobulin serum. On reacting with bound antibody, the antiglobulin will cross-link the particles and cause agglutination.

Passive Agglutination

Since agglutination is a much more sensitive technique than precipitation, it is sometimes considered desirable to convert a precipitating system to an agglutinating one. One way this may be done is by chemically linking soluble antigen to inert particles such as erythrocytes, bacteria or latex, so that specific antibody will make the coated particles agglutinate. Erythrocytes are among the best carrier particles for this purpose, and tests that employ coated erythrocytes are called passive hemagglutination tests. Some antigens such as the lipopolysaccharides from gram-negative bacteria, adsorb naturally to erythrocytes. This can be useful in establishing a hemagglutination test for antibodies to lipopolysaccharide. Unfortunately, these lipopolysaccharides are also adsorbed to erythrocytes *in vivo* so that the erythrocytes are destroyed by the antibacterial immune response; as a result, anemia is a feature of many diseases caused by gram-negative organisms (Chapter 15).

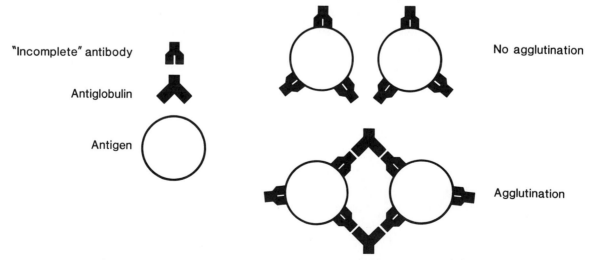

"Incomplete" antibody

Antiglobulin

Antigen

No agglutination

Agglutination

Figure 11–20. The direct antiglobulin test. The presence of the antiglobulin is required to agglutinate particles coated with "incomplete" antibody.

Complement Fixation Tests

As discussed in Chapter 10, the activation of the classical complement system by immune complexes results in the generation of factors capable of disrupting cell membranes. If the immune complexes are generated on erythrocyte surfaces, then the erythrocyte membranes are disrupted and hemolysis occurs. It is possible to use this reaction to measure serum antibody levels. The test is called the complement fixation test (CFT). The CFT is one of the most widely applicable serologic techniques. Once the required reagents are prepared and standardized, the CFT may be used to detect many immune interactions. The end point is very easily read and, unlike the hemagglutination tests, does not depend upon the settling of the erythrocytes and is less affected by prozones. In addition, this test does not depend upon the availability of pur-

ified suspensions of antigens and is therefore commonly used in the diagnosis of viral diseases. The most significant disadvantage of this test is its complexity, particularly with regard to the standardization and preparation of the required reagents.

The hemolytic complement fixation test is performed in two parts (Fig. 11–21). First, antigen and the serum being tested (deprived of its complement by heating at 56° C) are mixed and incubated in the presence of normal guinea pig serum, which provides a source of complement. (Guinea pig serum is most commonly used because its complement lyses sheep erythrocytes well.) After allowing the antigen-antibody-complement mixture to react for a short period, the amount of free complement remaining in the mixture is measured by adding an indicator system, consisting of antibody-coated sheep erythrocytes. Lysis of these erythrocytes (seen as the development

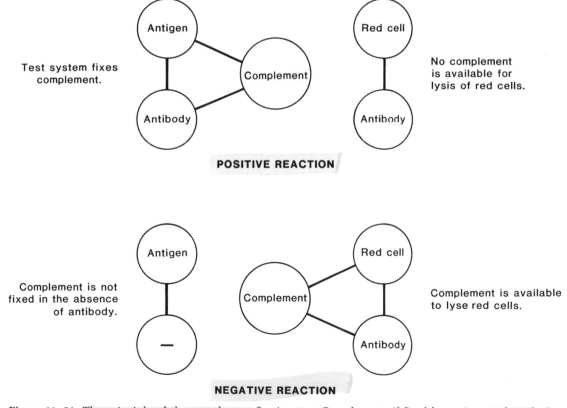

Figure 11–21. The principle of the complement fixation test. Complement, if fixed by antigen and antibody, will be unavailable to lyse the target cells in the indicator system. In the absence of antibody, the complement will remain unfixed and will be available to lyse the indicator system. (Modified from Roitt I. (1974) Essential Immunology, 2nd ed. Blackwell Scientific Publications, Oxford.)

of a transparent red solution) is a negative result, since it indicates that complement was not fixed and that antibody was therefore absent from the test serum. Absence of lysis (seen as a cloudy red cell suspension) is a positive result. It is usual to titrate the serum being tested so that if antibodies are present, as the serum is diluted the reaction in each tube will change from no lysis (i.e., positive) to lysis (i.e., negative). The titer may be considered to be the highest dilution of serum in which no more than 50 per cent of the red cells are lysed.

Before a hemolytic complement fixation test is performed, all reagents, antigen, complement, sheep erythrocytes and antibody against the erythrocytes (hemolysin) must be carefully standardized. The hemolysin should be heated at 56° C for 30 minutes in order to destroy its complement. Addition of the correct amount of complement is critical, since too little complement results in incomplete lysis, whereas excessive complement may not be completely fixed by immune complexes and may lead to false-negative results. Excessive antigen interferes with complement fixation, whereas insufficient antigen may fail to fix complement in demonstrable amounts.

Anticomplementary Effects

One problem commonly encountered when performing complement fixation tests is the presence of anticomplementary activity in the serum being tested. That is, the test serum appears to fix complement in the absence of antigen. There are several possible reasons for this. In serum taken from infected animals, any immune complexes present will effectively bind some complement. Similarly, the presence of bacterial contaminants in serum may activate complement through the alternate pathway. For these reasons the CFT must be accompanied by the use of a complete series of controls.

Pig serum has the curious property of possessing procomplementary activity—that is, it accentuates the hemolytic activity of the added complement. As a result, it is difficult to perform complement fixation tests on pig serum.

Modifications of Complement Fixation Tests

Various modifications of the CFT have been devised to overcome some of its limitations. For example, avian antibodies cannot fix mammalian complement. This disadvantage may be overcome either by using avian complement or, alternatively, by adding to the usual CF test system a complement-fixing indicator antibody against the antigen (Fig. 11–22). If the test serum is from an infected bird (i.e., contains antibodies), then on mixing with antigen, immune complex formation will occur. As a result, when indicator antibody and complement are subsequently added they will not be fixed. Addition of a second indicator system consisting of antibody-coated sheep erythrocytes consequently results in lysis. If, on the other hand, the test serum is negative, then the antigen remains free to bind to the indicator antibody and fix complement; as a result, the indicator system does not lyse. As can be imagined, because of its complexity this is not a widely employed test.

Some complement, such as that from the horse, is not hemolytic. The fixation of this type of complement, however, can be measured by estimating its ability to clump erythrocytes in the presence of immunoconglutinin. Immunoconglutinin is a natural autoantibody directed against epitopes on fixed C3 (Chapter 10). The test is performed in the same way as the hemolytic complement fixation test except that the indicator system contains a source of immunoconglutinin in addition to antibody-coated erythrocytes. The test is read by measuring immunoconglutination, a very strong agglutination, not hemolysis. This test has been used for the diagnosis of glanders in horses.

Complement fixation tests may also be modified by supplementing the guinea pig complement with homologous complement. Tests of this type have been employed successfully in detecting antibodies to vesicular stomatitis, bluetongue and other viruses in bovine and swine sera. The mechanism of this test is in some doubt, but it is possible that homologous C1q is required for activation of the guinea pig complement.

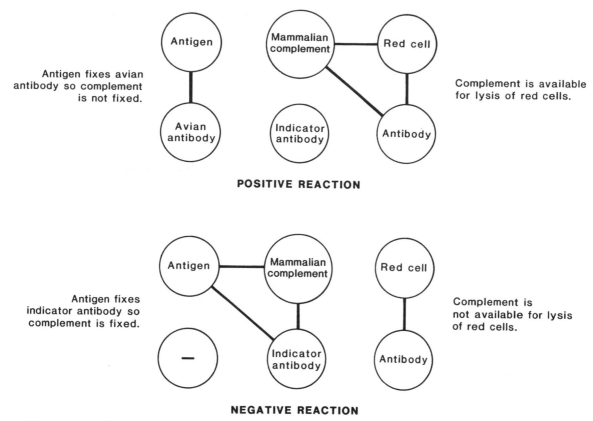

Figure 11–22. The principle of the indirect complement fixation test. In the presence of avian antibody, complement is not fixed and remains available to lyse the indicator system. In the absence of avian antibody, complement is fixed by the indicator antibody and the indicator system is not lysed. Lysis is therefore evidence of a positive reaction, and the absence of lysis is a negative reaction.

Cytotoxicity Tests

Complement may cause membrane damage, not only to erythrocytes but also to nucleated cells and to protozoa. Antibodies against cell surface antigens may thus be measured by reacting target cells with antibody in the presence of complement and estimating the resulting cell death. A simple method of doing this is to add a dye such as trypan blue or eosin-Y to the cell suspension. Living cells do not take up these dyes; dead cells stain intensely. This form of assay is employed in the identification of class I histocompatibility antigens (Chapter 8). A modification of this technique, known as the Sabin-Feldman dye test after its originators, is used in the diagnosis of toxoplasmosis.

Tests Involving Viral Hemagglutination and Its Inhibition

Certain viruses are capable of binding and agglutinating mammalian and avian erythrocytes. Antibodies directed against these viruses may inhibit this hemagglutination by blocking their binding sites. The detection of virus-induced hemagglutination may be used as a preliminary test when attempting to identify a virus, whereas inhibition of this phenomenon by antibody may be employed either as a method of identifying a specific virus or to measure antibody levels in serum. Hemagglutinating organisms include ortho- and paramyxoviruses, alpha-, flavi- and bunyaviruses as well as some adeno-, reo-, parvo- and coronaviruses. They also include some mycoplasma such as *Mycoplasma gallisepticum*.

Hemagglutination inhibition tests are performed in two general ways. In the first (sometimes called the alpha procedure), the amount of virus added to each tube is kept constant while the serum to be tested is serially diluted. (It is first necessary to titrate the virus in order to determine its hemagglutinating activity. It is common to employ four or eight times the minimal hemagglutinating dose, i.e., four or eight hemagglutinating units, in a test.) After virus and antibody are mixed, they are allowed to stand for a designated period of time before a suspension of washed erythrocytes is added to each tube. The hemagglutination inhibition (HI) titer of the serum is obtained by multiplying the highest dilution of serum that inhibits hemagglutination by the number of hemagglutinating units of virus involved.

An alternative method of estimating antibody levels by hemagglutination inhibition is to add a standard amount of antiserum to each tube while serial dilutions are made of a virus suspension of known hemagglutinating activity (the beta procedure). This is a useful technique in laboratories in which very large numbers of sera must be tested, since virus dilutions need be made only once, at the beginning of each day's testing, and there is no need to perform serial dilutions on each serum to be tested. By comparing the hemagglutinating titer of the virus in the presence of both a normal and a test serum, it is possible to arrive at an estimate of the inhibitory effect of that test serum.

While hemagglutination inhibition tests are technically relatively simple, problems may be encountered as a result of the presence in test serum of nonantibody hemagglutination inhibitors. Some of these are carbohydrates that may be destroyed by treatment of the test serum with bacterial neuraminidase (receptor-destroying enzyme, RDE). Others are lipoproteins that may be removed either by absorption of serum with washed kaolin or destroyed by trypsin treatment. It is also generally necessary to absorb the test serum with erythrocytes in order to remove natural hemagglutinins. Some myxoviruses possess

their own RDE, permitting them to spontaneously elute from red cells after incubation and also rendering these red cells inagglutinable. For this reason, a false-positive result may be obtained if there is excessive delay in reading some hemagglutination inhibition tests.

TESTS INVOLVING ASSAYS IN LIVING SYSTEMS

If an organism or antigen possesses biological activity, it is possible to assay antibody by its ability to neutralize this activity. The activities that may be neutralized include hemolysis of erythrocytes, lysis of nucleated cells and disease or death in animals. Unfortunately, reactions such as these are subject to a high degree of variability since they tend to change gradually over a wide range of doses of organism or antigen. For this reason, results obtained from a single positive or negative neutralization test are usually meaningless. For example, 0.003 mg of tetanus toxin may kill some mice in a test group, but about five times that dose is required to kill all mice in the same group. In addition, if an attempt is made to assess the lowest dose of tetanus toxin that will kill all the animals in a group (the minimum lethal dose, MLD), it is found to be extremely variable (Fig. 11–23). It is equally difficult to estimate with precision the highest dose of toxin that will just fail to kill all test animals. The most exact method of measuring the lethal effects of a toxin has been to estimate the dose that will just kill 50 per cent of a group of test animals. In practice, it is usually not possible to arrive at this 50 per cent endpoint by direct experimentation. For this reason, it is usually necessary to calculate it by plotting the results against the dose of toxin given and arriving at the 50 per cent end point by statistical evaluation.

In the example cited in the previous paragraph, the lethality of the toxin was estimated by measuring the dose required to kill 50 per cent of a group of experimental animals. This is known as the LD_{50}. Similarly, the dose of complement that just lyses 50 per cent of a red cell suspension is known as the CH_{50}. The

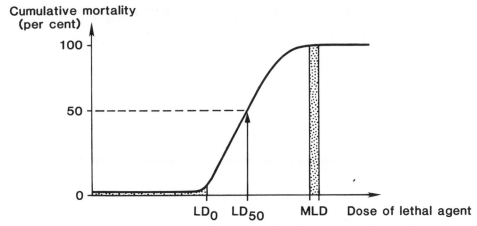

Figure 11–23. A cumulative mortality curve showing how the LD_{50} provides a more accurate estimate of the lethal effects of a toxin than either the LD_0 or the minimum lethal dose (MLD).

dose of organisms that infects 50 per cent of animals is the ID_{50}, the dose that just infects 50 per cent of tissue cultures is the $TCID_{50}$, and the dose of antiserum or vaccine that protects 50 per cent of challenged animals is the PD_{50}.

Neutralization Tests

Neutralization tests estimate the ability of antibody to neutralize the biological activity of antigen when mixed with it *in vitro*. These tests may be used to identify bacterial toxins such as *Clostridium perfringens* α toxin, which is a phospholipase that causes the development of an opaque white zone around colonies of this organism when grown on agar containing either serum or egg yolk. Antiserum to the α toxin prevents the formation of this zone. This reaction, known as the Nagler reaction, may therefore be employed to identify organisms producing this toxin. A similar type of test may be used to identify the presence of staphylococcal α toxin by inhibiting its hemolytic activity with specific antiserum (Fig. 11–24).

Viruses may be prevented from infecting cells after specific antibody has combined with and blocked their critical attachment sites. This reaction is the basis of the neutralization tests that are employed either for the identification of unknown viruses or for the measurement of specific antiviral antibody. Neutralization tests are highly specific and extremely sensitive. Thus, antiserum to coliphage T4 will neutralize phage-induced lysis of *Escherichia coli* because antibodies can block the receptor on the phage tail, thus preventing its attachment to a bacterium. A single antibody molecule is sufficient to cause this blockage, and a phage neutralization test may therefore detect as little as 0.00005 mg of antibody.

All neutralization tests require that the virus first be titrated so that its infectivity is known. This may be done by measuring its ID_{50} in animals or embryonated eggs or its $TCID_{50}$ in cell cultures. Given a virus suspension of known infectivity, it is possible to measure the neutralizing activity of a serum by two methods. In one, the virus concentration is kept constant while antiserum is diluted. In this way it is possible to estimate the neutralizing titer of an antiserum directly. Alternatively, the antiserum concentration may be kept constant and the virus diluted. This technique provides another measure of the neutralizing power of an antiserum, which can be expressed as a neutralization index. The neutralization index is the difference between the number of ID_{50} or $TCID_{50}$ neutralized by the test serum and by a known negative serum. In general, an index of more than 50 is required before a serum is considered to be positive. Similarly, the difference between the

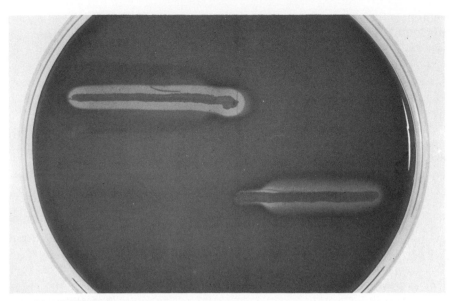

Figure 11–24. A blood agar plate, the center of which has been impregnated with antiserum to staphylococcal α toxin. The presence of this antiserum in the agar neutralizes the toxin produced by the staphylococcus and so inhibits hemolysis. (Courtesy of Mr. E. L. Thackeray.)

neutralization indices of two viruses must be less than 20 when tested against a standard antiserum before they can be considered identical.

Neutralization tests in tissue cultures are especially suitable for use with viruses that produce either readily identifiable cytopathic effects or hemadsorption, since both of these reactions may be inhibited by prior exposure of the virus to antibody. In general, if a serum is to be titrated, increasing dilutions of antibody are mixed with a constant amount of virus (usually 100 $TCID_{50}$) for a specified period of time and then each virus-antiserum mixture is used to inoculate a set of culture tubes. After incubation, the dilution of antiserum at which 50 per cent of cultures show signs of infection, multiplied by the number of $TCID_{50}$ neutralized, is taken to be its titer.

Although cytopathic effects are normally observed microscopically, other alternative techniques for assessing infection are also available. In the metabolic inhibition test use is made of the change in pH that occurs when healthy cells are grown in tissue culture. Normal, actively metabolizing cells produce acid that turns phenol red, the indicator dye, yellow. When cell metabolism ceases in infected cultures, this acid production does not occur.

As a result, either the phenol red does not change color or the medium turns alkaline (red) as a result of the accumulation of cell breakdown products. This color change may be employed to determine the presence or absence of infected cells.

A second technique for identifying virus-infected cells makes use of the phenomenon of hemadsorption. Certain viruses are able to induce the development of "hemagglutinins" on the surface of infected tissue culture cells. If a dilute suspension of washed erythrocytes is added to these cultures and examined 15 minutes later, the erythrocytes may be seen to be adherent to the infected cells. While many hemadsorbing viruses are also hemagglutinating, this is not an absolute relationship. For example, African swine fever virus is nonhemagglutinating, but it is hemadsorbing. The prevention of hemadsorption may be used as an indication of virus neutralization, especially with viruses that do not produce a significant cytopathic effect.

A third method of assessing virus cytopathogenicity is through inhibition of plaque formation. In this technique a confluent cell monolayer is infected by a dilute suspension of virus before being covered by a layer of agar. Because of the presence of the agar, virus particles are not free to diffuse but can only infect nearby cells. As a result, localized areas of cytolysis, revealed as clear plaques, develop in the monolayer. Each plaque develops as a result of the cytotoxic effects of a single virus particle. Antiserum that neutralizes the virus therefore reduces the number of plaques formed. This activity may be detected in several ways. In the plaque neutralization test, the virus is incubated in antiserum before infecting the cell monolayer. In the plaque reduction test, antiserum is incorporated into the agar used to cover the infected monolayer. In the plaque suppression technique, the monolayer is covered with agar-containing antiserum and virus is placed on top of this in a second layer of agar. Only virus that is not neutralized by antibody succeeds in diffusing through the antiserum-agar layer to cause plaque formation.

Although virus neutralization tests utilizing cell cultures are the most widely applicable serologic tests for virologic work, it is also possible to assay antibody by measuring virus neutralization *in vivo*. For example, antiserum to pox viruses may be assayed for its ability to inhibit pock formation on the chorioallantoic membrane of embryonated eggs. Antiserum to the equine encephalitis viruses may be titrated by measuring its ability to neutralize virus and so prevent death in mice injected intracerebrally with the virus-antibody mixture.

Protection Tests

Protection tests are a form of neutralization test carried out entirely *in vivo*. It is possible to measure the protective properties of a specific antiserum by administering it in increasing dilutions to a group of test animals, which may then be challenged with a standard dose of pathogenic organisms or toxin. Protection tests may therefore be classified as tertiary tests, since they measure not only the interaction between antigen and antibody *in vivo* but also the results of this in relation to disease resistance. Although protection tests provide a direct measure of the therapeutic efficacy of an antiserum, they are also subject to great

experimental variation because of the difference among animals in their susceptibility to infection and in a number of other factors, such as the rate of absorption of antiserum, the level of activity of the mononuclear-phagocytic system and the catabolic rate of the passively administered immunoglobulin. As in neutralization tests, meaningful results can be obtained only if relatively large numbers of animals are employed and if the challenge dose is carefully standardized. It is usual to use a dose of organisms or toxin containing a known number of LD_{50} or ID_{50}. Similarly, the protective effect of an antiserum may be expressed in PD_{50}, the dose required to protect 50 per cent of a group of animals.

DIAGNOSTIC APPLICATIONS OF IMMUNOLOGICAL TESTS

The immune responses of animals can be utilized in two general ways in the diagnostic laboratory. First, specific antibody may be used to detect or identify an antigen. Second, by detecting specific antibody in serum, it is possible to determine whether an animal has been exposed to a specific antigen and therefore assist in establishing a diagnosis or determining the degree of exposure of the population to that antigen.

Obviously, the presence of antibodies to a specific organism in a serum indicates previous exposure to an epitope present on that organism. It does not, however, automatically provide proof that infection exists or that any concurrent disease is actually caused by the organism in question. For example, although the sera of most healthy horses contain antibodies to *Salmonella typhimurium*, this does not prove that most horses have salmonellosis. Because of this problem, it can be stated that the presence of antibodies to an organism in a single serum sample is of little diagnostic significance. Only if at least two samples are taken one to three weeks apart, and at least a fourfold rise in titer is shown, can a diagnosis be made; and this should be done only in conjunction with careful analysis of clinical factors.

A second feature that must be considered

in the interpretation of serologic results is the possibility of errors. Technical errors are usually prevented by incorporation of appropriate controls into the test system. Other errors, however, are largely unavoidable. These may be of two types: false-positive results and false-negative results. A test in which a large proportion of the positive results is false is considered to be nonspecific, whereas one with a very high proportion of false-negative results is considered to be insensitive. In general, the level of such errors is set by the criteria used to differentiate positive from negative reactions. If these criteria are adjusted so that the number of false-positive results are reduced, then there will be an increasing proportion of false-negative results encountered, and vice versa (Fig. 11–25). Thus, highly sensitive tests

tend to be relatively nonspecific and highly specific tests are generally insensitive. The establishment of criteria in reading tests and, from this, the sensitivity and specificity of a test are determined both by the requirements of the test procedure and by the consequences of false-positive and false-negative reactions. In ideal tests, it would be desirable for the criteria used in interpreting the test results to be so obvious and absolute that each test would be absolutely sensitive and specific. Unfortunately, such ideal tests are uncommon.

As has been evident from the discussions earlier in this chapter, the advantages and disadvantages of each immunodiagnostic test vary according to the specific requirements of the investigator, the nature of the antigen

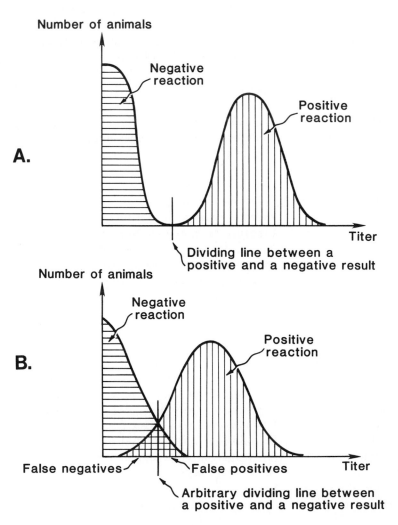

Figure 11–25. Schematic diagrams depicting the errors that are associated with immunological tests. A, An ideal test in which there is no ambiguity in interpreting test results. B, A more typical test in which an arbitrary line must be used to separate positive from negative results. By moving this dividing line the relative proportions of false-positive and false-negative results may be changed.

employed and the complexity, sensitivity and specificity of each method. In general, the selection of a diagnostic test represents a compromise between its sensitivity, its specificity and its complexity—that is, the number of steps involved, the degree of technical expertise required and the nature of the equipment needed to conduct the test. Although precise guidelines cannot be drawn up, it is usually most appropriate to use the most sensitive and specific test that can be satisfactorily performed with the available technical assistance and equipment.

ADDITIONAL SOURCES OF INFORMATION

Bolton AE. 1981. Antisera for radioimmunoassay. Irish Vet. J. 35 143–153.

Boto WMO, Powers KG and Levy DA. 1984. Antigens of *Dirofilaria immitis* which are immunogenic in the canine host: detection by immuno-staining of protein blots with the antibodies of occult dogs. J. Immunol. 133 975–980.

Carter GR and Moojen V. 1981. A summary of serologic tests used to detect common infectious diseases of animals. Vet. Med. (Small Anim. Clin.) 76 1725–1730.

Cripps AW, Husband AJ, Scicchitano R and Sheldrake RF. 1985. Quantitation of sheep IgG$_1$, IgA and IgM and albumin by radioimmunoassay. Vet. Immunol. Immunopathol. 8 137–147.

Delaat ANC. 1976. Primer of Serology. Harper & Row, New York.

Diamond BA, Yelton DE and Scharff MD. 1981. Monoclonal antibodies: a new technology for producing serologic reagents. N. Engl. J. Med. 304 1344–1349.

Friedman H, Linna TJ and Prier JE. (eds). 1979. Immunoserology in the Diagnosis of Infectious Diseases. University Park Press, Baltimore.

Gerstman BB and Cappucci DT. 1986. Evaluating the reliability of diagnostic test results. JAVMA 188 248–251.

Lennette EH and Schmidt NJ. (eds). 1979. Diagnostic Procedures for Viral, Rickettsial and Chlamydial Infections. 5th Ed. American Public Health Association, Washington, DC.

Milstein C. 1980. Monoclonal antibodies. Sci. Am. 243 66–74.

Pollack W and Reckel RP. 1977. A reappraisal of forces involved in hemagglutination. Int. Arch. Allergy Appl. Immunol. 54 29–42.

Rice CE. 1968. Comparative serology of domestic animals. Adv. Vet. Sci. 12 105–162.

Rose NR and Friedman H. (eds). 1980. Manual of Clinical Immunology. 2nd Ed. American Society of Microbiology, Washington, DC.

Schultz RD and Adams LS. 1978. Immunologic methods for detection of humoral and cellular immunity. Vet. Clin. North Am. (Small Anim. Pract.) 8 721–753.

Sutherland SS. 1980. Immunology of bovine brucellosis. Vet. Bull. 50 359–368.

Voller A and deSavigny D. 1981. Enzyme-Linked Immunosorbent Assay (ELISA). *In* Thompson RA. (ed). Techniques in Clinical Immunology. Blackwell Scientific Publications, London.

Whittaker RG, Spencer TL and Copeland JW. 1982. Enzyme-linked immunosorbent assay for meat species testing. Aust. Vet. J. 59 125.

Wilchek M and Bayer EA. 1984. The avidin-biotin complex in immunology. Immunol. Today 5 39–43.

Worthington RW. 1982. Serology as an aid to diagnosis: uses and abuses. N.Z. Vet. J. 30 93–97.

III
PROTECTIVE IMMUNITY

12

Immunity at Body Surfaces

Although animals possess an extensive array of defense mechanisms within the body, it is at the surface of an animal that invading micro-organisms are first encountered and largely repelled or destroyed. The protective systems at body surfaces achieve this by establishing, through physical and chemical mechanisms, environments suitable for only the most adapted micro-organisms. These surfaces are populated by an extensive microbial flora that, because it is well adapted, is also of low pathogenicity and effectively prevents the establishment of other, more poorly adapted and potentially pathogenic organisms. This environmental defense system is supplemented by immunological mechanisms in areas where the physical barriers to invasion are relatively weak.

NONIMMUNOLOGICAL SURFACE-PROTECTIVE MECHANISMS (Fig. 12–1)

The skin serves a number of functions one of which is to present a barrier to invading micro-organisms. The skin carries a dense and stable resident bacterial flora whose composition is regulated by a number of factors, including continuing desquamation, desiccation and a relatively low pH that is due, in part, to the presence of fatty acids in sebum. If any of these factors is altered, then the composition of the skin flora is disturbed, its protective properties are reduced and microbial invasion may occur. Thus, skin infections tend to occur in areas such as the axilla or groin where both pH and humidity are relatively high. Similarly, animals forced to stand in water or mud show an increased frequency of foot infections; as the skin becomes sodden its structure breaks down and its resident flora changes in response to alterations in the local environment. The importance of the resident flora is seen to much greater effect in the digestive tract, since it is essential not only for the control of potential pathogens but also for the digestion of some foods, such as cellulose in the diet of herbivores. In addition, the natural development of the immune system depends upon the continuous antigenic simulation provided by intestinal bacteria. Because they

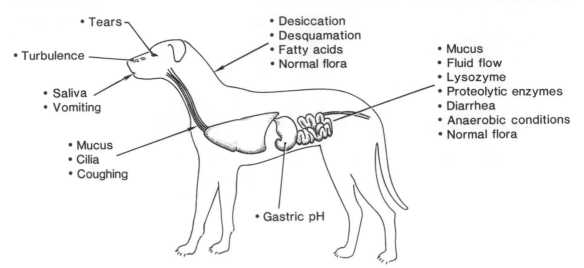

Figure 12–1. The nonimmunological surface protective mechanisms.

have no bacterial flora, gnotobiotic (germ-free) animals have hypoplastic secondary lymphoid organs that do not develop such features as secondary follicles, and their immunoglobulin levels are only about 2 per cent of normal. If the natural flora of the intestine is eliminated or its composition drastically altered (by aggressive antibiotic treatment, for example), then an overgrowth of potential pathogens may occur. The flora of the digestive tract normally acts competitively against potential invaders through a number of mechanisms that supplement the other physical defenses of this system. Thus, in the mouth the flushing activity of saliva is complemented by the generation of peroxidases from streptococci. In simple-stomached animals the gastric pH may be sufficiently low to have a bactericidal or viricidal effect, although this varies greatly between species and between meals. The dog, for instance, has a relatively low gastric pH relative to that of the pig. Similarly, the pH in the center of a mass of ingested food may not necessarily drop to low levels, and some foods such as milk are known to be potent buffers.

Farther down the intestine the resident bacterial flora ensures that the pH is kept low and the contents slightly anaerobic. The intestinal flora is also influenced indirectly by the diet; for instance, the intestine of milk-fed animals is colonized largely by lactobacilli,

which produce large quantities of bacteriostatic lactic and butyric acids. These acids inhibit colonization by potential pathogens such as *Escherichia coli*, so that young animals that are suckled naturally tend to have fewer digestive disturbances than animals weaned early in life. In the large intestine the bacterial flora is composed largely of strict anaerobes.

Lysozyme (Chapter 15), the antibacterial and antiviral enzyme, is synthesized in the gastric mucosa and in macrophages within the intestinal mucosa. It is therefore found in large quantities in all the intestinal fluids. The role of phagocytic cells in the intestine is not clear, but macrophages do move out through the intestinal wall and may be active for a short time within the lumen.

In the urinary system, the flushing action and low pH of urine generally provide adequate protection; however, when urinary stasis occurs, urethritis resulting from the unhindered ascent of pathogenic bacteria is not uncommon. In adult female animals, the vagina is lined by a squamous epithelium composed of cells rich in glycogen. When these cells desquamate, they provide a substrate for lactobacilli that, in turn, generate large quantities of lactic acid, which protects the vagina against invasion. Glycogen storage in the vaginal epithelial cells is stimulated by estrogens and thus occurs only in sexually mature animals. Because of this, vaginal infections in humans tend to be commonest prior to puberty and after the menopause.

The protective mechanisms of the udder are, presumably, not of the most effective kind, at least in that biological anomaly the modern dairy cow. The flushing action of the milk serves to prevent invasion by some potential pathogens while milk itself contains bacterial inhibitors. These antibacterial substances in milk are called lactenins. Lactenins include complement, lysozyme, the iron-binding protein lactoferrin and the enzyme lactoperoxidase. Lactoferrin competes with bacteria for iron and therefore renders it unavailable for their growth (see Chapter 15). Milk contains high concentrations of lactoperoxidase and thiocyanate (SCN^-) ions. In the presence of exogenous hydrogen peroxide, the lactoperoxidase can oxidize the SCN^- to bacteriostatic products such as sulfur dicyanide. The exogenous hydrogen peroxide may be produced by bacteria such as streptococci or, alternatively, by the oxidation of ascorbic acid. Some strains of streptococci are resistant to this bacteriostatic pathway, since they possess an enzyme that reduces the SCN^-. The phagocytic cells released into the udder in response to irritation may also contribute to antimicrobial resistance not only through their phagocytic

efforts but also by providing additional lactoferrin and myeloperoxidase.

The respiratory tract differs from the other body surfaces in that it is in intimate contact with the interior of the body and it is required by its very nature to allow unhindered access of air to the alveoli. The system obviously requires a filter. In fact, air entering the respiratory tract is largely cleared of suspended particles by turbulence that directs them onto its mucus-covered walls, where they adhere. The turbulence is brought about by the conformation of the turbinate bones, the trachea and the bronchi. This "turbulence filter" serves to remove particles as small as 5 μm in size before they reach the alveoli (Fig. 12–2).

The walls of the upper respiratory tract are covered by a layer of mucus produced by goblet cells and provided with "antiseptic" properties through its content of lysozyme and IgA. This mucus layer is in continuous flow, being carried from the bronchioles up the bronchi and trachea by ciliary action or backward through the nasal cavity to the pharynx. Here the "dirty" mucus is swallowed and digested in the intestinal tract. Particles smaller than 5 μm that can by-pass this mucociliary escalator and reach the alveoli are

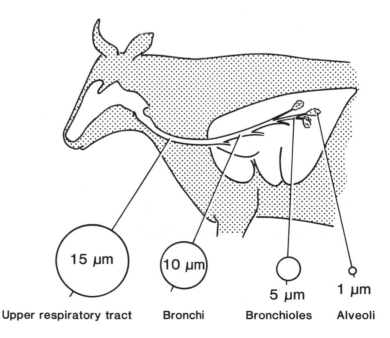

Figure 12–2. The influence of particle size on the site of deposition of particles within the respiratory tract. Only the smallest particles gain access to the alveoli.

15 μm   10 μm   5 μm   1 μm

Upper respiratory tract   Bronchi   Bronchioles   Alveoli

Table 12–1 APPROXIMATE IgA LEVELS IN THE SERUM AND VARIOUS SECRETIONS OF THE DOMESTIC ANIMALS

Animal	Serum	Colostrum	Milk	Nasal Secretions	Saliva	Tears
Horse	170	1000	130	160	140	150
Cow	30	400	10	200	56	260
Sheep	30	400	10	50	90	160
Pig	200	1000	500	*	*	*
Dog	50	1500	400	*	*	*
Chicken	50			*	20	15

*Figures not currently available to the author.

phagocytosed by alveolar macrophages. This material may remain in the alveoli for many months after being ingested. Normally, however, the lungs remain almost sterile since inhaled organisms are either removed by mucociliary action or destroyed by macrophages.

IMMUNOLOGICAL SURFACE-PROTECTIVE MECHANISMS

Immunoglobulins

Immunoglobulin A

In addition to the environmental and chemical factors that protect body surfaces, IgA is found in high concentrations in saliva, intestinal fluid, nasal and tracheal secretions, tears, milk and colostrum, urine and the secretions of the urogenital tract (Table 12–1).

The IgA monomer is a 6.8 S molecule with a molecular weight of about 160,000 daltons, having a typical four-chain Y-shaped structure and a higher carbohydrate content than the other immunoglobulin isotypes. It is usually found as a 9.3 S dimer with the subunits bound together by a J chain. The Fc region is tightly folded, with many interchain disulfide bonds. IgA is therefore relatively resistant to proteolytic digestion.

After IgA is synthesized by plasma cells in the intestinal mucosa it binds to a receptor on the interior surface of epithelial cells. The complex of IgA and the receptor is then endocytosed into a vesicle and transported across the epithelial cell (Fig. 12–3). When it reaches the exterior surface of the epithelial cell, the

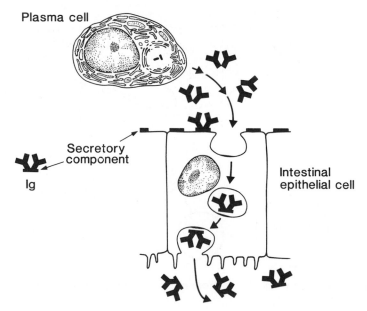

Figure 12–3. The passage of IgA through an intestinal epithelial cell by means of the secretory component–receptor.

vesicle fuses with the plasma membrane and exposes the IgA to the gut lumen. The IgA receptor is then cleaved by a protease in order to release the dimeric IgA, with about 75 per cent of the receptor still attached. This receptor fragment is called secretory component. Secretory component has a molecular weight of 71,000 daltons. When bound with IgA the complex is called secretory IgA (SIgA). SIgA is a 10.8 S molecule with a molecular weight of about 400,000 daltons (Fig. 12–4).

Secretory component renders IgA resistant to digestion by intestinal enzymes, although this resistance does vary between IgA subisotypes. For example, porcine SIgA1 is more resistant than SIgA2 to pepsin digestion, but SIgA2 is more resistant than SIgA1 to some of the bacterial proteases found in the intestine. (It is of interest to note that pigs possess a subpopulation of circulating mononuclear cells with receptors for secretory component. The function of these cells or their receptor is unknown.)

IgA is not bactericidal, does not bind to macrophages or enhance phagocytosis and fixes complement only by the alternate path-

way. It can, however, neutralize some viruses and some viral and bacterial enzymes. Its most important mode of action is the prevention of the adherence of bacteria and viruses to epithelial surfaces. The importance of this adherence may be seen, for example, in diseases of the intestinal tract caused by strains of *E. coli* possessing the F4 (K88) antigen. The F4 antigen is a pilus by which the bacteria bind to intestinal epithelial cells, so preventing their expulsion and promoting proliferation and enterotoxin production. Antibodies made specifically against the F4 antigen can inhibit this bacterial adherence and hence protect animals against disease caused by these strains of *E. coli*.

IgA is synthesized by plasma cells located in the submucosa in response to local antigenic stimulation. Some of this IgA diffuses directly into the intestinal lumen, combining with secretory component as it does so. However, in some species, such as rats, rabbits and chickens, the IgA may diffuse into the portal circulation and is thus carried directly to the liver. Hepatocytes in these species synthesize secretory component and incorporate it into

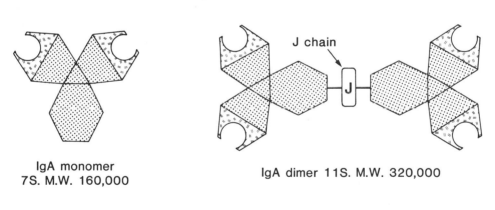

IgA monomer
7S. M.W. 160,000

IgA dimer 11S. M.W. 320,000

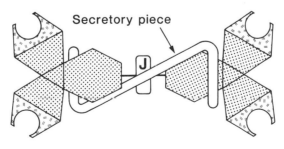

Secretory IgA (SIgA) 11.4S. M.W. 390,000

Figure 12–4. The structure of monomeric, dimeric and secretory IgA. The secretory piece effectively protects the Fc region of the IgA molecule from proteolytic digestion.

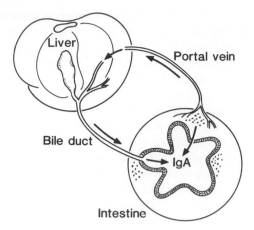

Figure 12–5. The circulation of IgA. In rats, rabbits and chickens, 35 to 75 percent of the IgA produced in the intestinal wall is carried to the liver and excreted in the bile. The remainder is secreted directly into the intestinal lumen. In humans, dogs and ruminants, less than 5 percent of the IgA excreted in bile.

their membrane, where it acts as an IgA receptor. The blood-borne IgA thus binds to hepatocytes and is carried across the hepatocyte cytoplasm to be released into the bile canaliculi. Bile is therefore extremely rich in IgA, and is a major route by which IgA reaches the intestinal lumen in these species (Fig. 12–5). It is also a route by which antigens bound to circulating IgA can be removed from the body. The reader should note, however, that the situation in ruminants, dogs and humans is different. There is very little IgA in the bile of these species.

The plasma cells in the gut-associated lymphoid tissue (GALT) arise from precursor B cells. These B cells, upon encountering antigen, respond in a manner similar to B lymphocytes elsewhere in the body—that is, they divide and differentiate either into plasma cells or into memory cells. However, many of these responding B cells leave the intestinal wall and migrate into the lymphatics, from which they reach the thoracic duct and the blood circulation (Fig 12–6). These recirculating cells have an affinity for mucosal surfaces in general. As a result, they lodge throughout the intestinal tract, the respiratory tract, the urogenital tract and the mammary gland. The movement of these IgA-producing B cells to the mammary gland is of major importance in veterinary medicine, since it provides a route by which cells stimulated by intestinal pathogens can secrete their IgA into milk and thus protect the intestines of newborn animals. Oral administration of an antigen to a pregnant animal will therefore result in the appearance of IgA antibodies to that antigen in its milk. In this way the intestine of its offspring will receive antibodies appropriate for any pathogenic organisms it may encounter.

Anamnestic immune responses are some-

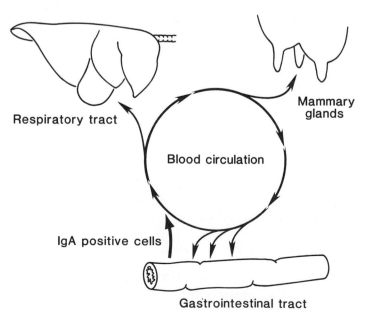

Figure 12–6. The circulation of IgA-producing cells following an immune response in the intestinal wall.

times difficult to induce in the surface immune systems. This is probably not due to any intrinsic defect but occurs because the IgA prevents antigen absorption and thus prevents sensitization. Multiple doses of antigen do not usually increase the intensity or duration of the local immune response to any significant extent. The reasons for this are unclear.

Immunoglobulin G

In ruminants, especially the bovine, IgG1 is the major secretory immunoglobulin and is therefore the predominant immunoglobulin in milk, intestinal contents and nasal washings. The presence of IgG1 in bovine bile suggests that it may also be transported through hepatocytes. (In sheep, very little immunoglobulin of any isotype is found in bile. IgG1 diffuses directly into the intestinal lumen in this species.)

Immunoglobulin M

IgM is only a minor component in secretions, although it can bind secretory component as it diffuses into the intestinal lumen and is therefore protected against proteolytic digestion.

Immunoglobulin E

IgE is mainly synthesized by plasma cells in the submucosa of the intestinal and respiratory tracts. Its production is associated with immunity to helminths and type I hypersensitivities and so will be discussed in Chapters 17 and 20.

Immunity in the Gastrointestinal Tract

The gastrointestinal tract is probably the major site of antigenic stimulation in animals. Antigenic particles such as bacteria can penetrate the intestinal mucosa relatively easily and in this way gain access to the lacteals and portal vessels. These organisms are consequently trapped in the mesenteric lymph nodes and liver, respectively. Bacterial endotoxins, exo-

toxins and antigens from protein-rich foods such as eggs or soy can be absorbed intact from the intestine and promote some antibody formation. Other antigens may enter the body via the surface lymphoid tissues. For instance, the tonsils possess a structural weakness in that the squamous epithelial covering at the bottom of the tonsilar crypts is very thin (Fig. 12–7). Viruses may enter the body by this route and multiply locally in the tonsil prior to the development of a viremia.

The tonsils and Peyer's patches are organized lymphoid tissues, possessing all the components required to mount an immune response, namely T cells, B cells and macrophages. The Peyer's patches are functionally heterogeneous. Some increase in size from birth to six months and then regress. Others remain throughout adult life. It is this latter population that probably plays a major role in intestinal defense. A calf normally has about 100 Peyer's patches, and these may cover as much as 50 per cent of the ileal surface. Collectively, the intestine contains more lymphocytes than the spleen. As described in Chapter 5, Peyer's patches are covered by highly specialized epithelial cells called M cells. These M cells can take up particulate or soluble antigens from the intestinal lumen and present them directly to the lymphocytes, which respond by producing IgA. (Some pathogens such as the salmonellae and the reoviruses may take advantage of the M cells and use them to gain access to the body.) Despite the size of the Peyer's patches, most IgA is formed in diffuse lymphoid nodules and in isolated plasma cells found in the walls of the intestine, in salivary glands and in the gallbladder. A significant population of T lymphocytes is also found within the intestinal epithelium. Their function is obscure.

If bacteria succeed in penetrating the intestinal wall, then in the ensuing inflammatory response capillary permeability will increase and IgG will be free to diffuse from the blood stream into the area of invasion. Thus, IgG may also act to protect body surfaces subsequent to an inflammatory reaction.

Because of the poor anamnestic response in the secretory immunoglobulin system, it is probably not possible to confer prolonged pro-

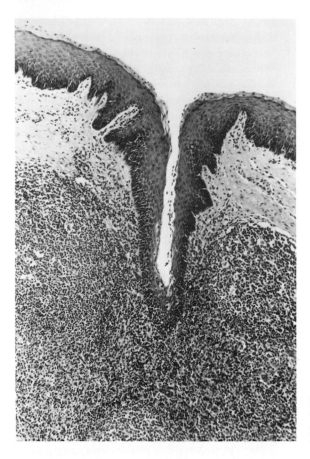

Figure 12–7. A section of pig tonsil showing a tonsillar crypt. Note how the epithelium thins out at the base of the crypt. × 150. (From a specimen kindly provided by Dr. S. Yamashiro.)

tection against intestinal infection using killed organisms as a vaccine. However, oral vaccination may be of use in protecting against those diseases to which an animal is susceptible for only a short period. Diets containing killed *E. coli* given to calves and pigs have resulted in a reduced incidence of diarrhea, a better feed conversion and an improvement in the overall health of the animals. Oral transmissible gastroenteritis vaccine containing live virus may also be given to pregnant sows in order to stimulate an intestinal IgA response and seed antibody-producing cells to the udder. This results in the appearance of specific antibodies in colostrum and in the protection of suckling piglets.

Immunity in the Mammary Gland

The mammary gland is protected in nonspecific fashion by the physical barrier of the teat canal, by the flushing action of the milk and by the presence of lactenins, of which the lactoperoxidase-thiocyanate system, lactoferrin and lysozyme are probably the most important. (It should be pointed out that lysozyme levels are very low in bovine milk.) In addition, milk also contains IgA, secretory component and IgG1 in low concentrations. The IgA and secretory component are closely associated with the milk fat globules. In animals with simple stomachs, IgA predominates, whereas in ruminants IgG1 is in highest concentration.

IgA is locally synthesized in the mammary tissue, although many of the IgA-producing cells in the mammary gland are derived from precursors originating in the intestinal tract. Once these cells colonize the gland they provide a source of antibodies against intestinal pathogens. IgG1, in contrast, is selectively transferred by an active transport mechanism from serum and only a small fraction is synthesized locally.

If antigen is infused into a lactating mammary gland, it tends to be promptly flushed out again in the milk. If it is infused into a nonlactating gland, then a local immune response develops in which IgA and IgG1 predominate. Unfortunately, because of the continuous removal of milk, antibody concentrations in this fluid remain relatively low even though, over a period of time, the amount of immunoglobulin secreted from the udder may be considerable. In cases of acute mastitis, the inflammatory response leads to the influx of actively phagocytic cells, especially neutrophils, and to the exudation of serum proteins. As a result, immunoglobulin levels in mastitic milk may rise to levels at which they can exert a protective influence. This phenomenon has led to the development of a plastic intramammary device that is inserted into the milk cistern and causes a low-grade irritation. The resulting emigration of neutrophils and effusion of immunoglobulins protects the gland against bacterial invasion and severe mastitis.

Because the local immune response in the udder is relatively ineffective in preventing infection, attempts at vaccination against mastitis-causing organisms have been generally unsuccessful. The difficulties encountered in attempting to vaccinate are also accentuated by the large number of potential mammary pathogens. For example, there are five different antigenic types of *Streptococcus agalactiae* alone. In addition there is antigenic cross-reaction between this organism and bovine tissues. Because of these difficulties, for a mastitis vaccine to be effective it should be autogenous and should be given either into the nonlactating gland toward the end of the dry period or into the supramammary lymph node. It may be anticipated that such a procedure will not totally prevent mastitis, but it may at least lessen the severity of acute infections.

Immunity in the Urogenital Tract

The predominant immunoglobulin in cervicovaginal mucus is IgA; within the uterus the predominant immunoglobulin is IgG. If bacteria such as *Campylobacter fetus* infect the genital tract, the vaginal IgA antibodies will immobilize the organisms and agglutinate them. If the mucus membrane becomes inflamed, IgG antibodies derived by transudation from serum will also assist in protection. *C. fetus* infections are associated with the presence of many mononuclear cells as well as with delayed skin reactions (type IV hypersensitivity), and it is therefore possible that cell-mediated immunity is also involved in resistance to this local infection. Preputial washings of bulls infected with *C. fetus* may also contain agglutinins, but these are largely IgG1, with some IgM and IgA. Similar local immune responses may also be directed against other organisms that cause infections of the cervix and vagina, and the presence of agglutinating antibodies in vaginal mucus may be used as a diagnostic test for brucellosis, campylobacteriosis and trichomoniasis. (The local immune response to trichomoniasis is largely mediated by IgE; see Chapter 17.)

IgA is present in small amounts in normal urine, produced presumably by lymphoid tissues in the walls of the urinary tract. If, however, a nephritis occurs, then IgG may also be found in relatively large amounts because of the breakdown in the glomerular barrier and defects in tubular reabsorption.

Immunity in the Respiratory Tract

In addition to the tonsils, the respiratory tract contains a considerable amount of lymphoid tissue in the form of nodules in the walls of the bronchi and as lymphocytes distributed diffusely throughout the lung and the walls of the airways. The immunoglobulin synthesized in these tissues is mainly secretory IgA, especially in the upper airways. In the bronchioles and alveoli, however, the secretions contain a large proportion of IgG, the concentration of which is intermediate between the levels in the trachea and in serum. IgE is also synthesized in significant amounts in the lymphoid tissues of the upper respiratory tract. As on other body surfaces, IgA in the respiratory tract is thought to protect by preventing adherence of antigenic particles including micro-organisms, whereas IgG is probably of major importance only when acute inflammation and transudation of serum protein occur. Severe inflammation will arise, for example, following an IgE-mediated hypersensitivity reaction, and it is tempting to suggest that a combination of IgA and IgE synthesis at mucosal surfaces is therefore not entirely fortuitous. It is possible that these immunoglobulins work in concert (Fig. 12–8), so that IgA prevents antigen adherence and penetration. If, in spite of the presence of this IgA, antigen gains access to the tissues, then the subsequent IgE-mediated hypersensitivity reaction will increase vascular permeability and make available large quantities of IgG in the resulting fluid exudate.

Large numbers of cells may be washed out of the lung by lavage with saline. These are mainly alveolar macrophages and T cells. It is possible to demonstrate the production of macrophage migration inhibition factor by these T cells under experimental situations and to show alveolar macrophage activation following infection with *Listeria monocytogenes*. It is likely, therefore, that cell-mediated immune reactions may be readily invoked among the cells within the lower respiratory tract.

When attempting to vaccinate animals against organisms that cause local infections of the upper respiratory tract, such as bovine viral rhinotracheitis or parainfluenza 3, it would appear logical to apply antigen locally.

In this way IgA production would be stimulated and invasion of the mucosa blocked. Systemic vaccination against these diseases gives some immunity, since small quantities of IgG may be transferred from serum to the mucous surface; nevertheless, complete protection by IgG cannot be achieved in this way until invasion, inflammation and exudation have occurred.

Immunity in the Skin

At the beginning of this chapter it was pointed out that the skin is the first line of defense against many microbial invaders. It carries out this function very effectively as judged by the infrequency of severe infections resulting from minor wounds. One way this is accomplished is through a local antigen trapping system that can present antigens to lymphocytes in a very efficient manner and thus provoke a rapid immune response. The antigen trapping system of the skin consists of a network of dendritic cells in the epidermis called Langerhans cells. These Langerhans cells carry class II MHC antigens on their surface and are able to present antigen to nearby helper T cells. The activities of these Langerhans cells are enhanced by keratinocytes. Keratinocytes also have class II antigens on their surface and are able to synthesize and secrete IL-1, stimulat-

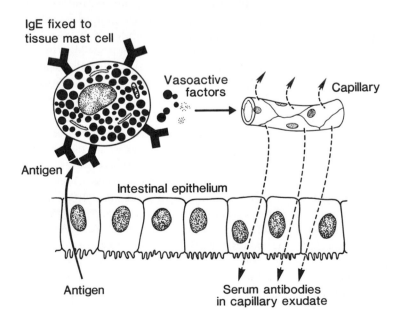

Figure 12–8. Antigen that penetrates the intestinal mucosa in a sensitized animal may encounter mast cell-fixed IgE. The resulting release of vasoactive factors causes an increase in vascular permeability and exudation of large amounts of IgG.

ing the T cells even further. There is also evidence to suggest that a T cell subpopulation selectively homes to the skin. Thus, if an antigen is injected intradermally, such as occurs when a tick bites an animal, for example, the antigen is trapped by Langerhans cells and presented to skin T cells thereby stimulating a rapid and effective immune response. A similar reaction occurs when reactive chemicals are painted on the skin (Chapter 23). If skin is subjected to severe ultraviolet irradiation, the Langerhans cells are destroyed and the protective mechanisms in the skin are effectively suppressed. Collectively the skin-associated lymphoid tissue has been called SALT.

ADDITIONAL SOURCES OF INFORMATION

Barratt MEJ, Twohig BMA, Hall H and Porter P. 1985. Hypersensitivity to dietary components in young farm animals. Immunization of calves for IgE antibody responses. Res. Vet. Sci. 39 62–65.

Bienenstock J and Befus AD. 1980. Mucosal immunology. Immunology 41 249–270.

Crago SS, Kulhary R, Prince SJ and Mestecky J. 1978. Secretory component on epithelial cells is a surface receptor for polymeric immunoglobulin. J. Exp. Med. 147 1832–1837.

Craven N and Williams MR. 1985. Defense of the bovine mammary gland against infection and prospects for their enhancement. Vet. Immunol. Immunopathol. 10 71–127.

Evans PA, Newby TJ, Stokes CR and Bourne FJ. 1982. A study of cells in the mammary secretions of sows. Vet. Immunol. Immunopathol. 3 515–528.

Fukimoto T and Brandon MR. 1982. Importance of the liver in immunoglobulin catabolism. Res. Vet. Sci. 32 62–69.

Husband AJ and Watson DL. 1978. Immunity in the intestine. Vet. Bull. 48 911–924.

Lascelles AK. 1979. The immune system of the ruminant mammary gland and its role in the control of mastitis. J. Dairy Sci. 62 154–160.

McDermott MR, Befus AD and Bienenstock J. 1982. The structural basis for immunity in the respiratory tract. Int. Rev. Exp. Pathol. 23 47–112.

McNabb PC and Tomasi TB. 1981. Host defense at mucosal surfaces. A. Rev. Microbiol. 35 477–496.

Newby TJ and Stokes CR. 1984. The intestinal immune system and oral vaccination. Vet. Immunol. Immunopathol. 6 67–105.

Newby TJ, Stokes CR and Bourne FJ. 1982. Immunological activities of milk. Vet. Immunol. Immunopathol. 3 67–94.

Reiter B. 1978. Review of the progress of dairy science: anti-microbial systems in milk. J. Dairy Res. 45 131–137.

Sheldrake RF, Husband AJ and Watson DL. 1985. Specific antibody-containing cells in the mammary gland of non-lactating sheep after intraperitoneal and intramammary immunization. Res. Vet. Sci. 38 312–316.

Solari R and Kraehenbuhl JP. 1985. The biosynthesis of secretory component and its role in the transepithelial transport of IgA dimer. Immunol. Today 6 17–20.

Tomasi TB, Larson L, Challacombe S and McNabb P. 1980. Mucosal immunity: the origin and migration patterns of cells in the secretory system. J. Allergy Clin. Immunol. 65 12–19.

13

Immunity in the Fetus and Newborn

When cows bear dizygotic twin calves, the blood vessels in their placentas commonly join together and the cells of the calves mingle freely. Circulating hematopoietic stem cells may therefore pass from one calf to the other. As a result each calf is born carrying blood cells derived from its twin. Despite being foreign, these cells persist throughout each animal's life. Thus, exposure to foreign blood cells during fetal life together with the persistence of these cells in the recipient calf leads to the development of tolerance. In the clonal selection theory, as first suggested by Burnet and Fenner, the dizygotic twin calf example was presented as evidence for the inability of the fetal animal to respond to foreign antigens. Burnet and Fenner sug-

gested that exposure of antigen-sensitive cells to potential antigens prior to birth resulted in tolerance and that this, therefore, accounted for the inability of the immune system to respond to self-antigens. Their theory seemed to be confirmed by the observation of Medawar that fetal mice injected with foreign mouse cells while *in utero* became tolerant to these cells and so could retain skin grafts from the donor strain indefinitely. In contrast, mice injected with the same cells after birth were able to mount an immune response as shown by prompt rejection of grafts from the donor strain.

In spite of the occurrence of calf chimeras (a chimera is an animal containing cells from different animals), the young of the domestic animals are very different from young rodents; their immune system is fully developed well before birth, and considerable difficulty is encountered in producing tolerance by fetal immunization. Newborn domestic animals are therefore susceptible to microbial invasion not because of any inherent inability to mount an immune response but because of the un-primed state of their immune system.

ONTOGENY OF THE IMMUNE SYSTEM

The development of the immune system in the fetus appears to follow a consistent pattern. The thymus is the first lymphoid organ to develop and is followed closely by the secondary lymphoid organs. Immunoglobulin-containing cells develop soon after the appearance of the spleen and lymph nodes, but serum immunoglobulins are not usually found until late in fetal life if at all. The ability of the fetus to respond to antigens may develop very rapidly after the lymphoid organs appear,

but all antigens are not equally capable of stimulating fetal lymphoid tissue. It was once considered that the immune system developed in a series of steps, each step permitting the fetus to respond to more antigens. It is more likely, however, that the ability to respond to most foreign antigens develops within a fairly narrow time span. The ability to mount cell-mediated immune responses develops at about the same time as antibody production.

Calf

The immune system of the calf develops very early in fetal life. Although the gestation period of the cow is 280 days, the fetal thymus is recognizable by 40 days postconception (Fig. 13–1). The bone marrow and spleen appear at 55 days. Lymph nodes are found at 60 days, but Peyer's patches do not appear until 75 days. Peripheral blood lymphocytes are seen in fetal calves by day 45, IgM-carrying cells by day 59 and IgG-carrying cells by day 135. The time of the earliest detection of serum antibodies depends on the sensitivity

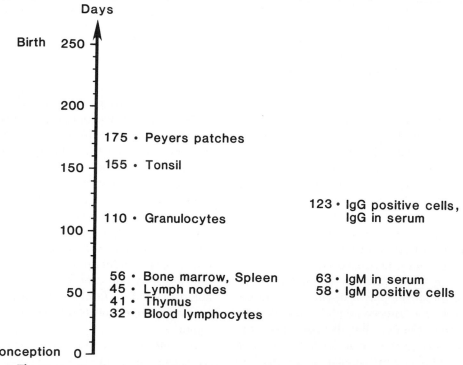

Figure 13–1. The progressive development of the immune system in the fetal calf. Each number indicates days post-conception.

of the techniques used. It is, therefore, no accident that the earliest detectable immune responses are those directed against viruses, for which exquisitely sensitive virus neutralization techniques are used. Calves have been reported to respond to rotavirus at 73 days and to parvovirus at 93 days. Calf peripheral blood lymphocytes can respond to phytohemagglutinin and pokeweed mitogen between 78 and 90 days, but this ability is temporarily lost around the time of birth as a result of elevated serum steroid levels.

Lamb

The gestation period of the ewe is about 145 days. The thymus and lymph nodes are recognizable by 35 and 50 days postconception, respectively, but the Peyer's patches appear only at 60 days. Peripheral blood lymphocytes are seen in fetal lambs by day 32. Fetal liver lymphocytes can respond to phytohemagglutinin by 38 days. Lambs can produce antibodies to phage φx 174 at day 41 and reject allogeneic skin grafts by day 77. Class II positive cells are detectable by 35 days and a few T6, T4 and T8 positive cells can be detected by 40 days. Cell surface Ig is seen at day 58. C3 receptors appear by day 120 but Fc receptors do not appear until the animal is born. Antibodies to SV40 virus can be provoked by day 90, to T4 phage by day 105, to bluetongue virus by day 122 and to lymphocytic choriomeningitis virus by day 140.

Piglet

The gestation period of the sow is about 115 days. The porcine thymus develops by 40 days postconception. Fetal piglets can produce antibodies to parvoviruses at 58 days and can reject allografts at approximately the same time. Their lymphocytes can respond to phytohemagglutinin between 72 and 90 days. NK cell activity does not develop until several weeks after birth. The number of circulating Ig-bearing cells rises dramatically between 70 and 80 days. The response to antigens in the fetus is essentially of the IgM type, but newborn and fetal piglets also produce a 4S immunoglobulin that may not have light chains.

Foal

The gestation period of the mare is about 340 days. Lymphoid cells are seen first in the thymus around 60 to 80 days postconception. They are found in the mesenteric lymph node and intestinal lamina propria at 90 days and in the spleen at 175 days. Peripheral blood lymphocytes appear at around 80 days. The equine fetus can respond to coliphage T2 at 200 days postconception and to Venezuelan equine encephalitis at 230 days. Normal newborn foals usually have a significant level of serum IgM prior to suckling. In spite of this, it is claimed that plasma cells are not normally seen until about 240 days.

Puppy

The gestation period of the bitch is about 60 days. The thymus differentiates around day 28 and fetal puppies can respond to phage φx 174 on day 40. Peripheral blood lymphocytes will respond to phytohemagglutinin by 45 days postconception, and these cells can be detected in lymph nodes around 45 to 50 days and in the spleen by 50 to 55 days. The ability to reject allografts also develops around day 45, although the rejection process is slow at this stage, and puppies may be made tolerant by intrauterine injection of antigen prior to day 42. Thymic seeding of T cells to the secondary lymphoid organs and the development of humoral immune responses therefore appears to be a relatively late phenomenon in the dog as compared with the other domestic animals.

Kitten

Data on the ontogeny of the kitten is limited. B cells with cytoplasmic Ig are seen in the fetal liver at 42 days postconception.

Chick

Stem cells arise in the yolk sac membrane and migrate under chemotactic influences to the thymus and bursa at between 5 and 7 days incubation. These cells differentiate within the bursa, and follicles develop within this organ by 12 days. Lymphocytes with surface IgM that are able to bind antigen may be detected in the bursa by 14 days, and antibodies to keyhole limpet hemocyanin and to sheep erythrocytes may be produced by 16 and 18 days incubation, respectively. Lymphocytes with surface IgG develop on day 21 around the time of hatching, whereas IgA-positive cells first appear in the gut by three to seven days after hatching.

Although the immune responses of marsupials are usually slower to develop than in the placental mammals, their immune system may develop remarkably early. Thus, the opossum is born after only 12 to 13 days gestation and can make antibodies to *Salmonella typhosa* and bacteriophage f2 after five days in the pouch (17 to 18 days post-conception!).

Development of Phagocytic Capability

In the fetal pig, peripheral blood leukocytes taken at 87 to 90 days postconception are fully capable of phagocytosing particles such as *Staphylococcus aureus.* They are, however, deficient in bactericidal capacity, which only reaches adult levels by 100 days. Near the time of birth the phagocytic and bactericidal capacity of these leukocytes declines as a result of an increase in fetal glucocorticoid synthesis. After birth, macrophages appear to have a depressed chemotactic responsiveness, and they are also able to support the growth of many viruses that macrophages from adult animals do not. Viricidal activity is gradually acquired, although this process appears to be under thymic influence. (The cells from neonatally thymectomized mice do not acquire this resistance, perhaps as a result of a deficiency of γ interferon.) The serum of newborn animals is also deficient in some complement components, resulting in a poor opsonic activity that is reflected in an increased susceptibility to infection.

Influence of the Ontogeny of the Immune System on Intrauterine Infection

Although the fetus is not totally defenseless, it is less capable than the adult of combating infection. It has been demonstrated that tissues taken from calves at 95 days postconception produce α and β interferon in amounts similar to those generated in adult tissues. It has also been shown, however, that the fetus is defective in production of γ interferon. Consequently, there are several diseases that may be mild or inapparent in the mother yet severe or lethal in the fetus. Examples of such diseases include bluetongue, infectious bovine rhinotracheitis (IBR), bovine virus diarrhea (BVD), rubella in humans and the protozoan infection toxoplasmosis.

In general, the response to these organisms is determined by the state of immunological development of the fetus. For example, if bluetongue virus vaccine, which is nonpathogenic for normal adult sheep, is given to pregnant ewes at 50 days postconception, it causes severe lesions in the nervous system of fetal lambs, including hydranencephaly and retinal dysplasia, whereas if it is given at 100 days postconception or to newborn lambs, only a mild glial response is seen. Bluetongue vaccine virus given to fetal lambs between 50 and 70 days postconception may be isolated from lamb tissues for several weeks, but if given after 100 days, re-isolation is not usually possible. Akabane virus acts in a similar fashion in lambs. If given prior to 30 to 36 days postconception, it causes congenital deformities such as hydranencephaly and arthrogryposis. If given to older fetuses, it provokes antibody formation and is much less likely to cause deformities.

Piglets that receive parvovirus before 55 days gestation will usually be aborted or stillborn. After 72 days gestation, however, piglets will normally develop high titers of antibodies to the parvovirus and survive.

Prenatal infection of calves with IBR virus produces an invariably fatal disease, in contrast to postnatal infection, which is relatively mild. The transition between these two types of infection occurs during the last month of pregnancy.

Infection of fetal calves with BVD prior to the development of their ability to mount an immune response to this virus (day 200) leads to fetal death as a result of the development of severe malformations involving the cerebellum and ocular tracts. If calves persistently infected with noncytopathic BVD *in utero* are later infected with cytopathic BVD virus, they develop mucosal disease. Fetal infections commonly lead to lymphoreticular hyperplasia and elevated immunoglobulin levels. For this reason the presence of significant levels of immunoglobulins in a newborn, unsuckled animal is generally considered to be indicative of intrauterine antigenic stimulation.

IMMUNE RESPONSE OF NEWBORN ANIMALS

After developing in the sterile environment of the uterus, newborn animals are launched into an environment rich in antigens. The young of the domestic animals are capable of mounting immune responses at birth. However, any immune response mounted by a newborn animal must, of necessity, be a primary response with a prolonged lag period and low concentrations of antibodies. Therefore, unless "immunological assistance" is provided, newborn animals may succumb rapidly to organisms that present little threat to an adult. This "immunological assistance" is rendered in the form of passive immunity by means of antibody transferred from the mother to her offspring through colostrum. Evidence suggests that maternal lymphoid cells may also be transferred to the fetus via the placenta or to newborn animals through colostrum and transintestinal migration, but the biological significance of this is unclear.

Transfer of Immunity From Mother to Offspring

The route by which maternal antibodies reach the fetus is determined by the nature of the placental barrier (Table 13–1). In humans and other primates, the placenta is hemochorial, the maternal blood is in direct contact with the trophoblast. This type of placentation allows maternal IgG but not IgM, IgA or IgE to transfer to the fetus. In this way, maternal IgG may enter the fetal blood stream and the newborn human infant may have circulating IgG levels comparable to those of its mother. As a result of this IgG transfer, the infant is protected against septicemic infection. Nevertheless, the intestine of the human infant is not protected by this circulating IgG, so that the IgA required to protect the intestine from infection must be provided from maternal milk. As a result, infants who are not breastfed are more likely to suffer from digestive disturbances than those who are.

Dogs and cats possess an endotheliochorial placenta in which the chorionic epithelium is in contact with the endothelium of the maternal capillaries. In these species a small amount of IgG (5 to 10 per cent) may transfer from

Table 13–1 RELATIONSHIP BETWEEN PLACENTAL TYPE AND TRANSFER OF IMMUNOGLOBULINS FROM MOTHER TO FETUS VIA PLACENTA OR COLOSTRUM

Species	Type of Placentation	Tissue Layers Intervening Between Maternal and Fetal Circulation	Placental Transfer of Immunoglobulin	Colostral Transfer of Immunoglobulin
Pig, horse, donkey	Epitheliochorial	6*	0	+ + +
Ruminants	Syndesmochorial	5	0	+ + +
Dog and cat	Endotheliochorial	4	+	+ + +
Primates	Hemochorial	3	+ +	+
Rodents	Hemendothelial	1	+ + +	+

*Maternal capillary endothelium, uterine tissue, uterine epithelium, chorionic epithelium, fetal connective tissue and fetal capillary endothelium

the mother to the puppy or kitten, but most is obtained through colostrum.

The placenta of ruminants is syndesmochorial, that is, the chorionic epithelium is in direct contact with uterine tissues; the placenta of horses and pigs is epitheliochorial, and the fetal chorionic epithelium is in contact with intact uterine epithelium. In animals with these types of placentation, the transplacental passage of immunoglobulin molecules is totally prevented, and the newborn of these species are thus entirely dependent on antibodies received through the colostrum.

Secretion and Composition of Colostrum and Milk

Colostrum represents the accumulated secretions of the mammary gland over the last few weeks of pregnancy together with proteins transferred from the blood stream under the influence of estrogens and progesterone. It is, therefore, rich in IgG and IgA but also contains some IgM and IgE (Table 13–2). The predominant immunoglobulin in the colostrum of most of the major domestic animals is IgG, which may account for 65 to 90 per cent of its total immunoglobulin content; IgA and the other immunoglobulins are usually minor but significant components. As lactation progresses and colostrum changes to milk, differences emerge between species. In primates and humans, IgA predominates in both colostrum and milk. In pigs and horses IgG predominates in colostrum but its concentration drops rapidly as lactation proceeds (Fig. 13–2) and IgA predominates in milk. In ruminants, IgG1 is the predominant immunoglobulin in both milk and colostrum.

All of the IgG, most of the IgM and about half of the IgA in bovine colostrum are derived from serum, but only 30 per cent of the IgG and 10 per cent of the IgA in milk are so derived, the rest being produced locally in the udder. Colostrum also contains secretory component both in the free form and bound to IgA.

Absorption of Colostrum

Young animals that suckle soon after birth take colostrum into their intestinal tracts. In these young animals, the level of proteolytic activity in the digestive tract is low, and is further reduced by trypsin inhibitors in colostrum. Therefore, colostral proteins are not degraded and used as a food source but instead reach the small intestine intact. In the ileum they are actively taken up by epithelial cells through pinocytosis and passed through these cells into the lacteals and possibly the intestinal capillaries. Eventually the absorbed immunoglobulin reaches the systemic circulation and newborn animals thus obtain a massive transfusion of maternal immunoglobulin.

The domestic animals differ in the selectivity and duration of their intestinal permeability. In the horse and pig, protein absorption is selective, IgG and IgM being preferentially absorbed while SIgA is left in the intestine. In ruminants, the intestine is unselectively permeable and all immunoglobulin isotypes are absorbed, although IgA is gradually re-excreted. Young pigs and probably other young animals possess large amounts of free secretory component within their intestinal tract. Colostral IgA and, to a lesser extent, IgM can bind to this secretory component, which may serve to inhibit their absorption.

The period for which the intestine is permeable to proteins varies between species and between isotypes. In general, permeability is

Table 13–2 COLOSTRAL IMMUNOGLOBULIN LEVELS IN DOMESTIC ANIMALS

| Species | Immunoglobulin (mg/100 ml) | | | | |
	IgA	IgM	IgG	IgG(T)	IgG(B)
Horse	500–1500	100–350	1500–5000	500–2500	50–150
Bovine	100–700	300–1300	3400–8000		
Sheep	100–700	400–1200	4000–6000		
Pig	950–1050	250–320	3000–7000		
Dog	500–2200	14–57	120–300		

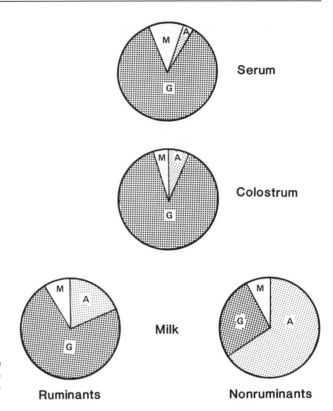

Figure 13–2. The relative concentrations of the major immunoglobulin isotypes in serum, colostrum and the milk of ruminants and nonruminants.

highest immediately after birth and declines after about six hours, perhaps because the intestinal cells that absorb immunoglobulins are replaced by a more mature cell population. The length of the absorptive period is a matter of debate among authorities. As a general rule, absorption of all immunoglobulin isotypes will have dropped to a relatively low level after approximately 24 hours. Feeding colostrum tends to hasten this closure while delaying feeding results in a slight delay of closure.

Unsuckled animals normally possess extremely low levels of immunoglobulin in their serum. The successful absorption of colostral immunoglobulin immediately supplies them with serum immunoglobulin (particularly IgG) at a level approaching that found in adults (Fig. 13–3). Because of the nature of the absorptive process, peak serum immunoglobulin levels are normally reached between 12 and 24 hours after birth. After absorption ceases, these passively acquired antibodies will immediately commence to decline through normal catabolic processes. The rate of decline depends upon the immunoglobulin

isotype involved (see Table 13–4), while the time taken for the immunoglobulins to decline to unprotective levels depends on their initial concentration.

As intestinal absorption takes place, a proteinuria is seen in young animals. This is due to the absorption from the intestine of proteins such as β lactoglobulin and polypeptides that are sufficiently small to be excreted in the urine. In addition, the glomeruli of newborn animals are permeable to macromolecules so that the urine of neonatal ruminants also contains intact immunoglobulin molecules. The proteinuria ceases spontaneously with the termination of intestinal absorption.

The secretions of the mammary gland gradually change from colostrum to milk. Milk is rich in both IgG1 and IgA in ruminants and in IgA in nonruminants (Table 13–3). For the first few weeks in life, while proteolytic digestion is poor, these immunoglobulins can be found throughout the length of the intestine and in the feces of young animals. As the digestive ability of the intestine increases, eventually only those IgA molecules protected

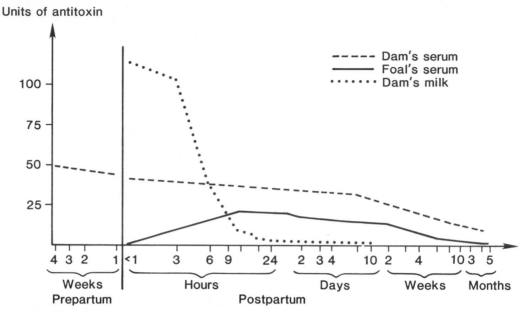

Figure 13–3. *Clostridium perfringens* antitoxin levels in serum, colostrum and milk of six pony mares and in the serum of their foals from birth to five months. (After Jeffcott L. B. 1974. J Comp Pathol 84 96. Used with permission.)

by secretory component are left intact. SIgA is therefore continuously present in the intestine of young animals and is the most important factor that protects them against enteric infection. The amount of IgA in the intestine can be relatively large; for instance, a three-week-old piglet may receive 1.6 g daily from the sow's milk.

The protective role of IgA has been discussed in Chapter 12. It must be pointed out here, however, that IgA may also serve to control the absorption of intact antigen molecules by neonates. Children who are fed cow's milk and lack IgA commonly develop IgE antibodies to bovine milk proteins. The IgA deficiency permits antigens to be absorbed and reach cells capable of mounting an IgE response. This is a good example of IgA serv-

ing as a primary defensive mechanism while IgE serves a secondary role (see Fig. 12–7).

CONSEQUENCES OF THE FAILURE OF PASSIVE TRANSFER (FPT)

The initial transfusion of IgG from colostrum is required for the protection of the young animal against septicemic disease. The continuous intake of IgA or IgG1 is required for protection against enteric disease. Failure of either of these processes predisposes a young animal to infection. In addition, for reasons unknown, it has been shown that colostrum-deprived lambs are neutropenic and that their few remaining neutrophils are relatively inef-

Table 13–3 MILK IMMUNOGLOBULIN LEVELS IN DOMESTIC ANIMALS

| Species | Immunoglobulin (mg/100 ml) | | | | |
	IgA	IgM	IgG	IgG(T)	IgG(B)
Horse	50–100	5–10	20–50	5–20	0
Bovine	10–50	10–20	50–750		
Sheep	5–12	0–7	60–100		
Pig	300–700	30–90	100–300		
Dog	110–620	10–54	1–3		

ficient at phagocytosis compared with neutrophils from colostrum-fed animals. The inflammatory responses of these animals are also depressed.

There are three major reasons for the failure of adequate colostral transfer. First, the colostrum may be insufficient or of poor quality. Second, there may be sufficient colostrum but inadequate intake by the newborn animal. The third possible reason for failure of passive transfer is due to a failure of absorption from the intestine despite an adequate intake of good quality colostrum.

Insufficient Colostrum

Since colostrum represents the accumulated secretions of the udder in late pregnancy, premature births may result in an insufficient quantity of colostrum being available for the offspring. Valuable colostrum may also be lost from animals in which there is excessive dripping of mammary secretions prior to birth.

Inadequate Intake

This may be due, in sheep or pigs for example, to too many offspring, since the amount of colostrum produced does not rise in proportion to the number of young. It may be caused by poor mothering, an important problem among young, inexperienced mothers. It also

may be due to weakness in the newborn or to physical problems such as damaged teats or jaw defects.

Failure of Intestinal Absorption

Failure of intestinal absorption is a major cause for concern in any species. It is especially important in the equine industry not only because of the value of many foals but also because even with good husbandry, about 25 per cent of newborn foals fail to obtain sufficient quantities of immunoglobulin.

Foals need to have at least 400mg/dl of IgG in their serum after receiving colostrum in order to ensure sufficient protection. Foals that receive less than this are at increased risk of infection. If their IgG level fails to reach 200 mg IgG/dl, severe infections are assured (Fig. 13–4.)

Diagnosis of FPT

The success of passive transfer cannot be evaluated in a foal until about 18 hours after birth, once antibody absorption is essentially complete. Several different assays for immunoglobulin are available. The most rapid and economic procedure is the zinc sulfate turbidity test. This involves the use of a zinc sulfate solution, which is mixed with the foal serum.

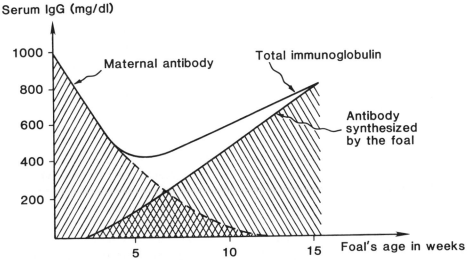

Figure 13–4. The levels of immunoglobulin in foal serum during the first 15 weeks of life, showing the relative contributions of maternal antibody and antibody synthesized by the foal.

Zinc sulfate causes globulins to precipitate out of solution so the result can be read visually or spectrophotometrically. In total failure of transfer, the reaction mixture remains clear. In sera containing IgG, the zinc sulfate precipitates the immunoglobulin and the mixture is turbid. Alternatively, the optical density of the mixture can be read in a spectrophotometer. The IgG concentration of the serum may then be read from a standard curve.

Single radial immunodiffusion is a more accurate method in that it is both quantitative and specific for IgG. As described in Chapter 11, known standards are compared with the test serum by measuring the diameter of precipitation produced in agar gel containing specific antiserum to equine IgG. A diagnosis of failure of passive transfer is made if IgG levels are less than 200 mg/dl and of partial failure of passive transfer if IgG levels are between 200 and 400 mg/dl. Unfortunately, radial immunodiffusion is expensive, and it takes 18 to 24 hours to get a result.

A third method of measuring IgG levels is by use of a latex agglutination test. The latex particles are coated with anti-equine IgG. In the presence of IgG they agglutinate. This test can be performed in about 10 minutes using either whole blood or serum. It appears to be reliable and rapid.

Other, less satisfactory techniques include serum protein electrophoresis, sodium sulfite precipitation and refractometry.

Treatment of FPT

Foals with immunoglobulin levels of more than 400 mg/dl will generally remain healthy and do not require treatment. Healthy foals more than three weeks old with IgG levels between 200 and 400 mg/dl may also remain healthy. However, they should be carefully watched and treated with antibiotics at the first signs of bacterial infection. Any foals with total failure of passive transfer or foals under three weeks of age with partial failure of passive transfer should be treated. The treatment given to foals with partial failure of passive transfer will also depend upon the cleanliness and general state of their environment.

Treatment for FPT involves administration of antibodies. If the foal is younger than 15 hours old, then it can be given oral colostrum. Two to three liters of colostrum should be given by bottle or nasogastric tube in three or four doses at hourly intervals. The colostrum must be free of antibodies to the foal's erythrocytes (see Chapter 21). Colostrum can be obtained from mares that have more than is needed for their own young. It can be stored frozen at $-15°$ to $-20°$ C for up to one year. If stored colostrum is unavailable, then fresh colostrum from primiparous mares can be used.

In foals that are older than 15 hours, an intravenous plasma infusion should be given. Ideally, the dose to be used can be calculated for each case; a level of 600mg IgG/dl is a minimal level to seek to attain. However, if this is not possible, then administration of 20 ml plasma/kg body weight or about 1 liter is usually sufficient.

The plasma to be used should be collected aseptically in large sterile bottles with heparin or sodium citrate. The plasma is collected after the erythrocytes are permitted to settle and stored frozen until used. The plasma must be checked for anti-erythrocyte antibodies and be free of bacterial contamination. The transfusion should be given slowly while the foal is monitored for untoward reactions.

Colostral transfer of immunity is essential for the survival of young animals, but it may also cause problems. If a mother becomes immunized against fetal red cells, colostral antibodies may cause massive erythrocyte destruction in the newborn animal, a condition known as hemolytic disease of the newborn, which is discussed at length in Chapter 21.

TRANSFER OF CELL-MEDIATED IMMUNITY IN MILK

Bovine milk contains up to a million lymphocytes per milliliter, about half of which are T cells. These milk lymphocytes may survive for up 36 hours in the intestine of newborn animals, and some penetrate the intestinal wall and reach the lacteal ducts and the mesenteric lymph nodes. There is evidence that cell-mediated immunity may be transferred to newborn animals in this way. Thus, tuberculin sensitivity, a cell-mediated hypersensitivity reaction, may be transferred to calves by tuberculin-positive cows, and it has been shown that the ability to reject skin grafts or induce tolerance may be transferred to newborn rats through the milk of sensitized mothers. Perhaps more importantly, these transferred cells may be vectors for the transmission of some viruses to the newborn.

DEVELOPMENT OF THE IMMUNE RESPONSE IN NEONATAL ANIMALS

Local Immune Response

By the time colostrum has converted to milk, the lymphoid tissues of the intestine of neonatal animals have become fully responsive to ingested antigen. For example, calves orally vaccinated with coronavirus vaccine at birth are resistant to virulent coronavirus by three to nine days, while piglets vaccinated orally three days after birth with transmissible gastroenteritis virus (TGE) vaccine develop neutralizing antibodies in the intestine 5 to 14 days later. Much of this early resistance is attributable to interferon, but there is an early intestinal IgM response that switches to IgA by about two weeks. In the growing animal, the SIgA response appears earlier and reaches adult levels well in advance of the other immunoglobulins. This ability of the unprimed intestinal tract to respond rapidly to antigens is also seen in germ-free pigs. In these animals, antibody synthesis in the intestinal tract can be detected by four days, and the intestine appears to become immunologically "normal" by ten days after infection with *E. coli*.

Systemic Immune Response

As described in Chapter 9, the level of the immune response is controlled in part by negative feedback, whereby specific antibody inhibits further production of more antibody of the same specificity. The passive immunization of the newborn animal by maternal antibody also inhibits the immune response of the young animal. The precise mechanisms of this suppression are not clear, but it is probably due both to central suppression and to antigen masking and sequestration. If calves fail to suckle and are therefore hypogammaglobulinemic, they will begin to synthesize their own immunoglobulin by about one week of age. In calves that have suckled and thus have serum immunoglobulins, immunoglobulin synthesis does not commence until about four weeks of age. Colostrum-deprived piglets respond well to pseudorabies (Aujesky's disease) virus by two days after birth, but if they are suckled immunoglobulin synthesis does not commence until they are five to six weeks old. Colostrum-deprived lambs synthesize IgG1 at one week and IgG2 by three to four weeks; if lambs are colostrum-fed, however, IgG2 synthesis does not occur until five to six weeks.

Not only does passively derived maternal antibody inhibit neonatal immunoglobulin synthesis, it also prevents the successful vaccination of young animals. This refractory period may persist for many months, its length depending on the amount of antibody transferred to the neonate and the half-life of the immunoglobulins involved.

This problem can be illustrated using the example of vaccination of puppies against canine distemper, but it must be emphasized that the same problems arise in the employment of all vaccines in young animals, including birds that receive antibodies from their mothers through the yolk.

Maternal antibodies, absorbed from the puppy's intestine on suckling, reach maximal levels in serum by 12 to 24 hours after birth. Thereafter, as homologous immunoglobulins, their levels will decline through catabolism. The catabolic rate of proteins is exponential and can therefore be expressed as a half-life (Table 13–4). Thus, the half-life of antibodies to distemper and canine infectious hepatitis is 8.4 days, and the half-life of antibodies to

Table 13–4 METABOLIC HALF-LIVES OF SERUM IMMUNOGLOBULINS IN DOMESTIC
ANIMALS AND MAN

| Species | IgG | Half-life (days) | | | |
		IgM	IgA	IgG(T)	IgE
Horse	11.5–23	*	*	20	*
Bovine	17(G1)–22(G2)	2.8	4.8		2.0
Sheep	14.5(G1)–10.6(G2)	1.8	4.1		*
Pig	6.5–22.5	2.3	3.5–6.5		*
Chicken	4.1	1.7	*		*
Human	23	6.0	5.0		2.7

*Figures not currently available to the author.

feline panleukopenia is 9.5 days (Fig. 13–5). On the average, the level of passively acquired antibodies to distemper in puppies will have declined to insignificant levels by about 10 to 12 weeks, although in extreme cases they may persist for as long as 16 weeks. In a population of puppies, the proportion of susceptible animals therefore increases gradually from a very few or none at birth, to almost all at 10 to 12 weeks. Puppies that are susceptible to the disease are also able to be vaccinated. Immediately after birth few puppies can be successfully vaccinated, but by 10 to 12 weeks almost all can. If canine distemper were not enzootic in Western Europe and North America, it would be sufficient to delay vaccination until all puppies were 12 weeks old, thus ensuring that all were capable of being successfully vaccinated. Unfortunately, a delay of this type would mean that an increasing proportion of puppies, fully susceptible to disease, would be without immune protection—an unacceptable situation. It is not feasible to vaccinate all puppies repeatedly at short intervals from birth to 12 weeks, a procedure that would ensure almost complete protection; a compromise must therefore be reached.

One possible protocol is to vaccinate puppies at 9 to 10 weeks when about 30 per cent of puppies are susceptible and capable of being effectively vaccinated, and then give a second dose at 16 weeks in order to boost the successfully vaccinated puppies and to protect those not protected by the first dose.

A simpler procedure is to vaccinate all puppies when presented and then revaccinate at 12 to 16 weeks. There are many similar alternative procedures, all aimed at conferring early protection while leaving as few puppies as possible unprotected. Colostrum-deprived orphan pups may be vaccinated at two weeks of age. Similar considerations apply in the case of cats being vaccinated with feline panleukopenia vaccine (Fig. 13–5).

An alternative method of overcoming the problems caused by maternal immunity to canine distemper is by the use of measles vaccine. Measles virus shares a major antigen, the F antigen, with canine distemper virus. The two viruses also possess distinctly different hemagglutinins (HA antigens). Generally, the presence of antibodies directed against both F and HA antigens is required for effective virus neutralization and complete protection, but antibodies to the individual antigens give partial protection. Thus, maternal antidistemper HA antibodies cannot prevent measles infection of puppy cells. The measles virus F antigen may then prime the puppy's immune system. As a result, measles vaccine given to puppies at six weeks of age may give puppies some protection against distemper in spite of the presence of a high level of antidistemper HA antibody.

Similar considerations apply when vaccinating large farm animals but it must be emphasized that there is tremendous variability in the persistence of maternal antibodies. The prime factor influencing this persistence will be the level of antibody in the mother at the time she is making colostrum. Thus maternally derived antibodies to equine influenza virus may be gone by two weeks after birth while antibodies to tetanus toxin can last for six months. Antibodies to bovine virus diarrhea may persist for up to nine months in calves.

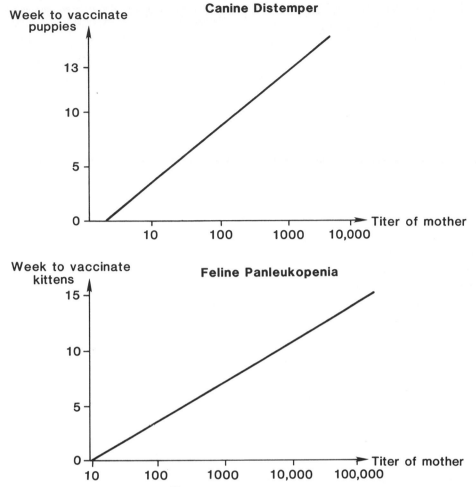

Figure 13–5. Nomographs showing the relationship between the antibody titer of the mother and the age at which to vaccinate her offspring with modified live virus vaccine. (Data from Scott *et al.* 1970. JAVMA *156* 439–453 [FPL] and from Baker *et al.* 1959. Cornell Vet *49* 158–167 [CB]. Used with permission.)

A safe rule is that calves and foals vaccinated before six months of age should always be revaccinated at six months or after weaning.

Specific antiserum may be given in circumstances of doubtful immunity when immediate protection is needed. This form of treatment tends to complicate analysis of these situations, since it prolongs the time required before passive immunity wanes and active immunization can be successfully initiated.

Passive Immunity in the Chick

Serum immunoglobulins are readily transferred from hen serum to the yolk while the egg is still in the ovary. In the fluid phase of the yolk, IgG is therefore found at levels equal to those in hen serum. In addition, as the egg passes down the oviduct, IgM and IgA from oviduct secretions are acquired with the albumin. As the chick embryo develops it absorbs some of the yolk IgG, which then appears in its circulation. The maternal IgM and IgA from the albumin diffuse into the amniotic fluid and are swallowed by the embryo, so that when the chick hatches it possesses IgG in its serum and IgM and IgA in its intestine. The newly hatched chick does not absorb all its yolk sac antibody until about 24 hours after hatching. These maternal antibodies effectively prevent successful vaccination until they disappear at between 10 and 20 days after hatching.

ADDITIONAL SOURCES OF INFORMATION

Campbell SG, Siegel MJ and Knowlton BJ. 1977. Sheep immunoglobulins and their transmission to the neonatal lamb. N.Z. Vet. J. 25 361–365.

Crawford TB and Perryman LE. 1980. Diagnosis and treatment of failure of passive transfer in the foal. Equine Pract. 2 17–23.

Fahey KJ and Morris B. 1978. Humoral immune responses in fetal sheep. Immunology 35 651–661.

Halliday R. 1978. Immunity and health in young lambs. Vet. Rec. 103 489–492.

Huh ND, Kim YB, Koren HS and Amos DB. 1981. Natural killing and antibody-dependent cellular cytotoxicity in specific pathogen-free miniature swine and germ-free piglets. Int. J. Cancer 28 175–178.

Kruse-Elliott K and Wagner PC. 1984. Failure of passive antibody transfer in the foal. Comp. Cont. Ed. Pract. Vet. 6 702–706.

Liu IKM, Pascoe DR, Chang LWS and Zee YC. 1985. Duration of maternally derived antibodies against equine influenza in newborn foals. Am. J. Vet. Res. 46 2078–2080.

Mackay CR, Maddox JF and Brandon MR. 1986. Thymocyte subpopulations during early fetal development in sheep. J. Immunol. 136 1592–1599.

Perryman LE, McGuire TC and Torbeck RL. 1980. Ontogeny of lymphocyte function in the equine fetus. Am. J. Vet. Res. 41 1197–1200.

Reynolds JD and Morris B. 1983. The evolution and involution of Peyer's patches in fetal and postnatal sheep. Eur. J. Immunol. 13 627–635.

Schultz RD. 1984. The effects of aging on the immune system. Comp. Cont. Ed. Pract. Vet. 6 1096–1105.

Sheldrake RF and Husband AJ. 1985. Intestinal uptake of intact maternal lymphocytes by neonatal rats and lambs. Res. Vet. Sci. 36 10–15.

Toivanen P, Asantila T, Granberg C, Leino A and Hirvonen T. 1978. Development of T cell repertoire in the human and sheep fetus. Immunol. Rev. 42 185–201.

Winters WD. 1981. Time dependent decreases of maternal canine virus antibodies in newborn pups. Vet. Rec. 108 295–299.

14

General Principles of Vaccination and Vaccines

The observation that individuals who had recovered from an infectious disease were resistant to subsequent reinfection long preceded the development of immunology and our understanding of the immune response. In fact, the attempts to reproduce this phenomenon in a controlled fashion by Jenner, Pasteur and Salmon provided the impetus for the early development of immunology. Their efforts to produce immunity by artificial exposure to infectious agents were so successful that many diseases, which had long been major scourges of mankind, were rapidly controlled. Vaccines were successfully developed against smallpox, rabies, tetanus, anthrax, cholera and diphtheria as well as against other diseases, and their success has been respon-

sible, in part, for the phenomenal increase in the world's population.

In general, vaccination involves giving antigen derived from an infectious agent to an animal so that an immune response is mounted and resistance to that infectious agent is achieved. Several criteria first must be satisfied in determining whether vaccination is either possible or desirable in controlling a specific disease. The first is the absolute identification of the causal organism. Although this appears to be an obvious requirement, it has not always been followed in practice. For instance, in the respiratory disease complex of cattle, it is possible to isolate *Pasteurella multocida* or *P. haemolytica* consistently from the lungs of cattle at autopsy. It is not possible, however, to reproduce the disease syndrome by the use of these organisms alone, and evidence suggests that the disease complex owes much to virus infections and immunopathological mechanisms. Nevertheless, pasteurella vaccines have been used in large quantities for many years in attempts to control this condition, despite their relative ineffectiveness.

Second, it must be established that an immune response can, in fact, protect against the disease in question. In some diseases, such as equine infectious anemia, feline infectious peritonitis and Aleutian disease in mink, the immune response is responsible for many of the disease processes. In other infections, such as foot-and-mouth disease in pigs and African swine fever, very poor or no protective immunity can be induced. In African swine fever, antibodies, in spite of being produced in large quantities and being capable of fixing complement or inhibiting viral hemadsorption *in vitro*, are unable to cause virus neutralization. In foot-and-mouth disease in pigs, the immune response is transient and relatively ineffective, so that animals that have been clinically infected become fully susceptible to reinfection as soon as three months later. Thus, for a vaccine to produce prolonged effective immunity against foot-and-mouth disease in pigs, it must induce an immune response superior to that produced by natural infection.

Finally, before using a vaccine we must be sure that the risks of vaccination do not exceed those associated with the chance of contracting the disease itself. A good example of this is pneumonic pasteurellosis of cattle, in which experimental and epidemiological data show that pasteurella bacterins may increase, not reduce, the severity of the lung lesions. In addition, because the detection of antibodies is a common diagnostic procedure, unnecessary use of vaccines may complicate diagnosis based on serological techniques and perhaps make final eradication of a disease impossible. Because of this, the decision to use vaccines for the control of any disease must be based on considerations not only of the severity of the problem but also of the prospects for its control by other techniques.

When vaccines are used to control disease in a population of animals rather than in individuals, the concept of herd immunity should also be considered. Herd immunity is the resistance of an entire group of animals to disease conferred by the presence in that group of a proportion of immune animals. Herd immunity acts by reducing the probability of a susceptible animal meeting an infected one so that the spread of disease is slowed or terminated. If it is acceptable to lose individual animals from disease while preventing epizootics, it may be possible to induce herd immunity by selective vaccination.

TYPES OF IMMUNIZATION PROCEDURES (Fig. 14–1)

There are two methods by which an animal may be rendered immune to infectious disease. One method, termed passive immunization, produces a temporary resistance by transferring antibodies from a resistant to a susceptible animal. These passively transferred antibodies give immediate protection, but, since they are gradually catabolized, this protection wanes and the recipient eventually becomes susceptible to reinfection.

As an alternative procedure to passive immunization, active immunization has much to commend it. This technique involves administering antigen to an animal so that it responds by mounting a protective immune response that may be either antibody- or cell-mediated or both. Reimmunization or exposure to infection will result in a secondary immune response. The disadvantage of this form of immunization is that protection is not conferred immediately. However, once established it is long-lasting and capable of restimulation (Fig. 14–2).

Passive Immunization

Passive immunization requires that antibodies be produced in a donor animal by active immunization and that these antibodies, after partial purification, be given to susceptible

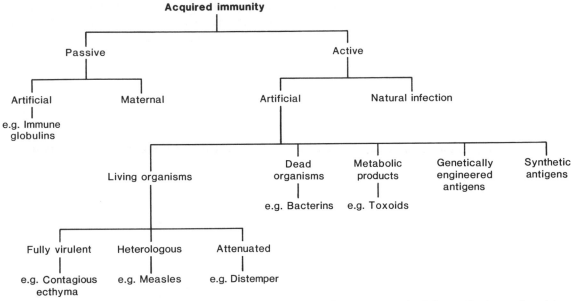

Figure 14–1. A classification of the different types of acquired immunity and of the methods employed to induce protection.

animals in order to confer immediate protection. These antisera may be raised against a wide variety of pathogens. For instance, they can be produced in cattle against anthrax, in dogs against distemper, in cats against panleukopenia and in humans against measles. Their most important role is in protection against toxigenic organisms such as *Clostridium tetani* or *Cl. perfringens*, using antisera raised in horses. Antisera made in this way are known as immune globulins and are generally produced in young horses by a series of immu-

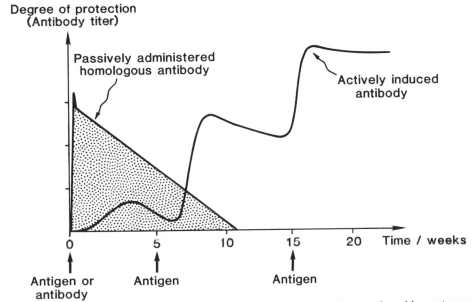

Figure 14–2. The levels of serum antibody (and hence the degree of protection) conferred by active and passive methods of immunization. Note that passive immunization confers immediate protection but wanes by about ten weeks. Active immunization is slow to develop but gives sustained immunity.

nizing inoculations. The toxins of the clostridia are proteins and can be made nontoxic by treatment with formaldehyde. Formaldehyde-treated toxins are known as toxoids. Initially, the horses are given toxoids, but once antibodies are produced, subsequent injections may contain purified toxin. The responses of these animals are monitored, and once their antibody levels are sufficiently high, the horses are bled. Bleeding is undertaken at regular intervals until the titer drops, when the animals are again "boosted" with antigen. Plasma is separated from the horse blood and treated with 48 per cent saturated ammonium sulfate in order to concentrate and purify the globulin fraction. The purified globulin fraction, rich in antibodies to the toxin, is then dialyzed, filtered, titrated and dispensed. It is known as tetanus immune globulin.

In order to check the potency of preparations of immune globulin, comparison must be made with an international biological standard. In the case of tetanus immune globulin, this is done by comparing the dose necessary to protect guinea pigs against a fixed dose of tetanus toxin with the dose of the standard preparation of immune globulin required to do the same. An alternative method of checking the potency of immune globulin preparations is to compare the ability of the test and standard antisera to flocculate a fixed amount of toxin. This method measures the power of the immune globulin to combine with toxin and has certain advantages, since toxins are relatively unstable and their toxicity may fluctuate while their antigenicity remains constant. The international standard immune globulin for tetanus toxin is a quantity held at the Statens Serum-Institute, Copenhagen; an International Unit (I.U.) of tetanus immune globulin is the specific neutralizing activity contained in 0.03384 mg of the international standard. The U.S. Standard Unit (A.U.) is twice the International Unit.

Tetanus immune globulin is given to animals in order to confer immediate protection against tetanus. At least 1500 I.U. of immune globulin should be given to horses and cattle; at least 500 I.U. to calves, sheep, goats and swine; and at least 250 I.U. to dogs. The exact amount should vary with the amount of tissue

damage, the degree of wound contamination and the time elapsed since injury. Tetanus immune globulin is of little use once clinical signs appear, although massive doses of up to 5000 I.U. may be of some assistance.

Although antisera give prompt immunity, certain problems are associated with their use. For instance, horse tetanus immune globulin may be given safely to horses, in which it is not regarded as foreign, and it will persist for a relatively long period of time, being removed only by catabolism. If, however, horse tetanus immune globulin is given to an animal of another species such as a cow or dog, then it is regarded as foreign, an immune response is mounted against it and it is rapidly eliminated. In order to reduce their antigenicity for other species of animals, immune globulins are usually treated with pepsin so as to destroy the immunoglobulin Fc region and leave intact only the portion of the immunoglobulin molecule required for toxin neutralization—the F(ab)'2 fragment.

If the amount of circulating horse serum protein is still relatively large at the time the recipient animal mounts an immune response, the immune complexes formed may participate in a type III hypersensitivity reaction known as serum sickness (Chapter 22). If repeated doses of horse immune globulin are given to an animal, there also exists the possibility of IgE production and the occurrence of a type I hypersensitivity reaction such as anaphylaxis (Chapter 20). Finally, the presence of high levels of circulating antibody may interfere with active immunization against the same antigen. This is a phenomenon similar to that seen in newborn animals passively protected by maternal antibodies.

Monoclonal antibodies represent another potential source of passive protection for animals. At the present time, however, these are mainly made by mouse-mouse hybridomas and thus consist of mouse immunoglobulins. They are therefore able to sensitize animals of other species. Nevertheless, mouse monoclonal antibodies against the F5 (K99) pilus antigens of E. coli can be given orally to calves to protect them against diarrhea caused by this organism. There is no doubt that monoclonal antibodies made by hybridomas derived from cells of the major domestic species would be very useful in veterinary medicine.

Active Immunization

The most important advantages of active immunization compared with passive protection are the prolonged period of protection achieved and the recall and boosting of this protective response by repeated injections of antigen or by exposure to infection. An ideal vaccine for active immunization (vaccination) should, therefore, give prolonged strong immunity. This immunity should be conferred on both the animal vaccinated and any fetus carried by it. In conferring this strong immunity, the vaccine should not cause adverse side effects. The ideal vaccine should be cheap, stable, adaptable to mass vaccination and, ideally, should stimulate an immune response distinguishable from that due to natural infection so that vaccination and eradication may proceed simultaneously.

Living and "Dead" Vaccines

Unfortunately, two of the prerequisites of an ideal vaccine, high antigenicity and absence of adverse side effects, tend to be mutually incompatible. Thus, living organisms stimulate the best immune response but may present hazards as a result of residual virulence, whereas "dead" organisms are relatively poor immunogens but are usually much safer (Table 14–1). The relative advantages and disadvantages of vaccines containing living or "dead" organisms may be seen, for example, in the

Table 14–1 THE RELATIVE MERITS OF LIVING AND DEAD VACCINES

Advantages of Living Vaccines	Advantages of Dead Vaccines
Few inoculating doses required	Stable on storage
Adjuvants unnecessary	Unlikely to cause disease through residual virulence
Less chance of hypersensitivity	Unlikely to contain contaminating organisms
Induction of interferon	
Relatively inexpensive	

vaccines available against *Brucella abortus* in cattle. *B. abortus* is the cause of contagious abortion in cattle, and in the absence of an effective eradication scheme, vaccination is required to control the disease. The organism, however, is a facultative intracellular parasite that is able to live within macrophages and must be controlled by a cell-mediated immune response, although antibodies also contribute to resistance. As a broad generalization, living organisms are much more capable of stimulating cell-mediated immunity than are "dead" organisms. For these reasons, a vaccine containing a living but avirulent strain of *B. abortus* is required for the control of this infection. The vaccine strain of *B. abortus* (strain 19) gives rise to a life-long immunity in cows and successfully prevents abortion, although it may not completely prevent infection (particularly in the udder). Strain 19 is "never" transmitted between cattle and is very stable; its biological properties have not changed since it was first isolated in 1930. In general, it may be regarded as an excellent vaccine.

However, strain 19 may cause systemic reactions, particularly in adult Jersey cows; local swelling at the injection site, high fever, anorexia, listlessness and a drop in milk yield have all been reported to occur following vaccination. Strain 19 may also cause abortion in pregnant cows and, while avirulent for heifers, can cause orchitis in bulls and undulant fever in humans. In addition, a small proportion of vaccinated cattle may remain persistently infected with strain 19 for many months. In order to eradicate brucellosis, it is necessary to employ serological tests to identify infected animals, and strain 19 gives rise to an antibody response that is only with difficulty distinguished from that seen in response to natural infection. One method used to assist in this differentiation is to ensure that strain 19 is given only to heifer calves between 4 and 10 to 12 months of age in the hope that the serum antibody response will have declined to low levels by the time the animal reaches breeding age and is tested for brucellosis. In areas where there is extensive brucellosis, it may be beneficial to use a reduced dose of strain 19 vaccine in adult cattle. In this procedure, adult cattle are given between 300 million and one billion organisms (calves are normally given about 6 billion organisms). This confers resistance to brucellosis, while the antibodies provoked usually decline rapidly. This technique reduces the losses due to the presence of positive serological reactors as well as hastening the elimination of brucellosis from herds. Its disadvantages include the occurrence of occasional persistent titers (reduced considerably by the use of the Rivanol test and the complement fixation test), a consistently positive milk ring test and, occasionally, persistent strain 19 infection. (For further details of the techniques available for distinguishing between *B. abortus* vaccinated and infected cattle, see Chapter 15.)

Because of the disadvantages associated with the use of strain 19, a dead vaccine utilizing a formolized rough strain of *B. abortus* has been developed. This organism (strain 45/20), which is administered in a water-in-oil adjuvant emulsion in two doses, will only protect cattle for less than a year. The immune response to this vaccine is readily distinguishable from that due to an infection, since it is devoid of antigens present on smooth virulent strains (Chapter 15). This vaccine is not permitted in North America but was used with some success in heavily infected herds in the United Kingdom, where slaughter would have been uneconomical. Uninfected animals were vaccinated with strain 45/20 and the infected animals were removed as soon as economics allowed.

The advantages of vaccines that contain dead organisms, such as strain 45/20, are that they are safe with respect to residual virulence and are relatively easy to store, since the organisms are already dead. These advantages of dead vaccines correspond to the disadvantages of live vaccines such as strain 19. That is, some live vaccines may possess residual virulence, not only for the animal for whom the vaccine is made but also for other animals. They may possibly revert to a fully virulent type or spread to unvaccinated animals—a feature not seen when strain 19 is used. The ability of a vaccine to spread can, in some circumstances, be advantageous. For example, the widespread use of living poliovirus vaccine

in humans in the developed countries has resulted in a replacement of the original virulent wild strain in the population by vaccine strains. Live vaccines always present the risk of contamination with unwanted organisms; for instance, outbreaks of reticuloendotheliosis in chickens in Japan and Australia have been traced to contaminated Marek's disease vaccines. It has been suggested, but is as yet unproven, that the adenovirus of poultry EDS 76 (egg drop syndrome 1976) and canine parvovirus may also have been distributed in contaminated vaccines. Contaminating mycoplasma may also be present in some vaccines. Finally, vaccines containing living attenuated organisms require care in their preparation, storage and handling in order to avoid killing the organisms.

The disadvantages of "dead" vaccines correspond to the advantages of living vaccines. Thus, the use of adjuvants to increase effective antigenicity can cause severe local reactions, while multiple dosing or high individual doses of antigen increase the risks of producing hypersensitivity reactions as well as adversely affecting costs. Most important, however, vaccines containing living organisms commonly give a better immunity than vaccines containing inactivated or "dead" organisms. One reason for this is that the living vaccine virus may invade host cells and induce interferon production, thus conferring early protection on susceptible animals. The increased efficacy of live vaccines is probably also due to the distribution of living organisms within the body as well as to the biochemical changes brought about by the killing process.

Inactivation and Attenuation of Organisms Used in Vaccines. If organisms are to be inactivated for use in vaccines, it is desirable that the "dead" organisms be as antigenically similar to the living organisms as possible. Therefore, a crude method of killing organisms such as heating, which causes extensive protein denaturation or lipid oxidation, is usually unsatisfactory. If chemicals are used, it is essential that they produce very little change in the antigens responsible for stimulating protective immunity. One compound used in this way is formaldehyde, which acts on amino and amide groups in proteins and on non-hydrogen bonded amino groups in the purine and pyrimidine bases of nucleic acids to form cross-links and so confer structural rigidity. Proteins can also be mildly denatured by acetone or alcohol treatment. In the case of louping-ill vaccine, alcohol treatment of the virus increases the antigenicity of the vaccine, although the mechanism involved is unknown. Alkylating agents that cross-link nucleic acid chains are also suitable for killing organisms, since by leaving the surface proteins of organisms unmodified, they do not interfere with antigenicity. Examples of alkylating agents include ethylene oxide, ethyleneimine, acetylethyleneimine and β-propiolactone, all of which have been used in veterinary vaccines.

Attenuation

Although the difference between living and "dead" organisms is, in the final analysis, only biochemical, it has a profound influence on the effectiveness of vaccines. As a compromise, therefore, it is possible to reduce the virulence of an organism until, although living, it is no longer capable of causing disease. This process of reduction of virulence is known as attenuation. Simple methods of attenuation include heating organisms to just below their thermal death point or exposing organisms to marginally sublethal concentrations of inactivating chemicals. Presumably, organisms injured by these processes are at a disadvantage when inoculated into an animal and, instead of multiplying rapidly and causing disease, may be phagocytosed and processed for the immune response.

The commonly used methods of attenuation involve adapting organisms to unusual conditions so that they lose their adaptation to their usual host. These techniques include culturing in unfavorable media or at an unfavorable temperature. For example, the BCG (Bacille Calmette-Guérin) strain of *Mycobacterium bovis* was rendered avirulent by being grown for 13 years on bile-saturated medium. The strain of anthrax currently used in vaccines was rendered avirulent by growth in 50 per cent serum agar under an atmosphere rich in CO_2 so that it lost its ability to form a capsule. Pasteur's fowl cholera (*Pasteurella multocida*)

vaccine was grown under conditions in which there was a shortage of nutrients.

Whereas bacteria can be rendered avirulent by culture under abnormal conditions, viruses may be attenuated by growth in species to which they are not naturally adapted. For example, rinderpest virus, which is normally a pathogen of cattle, was first attenuated by growth in goats, but this caprinized virus retained its virulence for some breeds of cattle. In an attempt to solve this problem, a rabbit-adapted (lapinized) vaccine was introduced, which had less residual virulence. In the course of further attempts to obtain a rinderpest vaccine devoid of residual virulence, a tissue culture-adapted vaccine was developed, which has proved extremely successful in controlling this disease in Africa. Similar examples include the adaptation of African horse sickness virus to mice and of canine distemper virus to ferrets.

As an alternative method of attenuation, mammalian viruses may be grown in eggs. This has been done for canine distemper, bluetongue and rabies vaccines. The Flury strain of rabies vaccine has been attenuated by repeated passage through eggs. The high egg passage vaccine (HEP) has been attenuated by 178 passages in eggs and appears to be completely safe for dogs and cats. In the case of some avian viruses, attenuation may be brought about by growth in eggs of another species; for instance, the virus of fowl influenza can be attenuated in pigeon eggs.

At present, the most commonly employed method of attenuation is by prolonged tissue culture, and most veterinary vaccines are now attenuated in this way. Although the tissue culture can be derived from many species, it is common to employ cultures of cells from the species to be vaccinated in order to reduce the side effects resulting from the administration of foreign tissues. In these cases virus attenuation may be accomplished by culturing the organism in cells to which they are not adapted. For example, virulent canine distemper virus preferentially attacks lymphoid cells. For vaccine purposes, therefore, this organism is cultured repeatedly in canine kidney cells, as a result of which its virulence is lost.

An example of attenuation by growth in

unusual species is the SAD (Street-Alabama-Dufferin) strain of rabies virus. This virus, originally isolated from a rabid dog in Alabama, was passaged through mice, hamster kidney tissue culture, chick embryos, porcine kidney tissue culture and, finally, canine kidney tissue culture. When grown on porcine tissue culture, the SAD strain can be used to vaccinate all species of domestic animals; a single dose provides protection for several years. When grown in canine tissue culture, it is used to vaccinate dogs. Unfortunately, SAD rabies vaccine may cause clinical rabies in cats and horses. It cannot, therefore, be used in those species.

Attenuation may be considered to be, in some ways, a primitive form of genetic engineering. The desired result is the development of a genetically stable agent that in some way lacks the ability to cause disease. This may be difficult to achieve, and reversion to virulence is an ever-present risk. It has become increasingly possible, however, to deliberately modify the genes of organisms so that they become effectively and irreversibly attenuated. For example, a pseudorabies vaccine is now available from which the thymidine kinase gene has been removed. Thymidine kinase is required by herpesviruses to replicate in nondividing cells such as neurons. Viruses from which this gene has been removed are able to infect nerve cells but cannot replicate and, therefore, cannot cause disease. As a result, this vaccine not only confers effective protection, but by blocking cell invasion by virulent pseudorabies viruses also prevents the development of a persistent carrier state.

Some vaccination processes use, instead of artificially attenuated organisms, antigenically related organisms normally adapted to another species. For example, measles virus can be used to protect dogs against distemper and bovine virus diarrhea virus can protect against hog cholera.

Finally, under some circumstances it is possible to use fully virulent organisms in vaccination procedures just as the Chinese did with smallpox, although this is generally done only if a better technique is not available. Vaccination against contagious ecthyma of sheep is of this type. Contagious ecthyma (orf) is a disease of lambs that, by causing massive scab formation around the mouth, prevents feeding and thus results in a failure to thrive. The disease has little systemic effect, and lambs recover completely within a few weeks and are immune thereafter. It is usual to vaccinate lambs by rubbing dried, infected scab material into scratches made in the inner aspect of the thigh. The local infection at this site has no untoward effect on the lambs, and they become solidly immune. Because the vaccinated animals may spread the disease, however, it is necessary to separate them from unvaccinated stock for a few weeks.

Some New Approaches to Vaccine Production

Although conventional vaccines have been very successful in controlling infectious diseases, there is always a need for improvement. The use of vaccines containing genetically modified agents such as the TK^- pseudorabies vaccine has already been discussed. Several other unconventional approaches are being studied in attempts to make vaccines more effective, cheaper and safer.

Subunit Vaccines

Recombinant DNA techniques can be employed to isolate genetic material coding for an antigen of interest. This DNA can then be placed in a bacterium, yeast or other cell and permitted to code for that protein. The first attempt to use gene cloning to prepare a veterinary vaccine was with foot-and-mouth disease virus. The purified VP1 gene was cloned into *E. coli* and after expression the VP1 antigen was purified and used in a vaccine for cattle.

Another example of a subunit vaccine is one directed against enteropathogenic *E. coli*. The heat labile enterotoxin of *E. coli* consists of two subunits. The α subunit of the enterotoxin is toxic while the β subunit is responsible for binding of the α subunit to enteric cells. Isolated β subunits are immunogenic and function as effective toxoids. A recombinant vaccine that consists of the cloned β subunit of *E. coli* enterotoxin has been prepared. In this case the β subunit gene was cloned, linked with a powerful promoter and transfected into a non-pathogenic strain of *E. coli*.

Attachment pili of enteropathogenic *E. coli*, for example F4 or F5, can be cloned and the purified pilus proteins incorporated into bacterins. The antipilus antibodies thus provoked will protect animals by preventing bacterial attachment to the intestinal wall.

Recombinant DNA techniques are very useful in any situation where protein antigens need to be synthesized in very large and pure quantities. Unfortunately, pure proteins such as these are often poor antigens because they are not effectively delivered to antigen sensitive cells. An alternative method is therefore to clone the genes of interest into an attenuated living carrier organism.

Subunit Vaccines in Attenuated Carrier Organisms. Genes coding for specific protein antigens may be cloned directly into a variety of organisms. The organism that has been most widely employed for this purpose is vaccinia virus. Vaccinia virus is very easy to administer by dermal scratching. It has a large genome that makes it relatively easy to insert a new gene and it can express high levels of the new antigen. Individuals vaccinated with genetically modified vaccinia virus make high levels of antibodies against the introduced antigen.

Alternative carriers that have been proposed include attenuated Salmonella strains. However, the use of attenuated carrier organisms has some intrinsic limitations and all the disadvantages of modified live vaccines.

Synthetic Peptides

Although globular protein molecules may be very large, they have a limited number of small epitopes. In addition, only a few epitopes are important in inducing protective immunity while others may promote suppression (see Chapter 9). Thus if the structure of a protective epitope is known, it may be chemically synthesized and used in a vaccine. The procedures involved include a complete sequencing of the antigen of interest, followed by identification of the important epitopes. This may be difficult, but the epitopes may be predicted by use of computer models of the protein or by the use of monoclonal antibodies to identify the critical protective components. Once identified, the protective peptides may be synthesized and used in a vaccine.

Attempts are underway to produce such a synthetic vaccine for foot-and-mouth virus protein VP1, since its complete sequence is known. Synthetic peptides based on the structure of VP1 have been synthesized and tested for their immunogenicity. One of these peptides can protect guinea pigs against foot-and-mouth disease and on a weight basis is much more immunogenic than intact VP1. Many other attempts are underway to produce synthetic peptide vaccines. None have yet reached the stage of clinical trials.

Anti-idiotype Vaccines

Antigens, injected into an animal, provoke the appearance of immunoglobulin molecules whose binding site (idiotype) has a complementary structure to that of the inducing epitope. The idiotype network concept suggests that these idiotypes provoke the formation of anti-idiotype antibodies. These anti-idiotype antibodies have a complementary structure to that of the idiotypic epitope. In other words, the binding site on an anti-idiotypic antibody has the same shape as the antigen that induced the idiotype. Thus if the anti-idiotype antibody is used to immunize an animal, the resulting anti–anti-idiotypes will be directed not only against the anti-idiotype but also against the original antigen. The use of an anti-idiotype vaccine, therefore, should provoke a protective response. This has in fact been shown to occur in several experimental situations. It may also provoke a T cell response and thus stimulate cell-mediated immunity. While the use of anti-idiotypes has not yet been used in the field, it presents an exciting new strategy for vaccination.

ADMINISTRATION OF VACCINES

Immunization by subcutaneous or intramuscular injection is the simplest and most usual method of administration of vaccines. This approach is obviously excellent for relatively small numbers of animals and for diseases in which systemic immunity is important. However, in some conditions, systemic immunity is not as important as local immunity, and it is perhaps more appropriate to administer the vaccine at the site of potential invasion. Therefore, intranasal vaccines are available for infectious bovine rhinotracheitis of cattle, for feline rhinotracheitis and calicivirus infections and for infectious bronchitis and Newcastle disease in poultry. Unfortunately, these techniques require that each animal be dealt with on an individual basis. When their numbers are very large, other methods must be employed. Aerosolization of vaccines enables them to be inhaled by all the animals in a flock. This technique is employed in vaccinating against canine distemper and mink enteritis on mink ranches, and against Newcastle disease in poultry. Alternatively, the vaccine may be put in the feed or drinking water; this is done with *Erysipelothrix rhusiopathiae* vaccines in pigs and against Newcastle disease, infectious laryngotracheitis and avian encephalomyelitis in poultry. Fish and shrimp may be vaccinated by adding antigen to the water in which they live.

Adjuvants

In veterinary medicine, adjuvants are usually required to potentiate the immunogenicity of dead vaccines and toxoids (Table 14–2). One

exception to this is the use of saponin in anthrax vaccines, where it is required to destroy tissue at the site of injection so that the anthrax spores may germinate. Saponin is also employed as an adjuvant for foot-and-mouth disease vaccines in which it appears to stimulate T cell activity. Unfortunately saponin is very destructive. Diethylaminoethyl (DEAE) dextran may be an effective substitute for it. Oil-based adjuvants are not usually appropriate for use in animals intended for human consumption, since the oil may track through fascial planes and spoil the meat. Freund's complete adjuvant is quite unacceptable in food animals, not only because of the mineral oil, but also because the mycobacteria in the adjuvant will render animals positive to tuberculin, a critical drawback in any area where tuberculosis is under control. There is also evidence to suggest that Freund's complete adjuvant may be carcinogenic. By far the most widely employed adjuvants in commercial veterinary vaccines are those that employ insoluble salts such as aluminum hydroxide, aluminum phosphate or aluminum potassium sulfate (alum). These adjuvants are produced in the form of a colloidal suspension to which the antigenic material is adsorbed. They are stable on storage, a feature not generally found in the oil-based adjuvants, and while they produce a small local granuloma on inoculation, they do not track nor make large parts of the carcass unsuitable for consumption. This type of adjuvant may therefore be considered to be the most suitable type for animals at present. (For more information on adjuvants see Chapter 27.)

Mixed Vaccines

Because of the complexity of many animal disease syndromes, it has become commonplace to employ complex mixtures of organisms in single vaccines. For respiratory diseases of cattle, for example, vaccines are available that contain infectious bovine rhinotracheitis (IBR), bovine virus diarrhea (BVD), parainfluenza 3 (PI3) and even *P. multocida*. Such a mixture may be of use in outbreaks of respiratory disease in which exact diagnosis is not possible, and may protect animals against several diseases with economy of effort. It can

Table 14–2 SOME EXAMPLES OF ADJUVANTS EMPLOYED IN VETERINARY MEDICINE

Adjuvant	Vaccine
Aluminum hydroxide	Leptospira
	Campylobacter
	Pasteurella
	Erysipelas
	Clostridia
	Anaplasma
Aluminum phosphate	Fusobacterium
Water-in-oil	Foot-and-mouth disease
	Brucella 45/20
Saponin	Foot-and-mouth disease
	Anthrax
DEAE dextran	Foot-and-mouth disease

be considered extremely wasteful, however, to use vaccines against organisms that may not be causing problems. Dogs may be given vaccines containing up to six of the following organisms—canine distemper virus, canine adenovirus 1, canine adenovirus 2, canine parvovirus, canine parainfluenza virus, leptospira bacterin and rabies vaccine—with a considerable saving in time and effort. When different antigens in a mixture are inoculated simultaneously, competition occurs between antigens. Manufacturers of mixed vaccines take this into account and modify their mixtures accordingly. However, vaccines should never be mixed indiscriminately, since one component may dominate the mixture and interfere with the response to the other components.

Vaccination Schedules

Although it is not possible to give exact schedules for each of the veterinary vaccines available, certain principles are common to all methods of active immunization.

Since newborn animals are passively protected by maternal antibodies, it is not usually possible to vaccinate animals successfully early in life. If simulation of immunity is deemed necessary at this stage, the mother may be vaccinated during the later stages of pregnancy, the vaccinations being timed so that peak antibody levels are achieved at the time of colostrum formation.

Once an animal is born, successful active vaccination is usually possible only after passive immunity has waned. Since it is rarely possible to predict the exact time of loss of maternal immunity, it is necessary to vaccinate young animals at least twice. The second injection is given at about 15 weeks of age in small animals and at six months in larger animals to ensure successful vaccination.

The interval between doses of vaccines varies; "dead" vaccines, which produce weak immunity, may require frequent administration, perhaps as often as every six months, whereas living vaccines, which usually produce a long-lasting immunity, may require administration only once every two or three years. The interval between vaccination doses

is also determined by the disease. Some diseases are seasonal, and vaccines may be given prior to the time disease outbreaks are expected. Examples of these include the vaccine against the lungworm *Dictyocaulus viviparus* given in early summer just prior to the anticipated lungworm season, the vaccine against anthrax given in spring, and the vaccine against *Clostridium chauvoei* given to sheep before turning them out to pasture. Bluetongue of lambs is spread by midges (*Culicoides varipennis*) and is thus a disease of midsummer and early fall. Vaccination in spring will therefore protect lambs during the susceptible period.

FAILURES IN VACCINATION
(Fig. 14–3)

There are many reasons why a vaccine will fail to confer protective immunity on an animal. In some cases the vaccine may actually be ineffective. This could be because it contains the wrong strain of organisms or the wrong antigens. The method of manufacture may have destroyed the protective epitopes or there may simply be insufficient antigen in the vaccine. Problems of this type are relatively uncommon and can generally be avoided by only using vaccines from reputable manufacturers. Of much greater significance is the failure of an effective vaccine to stimulate protective immunity. In some cases this may be attributed to unsatisfactory administration. A live vaccine may have "died" as a result of either poor storage, the use of antibiotics in conjunction with live bacterial vaccines, the use of chemicals to sterilize syringes or the excessive use of alcohol while swabbing the skin. Sometimes, animals given vaccines by nonconventional routes may not be protected. When large flocks of poultry or mink are to be vaccinated, it is common to administer the vaccine either as an aerosol or in drinking water. If the aerosol is not evenly distributed throughout a building, or if some animals do not drink, they may receive insufficient vaccine. Animals that subsequently suffer from disease may be interpreted as cases of vaccine failure.

Even animals given an adequate dose of an

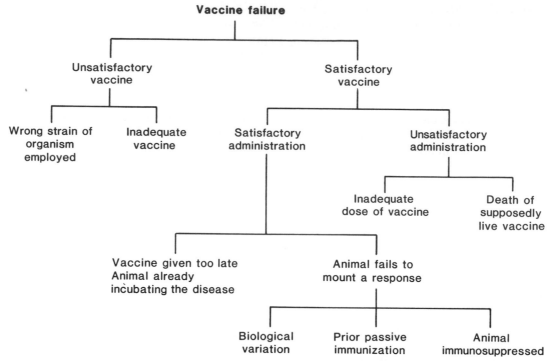

Figure 14–3. A classification of the ways in which a vaccine may fail to protect an animal.

effective vaccine may fail to be protected. If the vaccinated animal was incubating the disease prior to inoculation then the vaccine may be given too late to affect the course of the disease.

The immune response, being a biological process, never confers absolute protection and is never equal in all members of a vaccinated population. Since the immune response is influenced by a large number of genetic and environmental factors, the range of immune responses in a large random population of animals tends to follow a normal distribution (Fig. 14–4). This means that most animals tend to respond to antigens by mounting an average immune response, a few will mount an excellent response but a small proportion will mount a very poor immune response. This group of poor responders may not be protected against infection in spite of having received an effective vaccine. Therefore, it is impossible to protect 100 per cent of a random population of animals by vaccination. The size of this unreactive portion of the population will vary between vaccines, and its significance will depend on the nature of the disease. Thus,

for highly infectious diseases against which herd immunity is poor and in which infection is rapidly and efficiently transmitted, such as foot-and-mouth disease, the presence of unprotected animals could permit the spread of disease and would thus disrupt control programs. Likewise, problems can arise if the unprotected animals are individually important, for example companion animals. In contrast, for diseases that are inefficiently spread, such as rabies, 60 to 70 per cent protection may be sufficient to effectively block disease transmission within a population and may therefore be quite satisfactory from a public health viewpoint.

Another group of vaccine failures occur when the normal immune response is suppressed. For example, heavily parasitized or malnourished animals may be immunosuppressed and should not be vaccinated. Stress in general, including pregnancy, extremes of cold and heat, fatigue or malnourishment, may reduce a normal immune response, probably because of increased steroid production. This type of immunosuppression is discussed in detail in Chapter 26. The most important

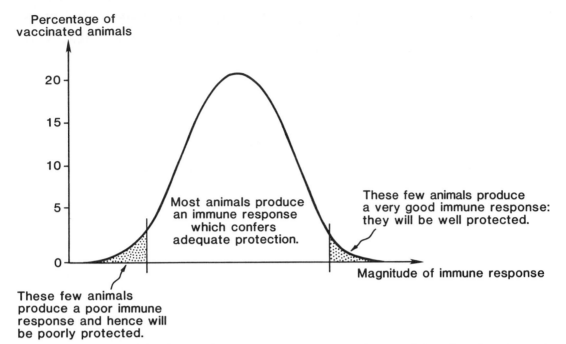

Figure 14–4. The normal distribution of protective immune responses in a population of vaccinated animals.

cause of vaccine failure of this type is due to the presence of passively derived maternal immunity in young animals as described in Chapter 13.

ADVERSE CONSEQUENCES OF VACCINATION

Residual virulence and toxicity, allergic effects, disease in immunodeficient hosts, neurological complications and harmful effects on the fetus are the most significant risks associated with the use of vaccines. For example, lesions of mucosal disease may be seen in calves vaccinated against bovine virus diarrhea (BVD). Vaccines containing killed gram-negative organisms may be intrinsically toxic owing to the presence of endotoxins, which can cause a "shock" with pyrexia and leukopenia. Although such a reaction is usually only a temporary inconvenience to male animals, it may be sufficient to provoke abortion in pregnant females. Thus, in general it may be prudent to avoid vaccinating pregnant animals unless the risks of not giving the vaccine are considered to be too great. Remember too, that

bluetongue vaccine has been reported to cause congenital anomalies in the offspring of ewes vaccinated while pregnant. The stress from this type of toxic reaction may also be sufficient to reactivate latent infections; for example, activation of equine herpesvirus has been demonstrated following vaccination against African horse sickness. One other form of toxicity is the "sting" produced by some inactivating agents such as formaldehyde. This can present problems not only to the animal being vaccinated but also, if the animal reacts violently, to the vaccinator.

One significant result of the use of some vaccines is a mild immunosuppression. For example, some modified live parvovirus vaccines may cause immunosuppression in puppies. As a result, they may become susceptible to modified live distemper vaccine virus.

In addition to the difficulties associated with virulence and toxicity, vaccines, like any antigen, may provoke hypersensitivity reactions. For example, type I hypersensitivity may occur in response not only to the immunizing antigen, but also to other antigens found in vaccines, such as egg antigens or antigens derived from tissue culture cells. All forms of hypersensitivity are more commonly associated with multiple injections of antigen and tend, therefore, to be associated with the use of "dead" vaccines.

Type III hypersensitivity reactions are also potential hazards. The clinical signs of this may include an intense local inflammatory reaction, or they may present as a generalized vascular disturbance such as purpura. A type III reaction can occur in the eyes of dogs vaccinated against infectious canine hepatitis (Chapter 22).

Type IV hypersensitivity reactions may occur in response to vaccination, but a much more common reaction is granuloma formation at the site of inoculation in response to the use of depot adjuvants. Some vaccines, however, are effective only because of these local tissue reactions. For instance, Vallee's vaccine for Johne's disease involves the administration of the living organism in a mixture of oil and pumice dust. This mixture, not surprisingly, is highly irritating and on injection produces a large granuloma that eventually opens to the surface and discharges its oily contents. The effect of this vaccine is to protect cattle against clinical Johne's disease, although it does not prevent infection. Because it makes an animal both tuberculin and Johnin positive, the use of this vaccine is prohibited in many countries (Chapter 23).

Amyloidosis is a problem seen in horses used for antiserum production. It is associated with excessive stimulation of interleukin 1 production (Chapter 19). Although amyloidosis is not uncommon in domestic animals, it does not usually occur as a result of normal vaccination procedures.

Under some circumstances autoimmune disorders may be provoked by vaccination. For example, an allergic encephalitis may be provoked by the use of vaccines, such as some of the rabies vaccines that contain central nervous tissue. An idiopathic polyneuritis (Guillain-Barré syndrome) has been associated with the use of certain virus vaccines (most notably "swine" influenza) in humans. The precise pathogenesis of this syndrome is unclear.

PRODUCTION, PRESENTATION AND CONTROL OF VACCINES

The production of veterinary biologicals is controlled by the Animal and Plant Health Inspection Service of the United States Department of Agriculture in the United States, by the Health of Animals Branch of the Canada Department of Agriculture in Canada and by the Ministry of Agriculture in the United Kingdom. In general, regulatory authorities have the right to license establishments where vaccines are produced and to inspect these premises to ensure that the facilities are appropriate and that the methods employed are satisfactory. All vaccines have to be checked for safety and potency. Safety tests include confirmation of the identity of the organism used and of the freedom of the vaccine from extraneous organisms (i.e., purity) as well as tests for toxicity and sterility. Because the living organisms found in vaccines normally die over a period of time, it is necessary to ensure that they will be effective even after storage. It is usual, therefore, to use antigen in generous excess of the dose required to protect animals under laboratory conditions, and potency is tested both before and after accelerated aging. Vaccines that contain inactivated organisms, although much more stable than living ones, also contain an excess of antigen for the same reason. Vaccines usually have a designated shelf life, and although properly stored vaccines may still be potent after the expiration of this shelf life, this should never be assumed and all expired vaccines should be discarded.

"Dead" vaccines are commonly available in liquid form and usually contain suspended adjuvant. These should not be frozen, and they should be shaken well before use. The presence of preservatives such as phenol or merthiolate in these vaccines will not control massive bacterial contamination, and multidose containers should therefore be discarded after partial use. Many vaccines containing modified live viruses are very susceptible to heat inactivation, but are much more resistant if lyophilized. Remember, however, that even lyophilized vaccines can be destroyed by intense sunlight and heat. They store well but should be kept cool and away from light and should only be reconstituted with the fluid provided by the manufacturer.

ADDITIONAL SOURCES OF INFORMATION

Anderson RM and May RM. 1985. Vaccination and herd immunity to infectious diseases. Nature *318* 323–329.

Bachrach HL. 1985. New approaches to vaccines. Adv. Vet. Sci. Comp. Med. *30* 1–38.

Beard CW. 1979. Avian immunoprophylaxis. Avian Dis. *23* 327–335.

Bennett BW. 1982. Efficacy of *Pasteurella* bacterins for yearling feedlot cattle. Bovine Pract. *3* 26–30.

Carmichael LE. 1983. Immunization strategies in puppies—Why failures? Comp. Cont. Ed. Pract. Vet. *5* 1043–1052.

Cornwell HJC and Thompson H. 1982. Vaccination in the dog. In Practice *4* 153–157.

Davidson I. 1975. Testing veterinary vaccines. Vet. Rec. *97* 389–392.

Equine Vaccination Guidelines Subcommittee, Council on Biologic and Therapeutic Agents. AVMA. 1984. Guidelines for vaccination of horses. JAVMA *185* 32–34.

Hennessen W and Huygelen C (eds). 1979. Immunization: benefits versus risk factors. Dev. Biol. Stand. *43* 1–476.

Kesel ML and Neil DH. 1983. Combined MLV canine parvovirus vaccine: immunosuppression with infective shedding. Vet. Med. (Small Anim. Clin.) *78* 787–691.

Lerner RA. 1983. Synthetic vaccines. Sci. Amer. *248* 66–74.

Liew FY. 1985. New aspects of vaccine development. Clin. Exp. Immunol. *62* 225–241.

Mitchison NA. 1984. Rational design of vaccines. Nature *308* 112–113.

Moss B. 1985. Vaccinia virus expression vector: a new tool for immunologists. Immunol. Today *6* 243–245.

Nervig RM, Gough PM, Kaeberle ML, and Whetstone CA. 1986. Advances in Carriers and Adjuvants for Veterinary Biologics. Iowa State Univ Press, Ames, Iowa.

Schultz RD and Scott FW. 1978. Canine and feline immunization. Vet. Clin. North Am. (Small Anim. Pract.) *8* 755–768.

15

Resistance to Bacteria and Related Organisms

Although animals live in an environment densely populated with bacteria, the vast majority of these organisms are capable neither of invading animal tissues nor of causing disease. This is not surprising, since successful organisms must survive and multiply. Illness or death of the host could interfere with the survival of the organism; therefore, this is normally avoided. Indeed, many of these bacteria are essential for the animal's well being, since they maintain an environment on body surfaces that is inimical to potential invaders and assist in the digestion of foods, particularly celluloses. Nevertheless, many of these "commensal" organisms are also potential pathogens. For example, *Clostridium tetani* and *Cl. perfringens* are commonly found among the intestinal flora of horses, while *Bordetella bronchiseptica* is found in the nasopharynx of many healthy swine. It is apparent, therefore, that bacterial disease is not an inevitable consequence of the presence on body surfaces of pathogenic organisms. The development of bacterial disease is related to many other factors, including the resistance of the host, the presence of damaged tissues, the exact location of the organism within the body and the disease-producing power (or virulence) of the organism. Only when the balance between host resistance and bacterial virulence is upset will disease or death result.

BACTERIAL STRUCTURE AND ANTIGENS

Bacteria are ovoid or spherical organisms consisting of a cytoplasm containing the essential

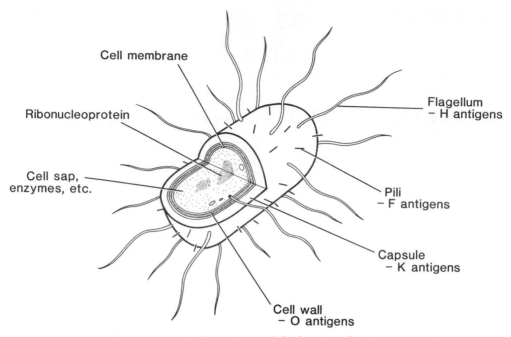

Figure 15–1. The structure of a bacterium and the location of its important antigens.

elements of cell structure surrounded by a cell membrane. The cell membrane is in turn covered by a cell wall that in some bacteria is enclosed by a capsule. From the cell there may extend flagella and pili (Fig. 15–1). The bacterial cytoplasm contains a complex mixture of enzymes and nucleoproteins, many of which are potentially antigenic. However, since these are confined to the interior of the organism, they are usually less important than the surface antigens in stimulating a protective immune response. The four major antigenic structures of the bacterial surface are the cell wall, the capsule, the pili and the flagellae. The cell wall of gram-positive organisms is largely composed of peptidoglycans (chains of alternating N-acetyl glucosamine and N-acetyl muramic acid cross-linked by small peptide side-chains), whereas that of gram-negative organisms is a polysaccharide-lipid-protein structure. The cell wall antigens of gram-negative organisms are toxic (they are called endotoxins) and are collectively classified as O antigens. Bacterial capsules may be polysaccharide or protein in nature. Because of their

hydrophilic properties, capsules may render organisms resistant to phagocytosis.

Encapsulated organisms such as *Klebsiella* spp. or *Streptococcus pneumoniae* are usually very poorly cleared from the blood stream unless antibody is present. For this reason, antibodies directed against these capsular or K antigens are essential for protection, and vaccines that do not contain K antigens tend to be relatively ineffective.

Pili or fimbriae are short, straight projections found on the surface of many gram-negative bacteria. They are classified as F antigens. Some pili serve to attach the bacteria to endothelial cells and prevent their expulsion from the body. Bacterial flagellae consist of protein and so are fully antigenic. Their antigens are known as H antigens. Two other significant groups of bacterial antigens are the porins and the exotoxins. The porins are highly antigenic proteins that form the pores on the surface of gram-negative organisms. Exotoxins are proteins secreted by or derived from the cytoplasm of bacteria, and they are responsible for some bacterial diseases. Exotoxins are highly immunogenic and are readily neutralized by antibodies (antitoxins).

PATHOGENESIS OF BACTERIAL INFECTIONS

Bacteria may cause disease by many different mechanisms but, in general, they either release toxins or, by invasion and multiplication, cause physical destruction of host cells. The toxins of bacteria may be divided into two groups: (1) toxins derived from the interior of organisms such as the clostridia and loosely called exotoxins, and (2) endotoxins derived from the cell walls of gram-negative organisms such as the Salmonellae. The differences between these two types of toxin are great (Table 15–1), and consequently the nature and significance of the immune response against toxigenic organisms varies according to the source of the toxin.

Pathogenesis of Disease Due to Exotoxigenic Organisms

Exotoxins are produced within bacterial cytoplasm. Some are secreted through the living cell wall and so are considered to be extracellular toxins, whereas others are released only by lysis of bacteria and so are termed protoplasmic toxins. One of the most significant diseases caused by an exotoxin is tetanus, which occurs as a result of the release from *Cl. tetani* of a powerful protoplasmic neurotoxin. *Cl. tetani* is strictly anaerobic and will, therefore, grow only in areas where oxygen tension is low, usually as a result of tissue destruction. The tetanus toxin, also known as tetanospasmin, is released from the bacteria as a prototoxin and is activated by proteolytic enzymes. It travels from the site of bacterial growth along nerve trunks to the spinal ganglia, where it interferes with the passage of the inhibitory transmitter and so blocks inhibitory synapses. As a result of this interference, tetanic spasm of voluntary muscles and, eventually, nerve block and paralysis occur. The ability to induce nerve blockage is also a property of the protoplasmic toxins of *Clostridium botulinum*. These toxins are absorbed intact following ingestion of contaminated food and cause death as a result of respiratory paralysis. The dose of botulinum toxin needed to block nervous activity is extremely small; only about eight molecules are required to block transmission by a neuron completely. A different type of exotoxin is the α toxin of *Cl. perfringens*, which is an extracellular phospholipase capable of causing hemolysis and tissue destruction and in this way facilitating bacterial growth and invasion.

Pathogenesis of Disease Due to Endotoxigenic Organisms

The walls of gram-negative bacteria consist of a complex of polysaccharides, lipids and pro-

Table 15–1 COMPARISON OF THE GENERAL PROPERTIES OF EXOTOXINS AND ENDOTOXINS

	Exotoxins	Endotoxins
Source	Secreted by living, usually gram-positive organisms or released from their cytoplasm on autolysis	Autolytic products from the cell walls of (usually gram-negative) bacteria
Chemical composition	Protein	Lipopolysaccharide-protein complexes
Lethality	Powerful toxins	Weak toxins
Stability	Heat labile	Heat stable
Activity	Each toxin has a specific pharmacological activity on a specific target	Stimulate interleukin 1 production
Antigenicity	Highly antigenic and readily neutralized by antibody	Weak antigen and poorly neutralized by antibody
Effect of formaldehyde	Forms toxoid	No effect

teins. These complexes, known as endotoxins, possess a number of important biological properties. Most of these activities are associated with the polysaccharide-lipid portions of the complex. The toxic properties, for example, are due to the lipid component known as lipid A. The polysaccharide component, however, is responsible for the characteristic antigenicity of O antigens. It consists of an oligosaccharide attached to the lipid A (which is itself part of the cell membrane). On the outer side of this complex are located a series of repeating trisaccharides (Fig. 15–2). These trisaccharides function as epitopes and therefore influence the antigenicity of the bacteria. As a result many organisms are classified according to this antigenic structure. For example, the salmonellae are a group of bacteria that have been classified into about 2100 serovars through the use of O and H antigens. Thus, O antigen number 1 is a trisaccharide with glucose as its terminal sugar, O antigen number 2 has paratose, O antigen number 3 has mannose, and so forth. The terminal sugar that confers the antigenic specificity is said to be immunodominant.

Gram-negative bacteria occur in two forms. One of these, known as the smooth form from the nature of its colonies, is fully virulent and possesses the entire surface structure described above. The other is known as the rough form. These rough forms lack the outer trisaccharides and part of the oligosaccharide. As a result, rough forms grown on agar form colonies with a matt rather than a shiny surface, and the organisms agglutinate spontaneously when suspended in saline. Rough forms tend to be avirulent organisms, and several have therefore been employed in vaccines. Examples of these variants include strain 45/20 of *Brucella abortus* and strain 51 of *Salmonella dublin*.

Endotoxins have the ability to stimulate the production of interleukin 1. As a result, they induce all the clinical effects of that protein. For example, when injected into animals they cause malaise, lethargy and temperature changes as well as a variety of other unpleasant effects that may contribute to the disease process. Some endotoxins also initiate the alternate complement pathway. The activated complement, particularly C3b, mediates extensive platelet aggregation and release of procoagulants. These procoagulants accelerate the coagulation cascade and thrombus formation while the endotoxin itself activates Hageman factor. If two spaced doses of endotoxin are given to a rabbit, one intradermally and the second intravenously several hours later, a violent hemorrhagic necrotic reaction will occur at the site of the first injection within two to three hours. This reaction is caused by local thrombosis and infarction at the intradermal injection site and is known as the local Shwartzman reaction. If both doses of endotoxin are given intravenously several hours apart, then disseminated intravascular coagulation and bilateral renal cortical necrosis may result. This is known as the generalized Shwartzman or the Shwartzman-Sanarelli reaction. Reactions of this type may contribute significantly to the development of lesions in infections caused by gram-negative organisms.

Pathogenesis of Disease Due to Invasive Organisms

Disease can be produced by bacterial invasion and subsequent destruction of tissues. This

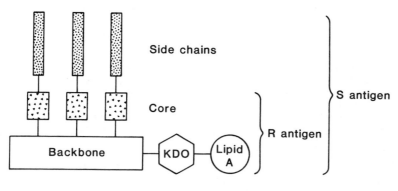

Figure 15–2. The basic structure of the lipopolysaccharide of the cell wall of gram-negative bacteria such as the salmonellae. KDO is ketodeoxyoctonic acid. The backbone consists of repeating heptose-phosphate units. The core consists of glucose and galactose attached to N-acetyl glucosamine.

tissue destruction may be due to vascular damage resulting in thrombosis and infarction, to the release of destructive bacterial enzymes or to local metabolic depletion. Some organisms may secrete hyaluronidase, which, by splitting hyaluronic acid in connective tissue, opens up intercellular spaces and so allows bacteria to spread through tissues. Other organisms secrete fibrinolytic enzymes (e.g., streptokinases), which cause clot disruption, and collagenases and elastases, which, through destruction of collagen and elastic fibers, serve to disrupt the structure of connective tissues. Some bacterial proteases may also digest immunoglobulins or complement components. Other organisms, particularly staphylococci, release coagulases, which, by causing clot formation, may establish a substrate for bacterial growth.

Whereas some bacteria invade intercellular tissue through the use of proteolytic enzymes, others are intracellular parasites and so live inside cells. The most notable bacterial examples of these include *Brucella abortus*, *Mycobacterium tuberculosis*, *Corynebacterium pseudotuberculosis*, *Listeria monocytogenes*, *Rhodococcus equi* and the Salmonellae. Although readily phagocytosed by macrophages, these organisms are resistant to intracellular destruction either by preventing lysosome-phagosome fusion or by being able to resist destruction by the enzymes found in normal macrophage lysosomes. These organisms may therefore multiply within macrophages and be distributed throughout the body within these cells. The macrophages eventually die as a result of the expanding physical bulk of the growing organisms, which leads to cell rupture.

MECHANISMS OF ANTIBACTERIAL RESISTANCE

Although immunologists tend to be preoccupied with the specific immune responses, it must be pointed out that these responses represent only a portion of the defenses available to an animal. Three general types of protection can, in fact, be identified. The first type is resistance as a result of species insusceptibility. An example of this is the resistance

of chickens to *B. abortus*. The second type of protection is due to the presence of nonimmunological inhibitory substances, and the third type is mediated by specific immune responses. The specific immune responses are probably the most important of these protective mechanisms, as demonstrated by the inevitably fatal consequences of the failure of an animal to develop a functioning immune system (Chapter 26).

General Factors Influencing Resistance

The most important general factors that influence disease resistance are genetic. Under natural conditions, disease is but one of the selective pressures that act on an animal population. The spread of disease through a population may initially eliminate all susceptible animals but leave a resistant residue to multiply and make use of the newly available resources such as food. By appropriate breeding programs it is therefore possible to develop strains of animals that are either highly resistant or highly susceptible to a specific disease. Thus, humped cattle (*Bos indicus*) are more responsive than European cattle (*Bos taurus*) to antigens administered by the conjunctival route. This is reflected by an enhanced resistance to ocular Moraxella infections in humped cattle. Resistance of this type is, in many cases, due to the activities of immune-response genes (Chapter 8).

A second group of nonspecific factors that influence disease resistance are hormones. Thus, thyroxine, low doses of steroids and estrogens may stimulate the immune response, whereas high doses of steroids, testosterone and progesterone are immunosuppressive. In stressed animals, increased steroid production may be immunosuppressive and so help precipitate disease. An example of this stress effect is seen when cattle are subjected to prolonged transportation under suboptimal conditions, as a result of which, these animals are liable to contract virus infection. This infection results in the development of a pneumonia characterized by secondary invasion with pasteurella organisms, which is known as shipping fever. A second example is salmonella enteritis in horses, a disease precipitated by stress such as surgery or transportation.

The last group of major nonspecific factors that influence disease resistance are nutritional. Malnutrition, which is discussed in detail in Chapter 26, significantly increases susceptibility to bacterial diseases. The negative protein balance incurred in heavily parasitized animals may also have an adverse effect on the immune response, so much so that as far as possible such animals should not be vaccinated until after their parasite burden is reduced. The stressful effect of surgery may also be magnified by the increase in protein catabolism that occurs following surgical intervention and results in a temporary immunosuppression.

Specific Chemical Factors Contributing to Resistance

Convincing evidence of the ability of animal tissues to discourage bacterial invasion is apparent in the relative infrequency of bacterial infections as a result of minor wounds. Some of this resistance is due to the presence of potent antibacterial factors in tissues (Table 15–2). The most important of these is lysozyme, a bactericidal enzyme first recognized by Sir Alexander Fleming, the discoverer of penicillin. Lysozyme is found in tissues and in all body fluids except cerebrospinal fluid, sweat and urine. It is said to be absent from bovine neutrophils but is found in high con-

centrations in tears and egg white. Lysozyme splits the acylaminopolysaccharides of the capsules of some gram-positive bacteria, killing them. It is also able to destroy some gram-negative organisms in conjunction with complement. Although many of the bacteria killed by lysozyme are considered to be nonpathogenic, it might reasonably be pointed out that this susceptibility could account for their lack of pathogenicity. Lysozyme is found in very high concentrations in the lysosomes of neutrophils and so tends to accumulate in areas of acute inflammation, including sites of bacterial invasion. The optimal pH for lysozyme activity, although somewhat low (pH 3 to pH 6), is easily achieved in inflammatory sites as well as within phagosomes, and as a result, it is here that its antibacterial activity is largely exerted. Finally, lysozyme may also act as a potent opsonin, facilitating phagocytosis in the absence of specific antibodies and under conditions in which its enzyme activity may be ineffective.

The observation that kidneys remain relatively unaffected in miliary tuberculosis led to the isolation of two tetra-amines called spermine and spermidine, which, in conjunction with a serum α globulin, form a bactericidal complex active against acid-fast organisms, cocci and *Bacillus anthracis*.

Free fatty acids are also inhibitory to bacterial growth under some circumstances. In general, unsaturated fatty acids such as oleic acid tend to be bactericidal for gram-positive

Table 15–2 SOME NONIMMUNOLOGICAL PROTECTIVE FACTORS FOUND IN BODY TISSUES AND FLUIDS

Group	Name	Major Sources	Activity Against
Enzymes	Lysozyme	Serum; leukocytes	Gram-positive and -negative bacteria; some viruses
Basic peptides and proteins	β-Lysin	Platelets	Gram-positive bacteria
	Phagocytin	Neutrophils	
	Leukin	Neutrophils	
	Plakin	Platelets	
Iron binding proteins	Transferrin	Serum	Gram-positive and -negative bacteria
	Lactoferrin	Leukocytes; milk	
Basic amines	Spermine; spermidine	Pancreas; kidney; prostate	Gram-positive bacteria
Complement components	—	Serum	Bacteria; viruses; protozoa
Peroxide splitting mechanisms	Myeloperoxidase; xanthine oxidase	Neutrophils; milk	Bacteria; viruses; protozoa
Interferon	—	Most cells but not neutrophils	Viruses; some intracellular protozoa

organisms, whereas saturated fatty acids are fungicidal. Because of this, scalp ringworm of children, which is somewhat refractory to conventional medical treatment, may resolve spontaneously at puberty when the amount of saturated fatty acids in sebum increases.

Several peptides and proteins rich in lysine and arginine and with potent antibacterial properties have been isolated from mammalian cells and tissues. They are commonly derived from proteins digested as a result of the release of proteolytic enzymes from neutrophils or platelets. β-Lysin, a polypeptide active against *B. anthracis* and the clostridia, is released from platelets as a result of their interaction with immune complexes.

One of the most important factors that influences the success or failure of bacterial invasion is the level of iron in body fluids. Many bacteria, such as *Staphylococcus aureus*, *Escherichia coli*, *Pasteurella multocida* and *Mycobacterium tuberculosis*, require iron for growth. Nevertheless, within the body, iron is largely associated with the iron-binding proteins transferrin, lactoferrin, haptoglobin and ferritin. Following bacterial invasion, intestinal iron absorption ceases. Interleukin 1 released from macrophages causes hepatocytes to release increased quantities of transferrin and haptoglobin, and there is increased incorporation of iron into the liver. The effect of these actions is to effectively hinder bacterial invasion. A similar situation occurs in the mammary gland when, in response to bacterial invasion, neutrophils release their stores of lactoferrin and so enhance the bactericidal power of milk. In spite of the sequestration of iron, some bacteria such as *M. tuberculosis* and *E. coli* succeed in invading the body because they can release potent iron-chelating compounds (mycobactin and enterochelin). These compounds may withdraw iron from serum proteins and make it available to the organisms. In conditions in which serum iron levels are elevated, such as in the hemolytic anemias, animals may become extremely susceptible to bacterial infection.

The production of reactive oxygen metabolites, which are important in bacterial destruction by neutrophils and macrophages, has been discussed in Chapter 2. Similarly, interferon is discussed in Chapter 7, and the alternate complement pathway in Chapter 10.

SPECIFIC IMMUNITY TO BACTERIA (Fig. 15–3)

There are four basic mechanisms by which the specific immune responses combat bacterial infections. These are (1) the neutralization of toxins or enzymes by antibody, (2) the killing of bacteria by antibodies, complement and lysozyme, (3) the opsonization of bacteria by antibodies (and complement), resulting in their phagocytosis and destruction, and (4) the phagocytosis and intracellular destruction of bacteria by activated macrophages. The relative importance of each of these processes

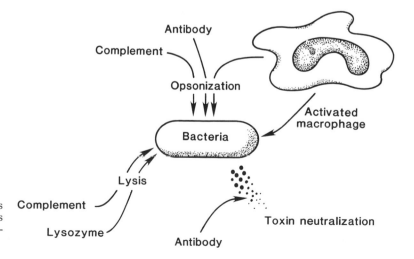

Figure 15–3. The mechanisms by which the immune responses can protect the body against bacterial invasion.

depends upon the organisms involved and on the mechanisms by which they cause disease.

Immunity to Exotoxigenic Organisms

In disease caused by exotoxigenic organisms such as the clostridia or B. anthracis, the function of the immune response must be not only to eliminate the invading organisms but also to neutralize any toxin produced by them. Unfortunately, destruction of these bacteria may be difficult, especially if they are embedded in a mass of necrotic tissue. On the other hand, antibodies can readily neutralize bacterial exotoxins. Neutralization occurs when the antibody prevents the toxin from binding to its receptor on a target cell. The neutralization process therefore involves competition between receptor and antibody for the toxin molecule, and it is apparent that once the toxin has combined with the receptor, antibody will be relatively ineffective in reversing this combination. This result is observed in practice, since the dose of antitoxin required to produce clinical improvement in a disease such as tetanus is greatly in excess of that required to prevent the development of clinical disease.

Immunity to Systemically Invasive Organisms

Protection against invasive bacteria is usually mediated by antibodies directed against the surface antigens of the bacteria. Antibodies against antigens in the interior of these organisms, such as ribonucleoprotein or enzymes, are usually only of limited usefulness in protection (although bacterial ribonucleoprotein may have a significant role in the development of cell-mediated immunity).

Antibody directed against capsular (K) antigens may serve to neutralize the antiphagocytic properties of the capsule, thus opsonizing the organism and permitting bacterial destruction by phagocytic cells to take place. In organisms lacking capsules, antibodies directed against O antigens also function as opsonins. A more subtle protective effect has been reported to occur when antibodies are produced against strains of E. coli carrying the pilus antigens F4 (K88) or F5 (K99). In this case, the antibodies interfere with the expression of the pilus antigens, and it has been claimed that they are eventually able to cause deletion of the genetic material (plasmid) that codes for these antigens. Once the adherence antigens are deleted these strains of E. coli cannot bind to the intestinal wall and are thus no longer pathogenic.

An example of the importance of bacterial capsules in immunity to disease is seen in anthrax. B. anthracis is an organism that possesses both a capsule and an exotoxin. Antitoxic immunity is protective in this disease but is slow to develop. In addition, toxin production tends to be prolonged, since the organism is encapsulated and phagocytic cells are therefore unable to eliminate the source of the toxin. As a result, death is usually inevitable in unvaccinated animals. The vaccine commonly employed against anthrax contains an unencapsulated but toxigenic strain of B. anthracis. Given in the form of spores that can germinate, the unencapsulated organisms are eliminated by phagocytic cells before dangerous amounts of toxin are synthesized but not before antitoxic immunity is stimulated.

Some bacteria are phagocytosed and destroyed by neutrophils or macrophages, or both; others are killed when free in the circulation. In sensitized animals, bacteria are destroyed by the actions of specific antibody and complement activated by the classical pathway. In unsensitized animals, the bacteria are destroyed by complement acting through the alternate pathway. Bacterial cell walls, lacking sialic acid, are capable of inactivating factor H and thus permitting the persistence of the alternate C3 convertase (C3bBbP). As a result, the bacteria are either opsonized or lysed. The importance of this pathway is seen in bovine mycoplasma infections, in which pathogenic and nonpathogenic organisms may be differentiated on the basis of their ability to activate the alternate pathway. Nonpathogenic mycoplasmas activate the pathway; pathogenic ones do not.

Activation of the terminal complement path-

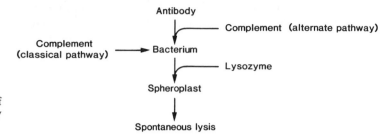

Figure 15–4. The mechanism of lysis of gram-negative bacteria by complement and lysozyme.

way leads to the development of a membrane attack complex consisting of poly C9. This complex alone is insufficient to kill many gram-negative bacteria. Once inserted in the bacterial wall, however, it reveals a substrate for the enzyme lysozyme. Lysozyme, therefore, acts on bacteria subsequent to complement to cause bacteriolysis (Fig. 15–4).

On a molar basis, IgM is about 500 to 1000 times more efficient than IgG in opsonization and about 100 times more potent than IgG in sensitizing bacteria for complement-mediated lysis. Therefore, during a primary immune response, the quantitative deficiency of the IgM response is compensated for by its quality, thus ensuring early and efficient protection.

Immunity to Facultative Intracellular Parasites

Certain organisms of major veterinary importance, particularly *Brucella abortus, Mycobacterium tuberculosis, Campylobacter jejuni, Rhodococcus equi, Listeria monocytogenes, Corynebacterium pseudotuberculosis, Chlamydia psittaci, Coxiella burnetii* and the Salmonellae, are engulfed by macrophages but are resistant to subsequent intracellular destruction. Several mechanisms are involved in permitting these bacteria to survive within macrophages (Table 15–3). Virulent mycobacteria, *B. abortus* and *Chlamydia psittaci*, prevent lysosomal fusion with the phagosome. As a result, the lysosomes remain distributed within the cytoplasm and the organisms continue to grow. Other mycobacteria can escape from the phagosome and persist free within the cytoplasm, whereas the cell wall waxes of *Corynebacterium pseudotuberculosis* can ren-

der it resistant to lysosomal killing. These facultative intracellular parasites can therefore replicate within macrophages in an environment free of antibody. As a result, the humoral immune response to these organisms is relatively ineffective.

Passively transferred antiserum will not confer significant protection against these bacteria, although passively transferred lymphocytes will. Therefore, protection against this type of organism is cell-mediated. Although macrophages from unimmunized animals are normally incapable of destroying these organisms, this ability is acquired about ten days after onset of infection. The changes that occur in these macrophages include increases in cell size, in metabolic activity and in the size and number of their lysosomes (see Fig. 7–7) and result in a significant increase in the bactericidal ability of the cells (see Fig. 7–8). The changes themselves are a reflection of a form of "acquired" cell-mediated immunity, which is mediated through γ interferon released by

Table 15–3 FACULTATIVE INTRACELLULAR BACTERIA AND THEIR MECHANISMS OF SURVIVAL

Organism	Method of Intracellular Survival
Brucella abortus	Resistant cell wall; Blocks phagosome-lysosome fusion
Corynebacterium pseudotuberculosis	Lipid cell wall; Lipid toxic for macrophages
Listeria monocytogenes	Neutralizes respiratory burst
Mycobacterium tuberculosis	Lipid cell wall; Blocks phagosome-lysosome fusion
Salmonella typhimurium	Lipopolysaccharide cell wall
Rhodococcus equi	?

sensitized T cells on exposure to bacterial ribonucleoprotein. The response of activated macrophages tends to be nonspecific, especially in listerial infections; these cells, therefore, are able to destroy a wide range of normally resistant bacteria. Thus, an animal recovering from an infection with *L. monocytogenes* shows increased resistance to infection by *M. tuberculosis*. The development of these activated macrophages often coincides with the appearance of delayed (Type IV) hypersensitivity to intradermally administered antigen. It has also been noted that protective immunity against these bacteria cannot be induced by the use of vaccines containing killed organisms, although vaccines containing living bacteria are protective. Acquired resistance to these facultative intracellular parasites is generally short-lived. The immunological memory seems to persist only as long as viable bacteria remain in the body. (One exception to this is in tuberculosis in which memory is prolonged.)

If, in a bacterial disease, it is observed that dead vaccines do not give good protection, that serum cannot confer protection, that antibody titers do not relate to resistance and that delayed hypersensitivity reactions can be elicited to the bacterial antigens, then the possibility that cell-mediated immunity may play an important role in resistance to the causative organism should be considered, and the use of vaccines containing living organisms should be contemplated.

Evasion of the Immune Response by Bacteria

Bacteria, like all parasites, are not well served either by the death of their chosen host or by their own immune elimination. They have thus evolved mechanisms by which the consequences of the immune responses may be evaded. We have already discussed such features as the use of antiphagocytic capsules and facultative intracellular parasitism, both of which delay bacterial destruction. Some organisms such as *E. coli*, *M. tuberculosis* and *Pseudomonas aeruginosa* secrete factors that can depress phagocytosis by neutrophils.

Staphylococcus aureus can also inhibit chemotaxis and phagocytosis by producing soluble toxins such as streptolysin O that can lyse neutrophil cell membranes. The most extreme form of this is shown by *Pasteurella haemolytica*, which secretes factors that kill ruminant alveolar macrophages and sheep lymphocytes and *Hemophilus pleuropneumoniae* which secretes a toxin that will kill porcine macrophages.

Other organisms can inhibit the bactericidal activities of cells in a more subtle fashion. For example, the carotenoid pigments responsible for the color of *S. aureus* can quench singlet oxygen and so survive the respiratory burst. *S. aureus* can also inhibit phagocytosis by means of a protein called protein A on its surface. Protein A attaches to the Fc region of IgG molecules, preventing the immunoglobulin from binding to the receptors on the phagocytic cell and preventing opsonization. *Taylorella equigenitalis* can bind equine IgG and IgM in a similar manner. *Pasteurella multocida* and *Haemophilus somnus* are also capable of inhibiting the respiratory burst, whereas strains of *E. coli* may carry a plasmid that confers resistance to complement-mediated lysis. Other protective devices employed by pathogenic bacteria include the production of proteolytic enzymes specific for IgA such as those produced by *Neisseria gonorrhoea*, *Haemophilus influenzae* and *S pneumoniae*.

Campylobacter fetus ssp. *venerealis*, an organism that normally colonizes the male and female genital tracts in cattle, shows cyclical antigenic variation. The successful destruction of a major portion of this bacterial population by a local immune response leaves a residual population of organisms that possess epitopes differing from those of the original population. This residual population may multiply and be largely eliminated in turn by a second immune response, leaving a residual population of a third antigenic type. This process may be repeated for a prolonged period, and, because of the poor memory in the surface immune system (Chapter 12), the organisms may reutilize antigens without stimulating a secondary immune response.

Mycoplasma mycoides evades the immune

response in a different fashion, by exerting a toxic effect on T cells. The mechanism of this effect is not clear but may involve competition with these cells for essential nutrients. Whatever the cause, the result is a depression of the immune response. The fungal toxin aflatoxin is also immunosuppressive, reducing the resistance of poultry to *P. multocida* and salmonellosis.

Adverse Consequences of the Immune Responses to Bacteria

Although the immune responses are generally considered to be beneficial in that they serve to eliminate invading bacteria, this is not always the case. The immune responses are capable of influencing the course of bacterial diseases without producing a cure, and in some situations may cause an increase in the severity of the pathological lesions. An example of the modulating influence of the immune responses is observed in human leprosy, in which two very different forms of disease occur, both due to the same organism, *Mycobacterium leprae*. In the tuberculoid form of the disease, the immune response is primarily cell-mediated and serum antibodies are low. The lesions, although almost devoid of organisms, consist of typical tubercle-like granulomas. In the lepromatous form of the disease, organisms are present in large numbers within invasive lesions, and little cellular response occurs. The affected individual has high serum antibody levels but no detectable cell-mediated response. A similar variation in disease types occurs in brucellosis, in which some species such as guinea pigs and swine tend to show local granulomatous lesions, whereas in cattle the disease is of a more invasive type.

The adverse consequences of the immune responses correspond in their mechanisms to the hypersensitivity types described in Chapter 19. Thus, it has been suggested that in chickens suffering from fowl typhoid (salmonellosis), death may be associated with a type I (anaphylactic) hypersensitivity reaction against bacterial products. A local type I hypersensitivity reaction is sometimes seen in

sheep vaccinated against foot rot by means of *Fusobacterium necrophorum* vaccine, but in this case it is felt that the hypersensitivity may assist in preventing reinfection.

Type II (cytotoxic) reactions may account for the anemia occurring in animals with salmonellosis. In these infections, bacterial lipopolysaccharides released from disrupted bacteria are readily adsorbed onto erythrocytes, and the subsequent immune response against the bacterium and its products results in erythrocyte destruction. Although a similar anemia is observed in leptospirosis, its mechanism is unknown, since antibodies produced by infected animals may agglutinate normal red cells taken from the same animal prior to infection (Chapter 25).

Type III (immune complex) reactions may contribute to the development of arthritis in *Erysipelothrix rhusiopathiae* infections in pigs or to the development of intestinal lesions in Johne's disease due to *Mycobacterium paratuberculosis*. In the former case, bacterial antigen tends to localize in joint tissues where local immune complex formation results in inflammation and arthritis. Therefore, passively administered antiserum may exacerbate the arthritis in these infected animals. In Johne's disease, type I or type III reactions occurring in the intestinal mucosa may result in an increased outflow of fluid and diarrhea. It is probable, however, that the intestinal lesions in this disease are etiologically complex, since diarrhea can be transferred to normal calves by either plasma or leukocytes, and antihistamines may reduce the diarrhea. The immune responses to *M. paratuberculosis* are also known to be, in large part, cell-mediated. Type III hypersensitivity reactions may be involved in purpura hemorrhagia of horses, in which a serum sickness-type of lesion may result from the immune response to *Streptococcus equi*.

Although cell-mediated immune responses are, in general, manifestly beneficial, they do contribute to the development of granulomatous lesions in some chronic infections (Chapter 23). The development of large granulomata, while serving to "wall off" invading organisms and so prevent their spread, may also involve uninfected tissues. If these granulomata involve essential structures such as airways in the lungs or large blood vessels, severe damage can occur.

Some Comments on Antibacterial Vaccines

Toxoids

The immunoprophylaxis of tetanus is essentially restricted to toxin neutralization. Tetanus toxoid in an aluminum hydroxide suspension is normally given for routine prophylaxis, and a single injection of this material will induce protective immunity in 10 to 14 days. Conventional immunological wisdom suggests that the previous use of immune globulin should interfere with the immune response to toxoid and must therefore be avoided. This is not true in practice, and both may be successfully administered simultaneously without problems. This may be because of the relatively small amount of immune globulin usually employed to protect animals.

Some other veterinary vaccines combine both toxoid and killed bacteria in a single dose by the simple expedient of formolizing a whole culture. These products are sometimes called anacultures. Anacultures are used to vaccinate against *Clostridium haemolyticum* and *Cl. perfringens*. Trypsinization of the anaculture is commonly performed, since this renders it more immunogenic. Toxoids, usually incorporated with an alum adjuvant, are available for most clostridial diseases and for diseases due to toxigenic staphylococci.

Bacterins

Bacterin is the term used to describe vaccines containing killed bacteria. It is usual to kill the organisms with formaldehyde and to incorporate them with alum or aluminum hydroxide adjuvants. Apart from the bacterins against pasteurellosis (shipping fever) and salmonellosis, which are of doubtful efficacy, most other bacterins are effective but somewhat limited in their usage. As with other dead vaccines, the immunity produced is relatively short-lived, usually lasting for not longer than a year and sometimes for a considerably shorter period. Thus, formolized swine

erysipelas (*E. rhusiopathiae*) vaccine protects for only four to five months, and *S. equi* bacterins give immunity for less than a year, even though recovery from a natural case of strangles may confer a lifelong immunity in horses.

Bacterins may be improved by adding purified immunogenic antigens to the killed bacteria. Thus, *E. coli* bacterins against enteric colibacillosis may be enriched and made much more effective by the addition of F4 (K88) or F5 (K99) pilus antigens to the mixture. Antibodies to these antigens block binding of *E. coli* to the intestinal wall and thus contribute significantly to the protective immune response.

One problem encountered, especially when using coliform and campylobacter bacterins, is strain specificity. Several different antigenic types of each organism commonly occur, and successful vaccination requires immunization with appropriate bacterial strains. This is sometimes not possible if a commercial bacterin must be employed. One method of overcoming this difficulty is to use autogenous bacterins. These are bacterins that contain either organisms obtained from infected animals on the farm where the disease problem is occurring or from the infected animal itself. These can be very successful if carefully prepared, since the bacterin will contain all the antigens required for protection in that particular location. As an alternative to the use of autogenous bacterins, some manufacturers produce polyvalent bacterins containing a mixture of antigenic types. For example, leptospirosis bacterins commonly contain up to five different serovars. This practice, although effective, is inefficient, since only a few of the antigenic types employed may be appropriate in any given situation.

As pointed out earlier, the use of bovine respiratory disease vaccines containing killed Pasteurella organisms together with viral components has been shown to be associated with increased mortality due to respiratory disease. The reasons for this are unclear.

Living Bacterial Vaccines

Perhaps the most successful of the living bacterial vaccines in current practice is strain 19 of *B. abortus* (see page 189). Another successful living vaccine is that employed for the prevention of anthrax. Older anthrax vaccines utilized Pasteur's technique of culturing the organisms at a relatively high temperature (42 to 43° C) so that their virulence is reduced. The anthrax vaccines currently available contain capsuleless mutants, which remain capable of forming spores. The vaccine is prepared as a spore suspension and is administered with saponin. A live avirulent vaccine is also employed against swine erysipelas. Unfortunately, the avirulence of this strain is not fully fixed and there has been some difficulty in preventing its reconversion to the virulent form. A rough strain of *S. dublin* (strain 51) is used in Europe to give good protection to calves when administered at two to four weeks of age. As discussed earlier, immunity to salmonellosis is cell-mediated and thus relatively nonspecific. For this reason, strain 51 may also give good protection against *Salmonella typhimurium*. Recently, modified live, avirulent *Pasteurella haemolytica* vaccines have been used for the prevention of bovine pneumonia.

Vaccines against contagious bovine pleuropneumonia (CBPP) usually contain living organisms of reduced virulence. The organisms are cultured in eggs, and good protection used to be obtained by injecting this avianized vaccine into the tip of the tail of cattle. Unfortunately, the reaction of cattle to this organism, even in vaccine form, can be extremely violent and the tail usually dropped off! Nevertheless, the severity of this toxic reaction tends to correlate well with the degree of immunity produced, weakly toxic vaccines giving poor protection and strongly toxic vaccines giving good protection. For this reason excellent immunity is now produced by giving the vaccine subcutaneously and, if necessary, controlling the subsequent reaction with tylosin.

THE SERODIAGNOSIS OF BACTERIAL INFECTIONS
(Table 15–4)

The agglutination test is widely employed in the diagnosis of bacterial infections, particularly those involving gram-negative organisms such as *Brucella* and *Salmonella*. The usual procedure in bacterial agglutination tests is to titrate serum (antibody) against a standard suspension of antigen. Bacteria are not, of course, antigenically homogeneous but are covered by a mosaic of many different antigens. Thus, motile organisms will have flagellar (H) antigens, and agglutination by the anti-flagellar antibodies will produce fluffy cottonlike floccules as the flagellae stick together, leaving the bacterial bodies only loosely agglutinated. Agglutination of the somatic (O) antigens results in tight clumping of the bacterial bodies so that the agglutination is finely granular in character. Many organisms possess several O and H antigens as well as capsular (K) and pilus (F) antigens. By means of a battery of specific antisera it is therefore possible to characterize the antigenic structure of an organism and consequently to classify it. It is, for instance, on this basis that the 2100 or so different serovars of salmonellae are classified.

Flagellar antigens are destroyed by heating, whereas O antigens are heat resistant and

Table 15–4 SOME TESTS COMMONLY USED IN THE DIAGNOSIS OF SELECTED BACTERIAL INFECTIONS

Disease	Tube Agglutination	Complement Fixation	Passive Hemagglutination	Skin Test	Vaginal Mucus Agglutination
Campylobacteriosis	+	−	−	−	+
Salmonellosis	+	−	−	−	−
Glanders	+	+	+	+	−
Erysipelas	+	+	+	−	−
Leptospirosis	+ *	+	+	−	−
Listeriosis	+	−	−	−	−
Johne's disease	−	+	−	+	−
Tuberculosis	−	−	−	+	−
Contagious equine metritis	+	−	+	−	−

*A microagglutination test is probably the best of the available tests for leptospirosis.

therefore remain intact on heat-killed organisms. K antigens vary in their heat stability. The L antigen of *E. coli*, which is a capsular antigen, is heat labile, whereas another K antigen, antigen A, is heat stable. *Salmonella typhi* possesses an antigen known as Vi, which, although heat stable, is removed from the bacterial cells by heating. The presence of K or Vi antigens on an organism may render them O-inagglutinable and thus complicate agglutination tests. It should also be pointed out that rough forms of bacteria (page 204) do not form stable suspensions and therefore cannot be typed by means of agglutination tests.

Bacterial agglutination tests may be performed by mixing drops of reagents on glass slides or by titrating the reagents in tubes or wells in plastic plates. Tube agglutination tests are commonly used for such diseases as salmonellosis, brucellosis, tularemia and campylobacteriosis. Slide agglutination tests are commonly used as screening tests. They include the brucella acid-antigen tests, in which organisms stained with the red dye rose-bengal are suspended in an acid buffer (pH 3.6). There are several different tests of this type. The tests employed in the United Kingdom and Australia are considered to be relatively sensitive but of low specificity and as such may be used as screening tests to remove negative animals from further consideration.

In contrast, the card test employed in the United States and Canada is considered to be of reduced sensitivity but is more specific than some of the other tests available.

One test for *Salmonella pullorum* infection in poultry is a slide agglutination test in which *S. pullorum* stained with gentian violet is mixed with whole chicken blood. Because of the stain, agglutination of the organisms is readily seen when the chicken carries antibodies to this organism. Leptospirosis is diagnosed by a "microscopic" agglutination test in which mixtures of living organisms and test serum are examined under the microscope for agglutination. This technique detects IgM antibodies preferentially and is thus an excellent test for detecting recent outbreaks as well as for distinguishing between infected and vaccinated animals.

It is not mandatory that serum be used as the source of antibody for diagnostic tests. The presence of antibodies in body fluids other than serum, such as milk whey, vaginal mucus or nasal washings, may be of more significance, especially if the infection is of a local or superficial nature. One such test is the milk ring test used to direct the presence of antibodies to *B. abortus* in milk (Fig. 15–5). Fresh milk is shaken with organisms stained with hematoxylin or triphenyl tetrazolium and is allowed to stand. If antibodies, especially

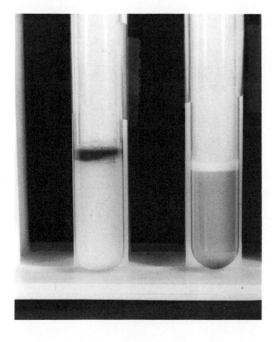

Figure 15–5. The milk ring test. Stained *Brucella* remains suspended in the milk in a negative test (*right*) but rises with the cream in a positive reaction (*left*). (Courtesy of Mr. E. L. Thackeray.)

Table 15–5 A COMPARISON OF THE TESTS USED IN THE DIAGNOSIS
OF BOVINE BRUCELLOSIS

Test	Isotype Detected	Comments
Serum agglutination test (SAT)	IgM, IgG2	Simple and standardized but failure to detect IgG1 is a significant disadvantage
Complement fixation test (CFT)	IgM, IgG1	Complex but it detects IgG1, an advantage
ELISA test	All isotypes	Requires specialized equipment but otherwise excellent
Card test	IgG1, IgG2	Failure to detect IgM antibodies reduces false-positive reactions
Milk ring test	Milk antibodies, especially IgA	Used for testing bulk milk samples

those of the IgM or IgA isotypes, are present, then the organisms will clump and adhere to the fat globules of the milk and rise to the surface with the cream. If antibodies are absent, then the stained organisms will remain dispersed in the milk and the cream, on rising, will remain white.

The Serodiagnosis of Bovine Brucellosis (Table 15–5)

In their attempts to eradicate brucellosis from their cattle, the countries of North America and Western Europe have employed vaccination of calves with strain 19 vaccine in conjunction with the serological detection and slaughter of infected animals. Unfortunately, since strain 19 of *Brucella abortus* is a living organism, the process of vaccination may be thought of as being nothing more than a controlled infection. It is therefore difficult to distinguish between the immune response to strain 19 and the response to natural infection. In order to assist in this differentiation, it has been usual either to restrict the practice of vaccination to calves so that their serum antibody response will have declined to low levels by the time of serological testing as adults or to vaccinate adult cattle with very low doses

of antigen. Consequently, if antibodies are present in adult animals, they may be present in high levels as a result of infection or recent vaccination or, alternatively, they may be present in low levels as a result either of very recent infection or of calfhood vaccination. In addition, some adult cattle possess a low level of antibrucella antibodies in spite of a complete absence of infection. Therefore, the correct interpretation of serological results from animals showing low levels of antibody is a matter of critical importance.

All of the serological methods used to detect antibodies to *Brucella abortus* suffer from defects as a result of the inability of some bovine antibody subisotypes, especially IgG1, to produce secondary reactions such as agglutination (Table 15–6). In addition, the antibodies that persist at low levels after vaccination tend to be of the IgM isotype. Thus strenuous efforts have been made to modify tests in an attempt to enhance the effects of IgG1 while at the same time reducing the effects of IgM. As a result, there has been a growing interest in the development of effective and practical primary binding tests in *Brucella* serology. The most convenient of the serological tests available for the diagnosis of brucellosis is the serum agglutination test (SAT) performed in tubes. Unfortunately, this agglutination test

Table 15–6 THE IMMUNOGLOBULINS OF IMPORTANCE IN BRUCELLA DIAGNOSIS

Isotype	Importance	Detected by	Missed by
IgG1	Very important	CFT, ELISA, card test	SAT
IgG2	Relatively less important	SAT, Card test, ELISA	CFT
IgM	Cause of false-positives	SAT, CFT, ELISA	Card test, Rivanol test

fails to detect IgG1 antibodies, since these antibodies cannot agglutinate antigen at pH values near neutrality and when in excess are liable to block the agglutinating activity of other isotypes, resulting in false-negative reactions. If the pH of the suspending fluid is dropped to 3.65, as occurs in the card test, IgG1 antibodies become agglutinating while IgM antibodies, readily detected by the tube test, become non-agglutinating. An alternative procedure is to treat serum with Rivanol (2-ethoxy-6,9-aminoacridine lactate) before testing. This chemical precipitates out the IgM, thus reducing the chances of getting false positive reactions. Other methods that have been used to remove the IgM from serum include treatment with 2–mercaptoethanol and heating the test serum to 56°C for 15 minutes prior to testing. The presence of a calcium chelating agent such as EDTA may also reduce some false-positive reactions.

In contrast to the agglutination tests, the complement fixation test (CFT) preferentially detects antibodies of the IgG1 subisotype, but is relatively insensitive to IgM antibodies and fails to detect IgG2 antibodies. As a result, the CFT has replaced the SAT in many countries in which eradication schemes are in progress. The CFT is much less likely to produce false-negative reactions than the SAT. In addition, CFT titers do not usually persist in vaccinated cattle. This is probably because heating of the test serum to destroy complement also effectively destroys any residual IgM antibodies. A related test that selectively detects antibodies of the IgG1 subisotype is hemolysis-in-gel. This test involves passive sensitization of sheep erythrocytes using purified *B. abortus* lipopolysaccharide. These erythrocytes are then incorporated in agarose gel in the presence of guinea pig serum as a source of complement. The mixture is then poured onto a plate, and, after cooling, wells are punched in the agarose. The serum being tested and the control serum are placed in the wells. After incubation overnight in the cold, the plates are incubated at 37°C for one hour. If antibodies are present, they will bind to the erythrocytes, activate the complement and a ring of clear hemolysis will develop. Its diameter provides a quantitative measure of the amount of IgG1 antibody in the serum. In contrast to the mixed performance of the secondary binding tests, a well standardized ELISA can be used to detect anti-*Brucella* antibodies of all four major isotypes at relatively low concentrations without ambiguity. It is probably the best of the currently available diagnostic tests for brucellosis.

Finally, it should be pointed out that infected cattle may occasionally have low antibody titers, and at times IgM may be the only isotype present. For this reason it is essential that the serological tests for brucellosis be interpreted with caution and in conjunction with careful analysis of the field situation.

IMMUNITY TO FUNGAL INFECTIONS

The first line of defense against invasive fungi such as *Candida* or *Aspergillus* includes activation of the alternate pathway of the complement system, attraction of neutrophils to the lesion and attempts by the neutrophils to ingest the invading hyphae or pseudohyphae. Because of their size, neutrophils cannot totally ingest the invading fungi. Nevertheless, by releasing their enzymes into the surrounding tissue fluid, the neutrophils may severely damage fungal hyphae. Very small fungal fragments or spores may be ingested and destroyed by macrophages or by NK cells.

Once established, fungal infections can only be destroyed by T cell–mediated mechanisms. Thus some species of *Aspergillus* are facultative intracellular parasites, and chronic or progressive fungal diseases are commonly associated with defects in the T cell system (Chapter 26). T cells primarily function in fungal infections by activating macrophages and by promoting epidermal growth and keratinization. It is not uncommon for recovered animals to develop a type IV hypersensitivity to fungal antigens.

ADDITIONAL SOURCES OF INFORMATION

Barton CE and Lomme JR. 1980. Reduced-dose whole-herd vaccination against bovine brucellosis: a review of recent experience. JAVMA *177* 1281–1220.

Collins FM and Campbell SG. 1982. Immunity to intracellular bacteria. Vet. Immunol. Immunopathol. *3* 5–66.

Elsbach P. 1980. Degradation of microorganisms by phagocytic cells. Rev. Infect. Dis. *2* 106–128.

Frenchick PJ, Markham JF and Cochrane AH. 1985. Inhibition of phagosome-lysosome fusion in macrophages by soluble extracts of virulent *Brucella abortus*. Am. J. Vet. Res. *46* 332–335.

Koenig EHW and Finger H. 1982. Failure of killed *Listeria monocytogenes* vaccine to produce protective immunity. Nature *297* 233–234.

Lehmann PF. 1985. Immunology of fungal infections in animals. Vet. Immunol. Immunopathol. *10* 33–69.

Liefman CE. 1980. Combined active-passive immunization of horses against tetanus. Aust. Vet. J. *56* 119–122.

Mims CA. 1982. The Pathogenesis of Infectious Disease. 2nd Ed. Academic Press, New York.

Nielsen K, Heck F, Wagner G, Stiller J, Rosenbaum B, Pugh R and Flores E. 1984. Comparative assessment of antibody isotypes to *Brucella abortus* by primary and secondary binding assays. Prev. Vet Med. *2* 197–204.

Reiter B. 1978. Antimicrobial systems in milk. J. Dairy Res. *45* 131–147.

Riley LK and Robertson DC. 1984. Ingestion and intracellular survival of *Brucella abortus* in human and bovine polymorphonuclear leukocytes. Infect. Immunol. *46* 224–230.

Segal AW. 1981. The antimicrobial role of the neutrophil leukocyte. J. Infect. *3* 3–17.

Simonsen RR and Maheswaran SK. 1982. Host humoral factors in natural resistance to *Haemophilus somnus*. Am. J. Vet. Res. *43* 1160–1164.

Tashjian JJ and Campbell SG. 1983. Interaction between caprine macrophages and *Corynebacterium pseudotuberculosis*: an electron microscopic study. Am. J. Vet. Res. *44* 690–693.

Widders PR, Stokes CR, Newby TJ and Bourne FJ. 1985. Nonimmune binding of equine immunoglobulin by the causative organism of contagious equine metritis *Taylorella equigenitalis*. Infect. Immunol. *48* 417–421.

Winter AJ. 1979. Mechanisms of immunity in bacterial infections. Adv. Vet. Sci. Comp. Med. *23* 53–69.

Woolcock JB. 1979. Bacterial Infection and Immunity in Domestic Animals. Developments in Animal and Veterinary Science series. Elsevier, North-Holland, New York.

16

Resistance to Viruses

Since viruses are obligate intracellular parasites, their very existence is threatened if they are completely eliminated from the body by the immune responses. Nor are they well-served by the death of their host as a result of virus-mediated disease. Because of these opposing factors, both viruses and their hosts have been subjected to a rigorous process of adaptation and selection. The viruses are selected for their ability to evade the hosts' immune responses, and host animals are selected for resistance to virus-induced disease. It is possible, therefore, to loosely classify viruses on the basis of their ability to evade the hosts' immune responses, a property that shows an inverse relationship to their virulence.

For example, in infections in which virus-host adaptation is poor, diseases tend to be very severe. Rabies in man, horses and cattle is an excellent example of this. Rabies is inevitably lethal in these species because they are unnatural hosts. In its natural hosts, especially bats and skunks, the virus persists and can be shed in saliva for a long period of time before or without causing disease. Transmission usually occurs following a bite. From the virus' point of view, infection of humans, cattle or horses is unprofitable since they never (or rarely) transmit rabies to skunk. Slightly less severe diseases of this type include feline panleukopenia, canine distemper and the hypervirulent forms of Newcastle disease. Vaccination tends to be relatively successful in this type of infection.

In situations in which the virus and host are better adapted, although the viral disease may be relatively severe, mortality may not necessarily be high and the virus may be persistent. In this type of disease, further attacks can occur as a result of infection by antigenic variants of the same virus. Examples of this type of virus infection include foot-and-mouth disease and influenza. Vaccination against diseases of this type is complicated by the antigenic diversity among viruses circulating in the population. Some even better-adapted viruses cause persistent infection, and the immune system appears to be incapable of eliminating the virus. Diseases of this type include equine infectious anemia, visna of sheep, AIDS virus in humans and Aleutian disease of mink. The virus may even change during the course of these infections and thus constantly elude the immune system. Vaccination against these diseases is essentially unsuccessful.

In studying the nature of the host responses to viruses, it is well to recognize that this continuing selective pressure on both host and virus exists and profoundly influences the outcome of all host-virus interactions.

VIRUS STRUCTURE AND ANTIGENS (Fig. 16–1)

Viruses are very small particles that consist of a nucleic acid core surrounded by a layer of repeating protein subunits. This protein layer is termed the capsid, and the constituent subunits are termed the capsomeres. Viruses may also be surrounded by an envelope containing lipoprotein and derived in part from the host cell. The complexity of viruses varies with the species; some such as pox viruses are complex, whereas others such as foot-and-mouth disease virus are relatively simple. Antibodies can be produced against all the proteins situated both inside and on the surface of the virus. Antibodies against the nucleoprotein components are not usually considered to be highly significant from a protective point of view, but they may be of some assistance in diagnostic procedures.

PATHOGENESIS OF VIRUS INFECTIONS

Viruses are obligate intracellular parasites that invade and alter the properties of cells. They invade cells by binding to cell membranes and are then internalized through pinocytosis. Some viruses bind to histocompatibility antigens on the cell membrane. The alterations in infected cells may be minimal, perhaps only detectable by the development of new antigens on the cell surface, or the changes may be extensive and result in either cell lysis or malignant transformation and the development of a tumor.

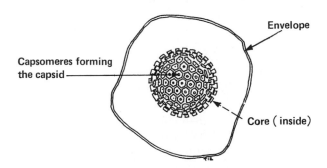

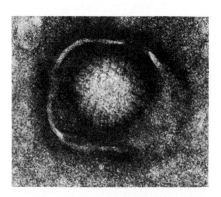

Figure 16–1. The structure of a virus (In this case equine herpesvirus type I. × 184,000) and the position of important viral antigens. (Courtesy of Dr. J. Thorsen.)

MECHANISMS OF ANTIVIRAL RESISTANCE

Nonimmunological Defense Mechanisms

Nonimmunological factors influence the outcome of many viral infections. Lysozyme, for example, is capable of destroying several viruses, as are many of the intestinal enzymes. Bile is a powerful neutralizer of some viruses, so much so that Koch first successfully vaccinated cattle against rinderpest with the bile of animals dying from that disease.

Interference and Interferons

Probably the most important of the nonimmunological antiviral defense mechanisms is interference. Interference is the name given to the inhibition of viral replication by the presence of other viruses. One cause of this inhibition is the production of interferons. Interferons are released from virus-infected cells within a few hours after viral invasion, and high concentrations of interferon may be achieved within a few days *in vivo*, at a time when the primary immune response is still relatively ineffective (Fig. 16–2). For example, in cattle that receive infectious bovine rhinotracheitis (IBR) virus intravenously, peak interferon levels in serum are reached two days

later and then decline, but they are still detectable by seven days. In contrast, antibodies are not usually detectable in serum until five to six days after virus administration.

Production of interferons is brought about by the association between viral genetic material and host cell ribosomes, resulting in derepression of target cell DNA coding for interferon production (Fig. 16–3). Interferon is released from infected cells and binds to receptors on other, nearby cells. It stimulates these cells to synthesize two compounds, a molecule called 2-5A and a protein kinase. 2-5A is an adenine trinucleotide that activates an endonuclease which destroys the mRNA used for viral protein synthesis. The protein kinase acts on double stranded RNA to prevent its elongation and also inhibits viral protein synthesis.

Virus-induced interferons are not species-specific, although bovine interferon appears to be most effective when acting on bovine cells. They are not virus-specific either, and interferon induced by one virus may be equally effective when acting against other, unrelated viruses. The ability of cells to produce interferon varies. Virus-infected leukocytes, especially macrophages and lymphocytes, produce the α interferons; virus-infected fibroblasts produce β interferon; and antigen-stimulated T cells are the major source of γ interferon (Chapter 7). Cells such as those from the

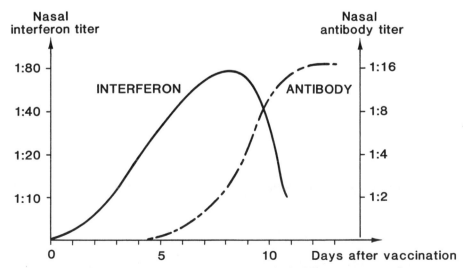

Figure 16–2. The sequential production of interferon and antibody following intranasal vaccination of calves with infectious bovine rhinotracheitis vaccine. (From data kindly provided by Dr. M. Savan.)

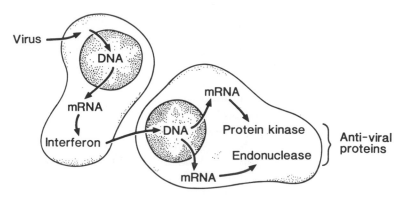

Figure 16–3. A simplified view of the mechanism by which interferon production is induced and its mode of action in protecting cells from virus infection.

kidney are relatively poor interferon producers, and neutrophils produce no interferon.

Although live or inactivated viruses are normally considered to be the most important stimulators of interferon production, interferons may also be produced under circumstances other than virus infection. For example, bacterial endotoxins can stimulate the release of interferon from target cells within a few minutes of exposure. This interferon differs both in size and in heat stability from that produced by virus-infected cells and is probably released from stores within cells. Other substances that can induce interferon production include some plant extracts such as phytohemagglutinin and synthetic polymers, which act by mimicking the action of viral RNA. One of the most potent of these synthetic polymers (Poly I:C) consists of inosinic and cytidilic acids. Poly I:C may increase survival in experimental virus infections (Chapter 27).

A second and probably much more important role for the interferons is the regulation of immune reactivity (Chapter 9). Interferons can influence the activities of T cells, B cells, macrophages and NK cells. They generally enhance the protective activities of these cells and promote antitumor and antivirus immunity.

Specific Immunity to Viruses
(Fig. 16–4)

Antibody-Mediated Immunity to Viruses

Being protein, the capsid of viruses is antigenic, and it is against this component and the envelope that antiviral immune responses

are largely mounted. Antibodies may destroy viruses or prevent infection of cells in many ways. The combination of antibody and virus need not be virucidal in itself, since the splitting of virus-antibody complexes may lead to the release of infectious virus. Antibody can, however, prevent cell invasion by blocking the adsorption of coated virus to its target cell, by stimulating phagocytosis of viruses by macrophages, by initiating complement-mediated virolysis or by causing clumping of viruses, thus reducing the number of infectious units available for cell invasion. Circulating antibody therefore may be capable of virus neutralization. Of course, this neutralizing ability is limited to areas reached by antibody, so that, for example, although chicks hatched from Newcastle disease-immune hens are resistant to systemic virus disease, they remain susceptible to local respiratory tract infection because they possess no local immunity.

Not only are antibodies active against the protein coat of free virions, but they are also active against cells that express viral antigens on their surface, so that these cells are also liable to be destroyed. Virus infections in which antibody-mediated destruction of infected cells is known to occur include Newcastle disease, rabies, bovine virus diarrhea, infectious bronchitis of birds and feline leukemia. Antibody may cause destruction of these infected cells not only through complement-mediated cytolysis but also through the activities of cytotoxic cells by antibody-dependent cell-mediated cytotoxicity (ADCC). These cytotoxic cells include lymphocytes, macrophages and neutrophils that possess Fc receptors, through which they can bind to antibody-coated target cells (Chapter 7).

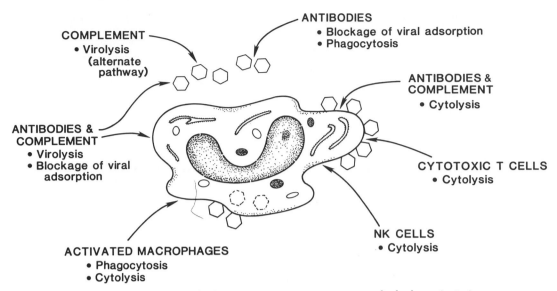

Figure 16–4. The ways in which an immune system can protect the body against viruses.

The immunoglobulins involved in virus neutralization include IgG and IgM in serum and IgA in secretions. It is possible that IgE also plays a protective role, since humans with a selective IgE deficiency have an increased susceptibility to respiratory infections. As in antibacterial immunity, IgG is quantitatively the most significant immunoglobulin, whereas IgM is qualitatively best at virus neutralization.

Cell-Mediated Immunity to Viruses

Although serum antibodies are able to neutralize viruses, it is probable that cell-mediated immune mechanisms are the most important pathways for the control of viral diseases in general. This can be readily seen in humans who are unable to mount antibody-mediated responses (Bruton-type agammaglobulinemia). These individuals suffer severely from recurrent bacterial infections but usually respond normally to smallpox vaccination and recover from mumps, measles, chickenpox, poliomyelitis and influenza. In contrast, humans who have a congenital deficiency in their cell-mediated immune response (thymic aplasia) are commonly resistant to bacterial infection but highly susceptible to virus diseases, and may die from generalized vaccinia if vaccinated against smallpox. In spite of this, it is probable that both antibodies and the cell-mediated immune response work together in most cases so that antibodies eliminate circulating virus while the cell-mediated immune system acts to eliminate infected cells. This may be seen in rabbit fibroma infections, in which antibody eliminates circulating virus while the cell-mediated immune response causes tumor regression.

Viral antigens may be expressed on the surface of infected cells long before progeny viruses are produced. These new antigens are found not only on cells from which virus particles bud, but also on virus-induced tumor cells, where viruses may code for tumor antigens on the cell surface. Virus-infected cells may therefore be recognized by the body as foreign and eliminated in a manner analogous to graft rejection. Although antibody and complement or ADCC can play a role in this process, T cell-mediated cytotoxicity is the major mechanism through which this destruction is achieved. Cytotoxic T cells recognize the virus antigen in association with class I histocompatibility antigen molecules. Evidence for this concept has been provided by studies showing that cytotoxic T cells will destroy canine distemper-infected cells only if both the cytotoxic cell and the virus-infected target cell have identical class I antigens.

NK cells also destroy virus-infected cells.

NK cells are a population of cytotoxic lymphocytes found in normal, nonimmunized animals (Chapter 18). Activated by the presence of interferon, they have the ability to recognize and destroy some abnormal cells.

Acquired cell-mediated immunity, mediated by macrophages that have been activated by T cell-derived interferon (Chapter 7), is also a feature of some virus diseases. For example, macrophages derived from birds immunized against fowlpox show an enhanced antiviral effect against Newcastle disease and will prevent the intracellular multiplication of *Salmonella gallinarum*, a feature that is not a property of normal macrophages.

Evasion of the Immune Response by Viruses

As discussed at the beginning of this chapter, the relationship between host and virus must be established on the basis of mutual accommodation so that the long-term survival of both is ensured. Failure to reach this accommodation will result in the elimination of either host or virus, and death of the host automatically eliminates the virus. One aspect of this adaptation involves the avoidance by the virus of the attentions of the immune system.

This evasion may be accomplished by several techniques, one of the simplest of which is antigenic variation. The most significant example of this is seen among the type A influenza viruses. These influenza viruses possess many different surface antigens, of which the hemagglutinins and neuraminidases are most important. There are 13 different hemagglutinins and nine neuraminidases among the type A influenza viruses, and they are identified according to a nomenclature system recommended by the World Health Organization (Table 16–1). Thus, the hemagglutinin of the swine influenza virus is classified as H1 and its neuraminidase as N1. The two equine influenza viruses are A/equine/Prague//56, which is H7N7, and A/equine/Kentucky//81, which is classified as H3N8.

Influenza viruses in a human population may show an antigenic "drift" as mutation and

Table 16–1 EXAMPLES OF INFLUENZA A VIRUSES AND THEIR ANTIGENIC STRUCTURES

Species	Virus Strain	Antigenic Structure
Human	A/Brazil/11/78*	H1N1
	A/Philippines/2/82	H3N2
	A/New Jersey//76 (Swine Flu)	H1N1
Equine	A/Equine/Prague/1/56	H7N7
	A/Equine/Kentucky//81	H3N8
Swine	A/Swine/Iowa/15/30	H1N1
Avian	A/Fowl Plague/Dutch//27	H7N7
	A/Duck/England//56	H11N7
	A/Turkey/Ontario/6118/68	H8N4

*The first number is the isolate number; the second is the year of isolation.

selection gradually change the structure of their hemagglutinins and neuraminidases in a seemingly random fashion. As a result, a significant antigenic change eventually occurs within each subtype. This drift permits the virus to persist in a human population for many years. In addition to drifting, influenza viruses sporadically exhibit a sudden, major antigenic "shift" in which a new strain develops whose hemagglutinins show no apparent relationship to the hemagglutinins of previously known strains. Such a major change cannot be produced by mutation and is probably due to recombination between two virus strains. It is the development of these influenza viruses with a completely new antigenic structure that accounts for the periodic pandemics of influenza in humans. In horses and pigs, in contrast, the rapid turnover of the population and the constant production of large numbers of susceptible young animals ensure the persistence of influenza without the necessity for extensive antigenic drift. As a result, the antigenic structure of equine and swine influenza viruses has changed only very slowly since they were first described. Nevertheless, the H3N8 equine influenza virus A/Kentucky//81 is now distinctly different from the original strain A/Miami/1/63.

A second form of virus adaptation is seen in equine infectious anemia (EIA), Aleutian disease (AD) of mink and African swine fever. Although infected animals mount an immune response to these viruses, the antibodies formed are incapable of virus neutralization.

Thus, virus-antibody complexes from AD-infected mink or EIA-infected horses are fully infectious. The precise reason for the inability of antibody to neutralize these viruses is not clear, although it is assumed that antibody must bind to a "noncritical" site on the virus. It has also been suggested that these viruses undergo some form of antigenic variation.

In contrast to the short-lived immune response against bacteria, antiviral immunity is, in many cases, very long lasting. The reasons for this are not completely clear, but they appear to be related to virus persistence within cells, perhaps in a slowly replicating or a nonreplicating form, as typified by the herpesviruses. It is usually very difficult, if not impossible, to isolate virus from an animal that has recovered from a herpesvirus infection. Some time later, however, especially when the individual is stressed, the herpesvirus may reappear and may even cause disease again. During the latent period, when it is present in the host but cannot be reisolated, the virus nucleic acid persists in host cells but its transcription is blocked and viral proteins are not made. The persistent virus may periodically boost the immune response of the infected animal and in this way generate long-lasting immunity to superinfection. The immune responses in these cases, although not capable of eliminating virus, may serve to prevent the development of clinical disease and therefore serve a protective role. Immunosuppression or stress may permit disease to occur in persistently infected animals. The association between stress and the development of some virus diseases is well recognized, and it is likely that the increased levels of steroid production occurring in stressful situations may be sufficiently immunosuppressive to permit activation of latent viruses or infection by exogenous ones.

Adverse Consequences of the Immune Responses Against Viruses

The immune response to viruses can, on occasion, be disadvantageous. For example, bovine respiratory syncytial virus (RSV) can induce a specific IgE response in infected cattle. This may result in the occurrence of a type I hypersensitivity reaction, since there is a direct relationship between this IgE level and the severity of disease caused by RSV in some animals.

The destruction of virus-infected cells by antibody is classified as a type II hypersensitivity reaction (Chapter 21) and although normally beneficial may exacerbate virus diseases. For example, passive administration of antibodies to animals suffering from Aleutian disease of mink may intensify the severity of the lesions. The demyelinating encephalitis commonly seen in canine distemper may be a form of type II hypersensitivity, since most animals suffering from this syndrome possess antibodies to myelin proteins, and the level of these antibodies is related to the severity of the lesions. The active participation of these antibodies in the demyelinating syndrome may be demonstrated in vitro, since some sera from affected dogs can cause demyelination in cultures of canine cerebellum. Old dog encephalitis, a disease of middle-aged dogs, is perhaps a variant of this postdistemper lesion.

Type III (immune complex) lesions (Chapter 22) are very commonly associated with viral diseases, especially those in which viremia is prolonged. For example, glomerulonephritis resulting from the deposition of immune complexes in glomeruli is a common complication of equine infectious anemia, Aleutian disease of mink, feline leukemia, chronic hog cholera, bovine virus diarrhea-mucosal disease, canine adenovirus infections and feline infectious peritonitis. A generalized vasculitis due to deposition of immune complexes throughout the vascular system is seen in equine infectious anemia, Aleutian disease of mink, malignant catarrhal fever and, possibly, equine viral arteritis.

If immune complexes are deposited in tissues, damage may occur as a result of cellular infiltration and subsequent lysosomal enzyme release. In feline infectious peritonitis, for example, the virus appears to multiply within macrophages of the peritoneal serosa. As a result of the cat's immune response, large quantities of non-neutralizing antibodies are produced and immune complexes are deposited within the serosa (Fig. 16–5). The resulting hypersensitivity reaction causes the severe peritonitis that is characteristic of this infection.

In dogs infected with canine adenovirus 1 (infectious canine hepatitis), an immune complex-derived uveitis has been reported in addition to a focal glomerulonephritis. This is known as blue-eye, a transient uveitis seen both in infected dogs and in dogs vaccinated with live attenuated adenovirus vaccine (Figs. 16–6 and 16–7). Blue-eye results from the formation of virus-antibody complexes in the anterior chamber of the eye and in the cornea with complement fixation and consequent neutrophil accumulation. The neutrophils release enzymes that damage the corneal epithelial cells and cause corneal edema and opacity. The condition resolves spontaneously in about 90 per cent of affected dogs.

Finally, many virus diseases are associated with the occurrence of rashes. The pathology of these is complex but may reflect type II, type III or even type IV hypersensitivity reactions occurring as the host responds to the presence of viral antigen in the skin.

Aleutian Disease of Mink (AD)

Although immune complex-mediated lesions are usually only of passing interest in many infectious diseases, they generate some of the major pathological lesions in Aleutian disease of mink. Aleutian disease is a persistent virus infection first recognized in mink with the "Aleutian" coat color. Although all strains of mink are susceptible to this virus, Aleutian mink are genetically predisposed to the development of severe lesions since they are also affected by the Chédiak-Higashi syndrome (Chapter 26). Infected mink develop a plasmacytosis, which has been compared to a myeloma-like neoplasm, since it results in a marked polyclonal or monoclonal gammopathy (see Fig. 26–9). They also develop lesions of systemic type III hypersensitivity (Chapter

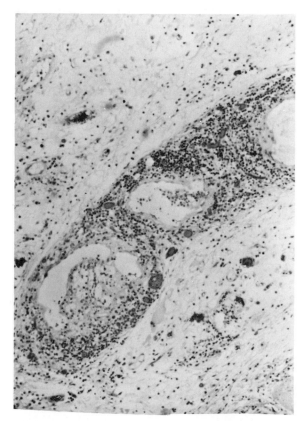

Figure 16–5. Granulomatous vasculitis of serosal blood vessels in a cat with feline infectious peritonitis. Note the marked mononuclear infiltration of the vessel adventitia and media. This reaction may be partially due to the deposition of virus-antibody complexes in the vessel walls.

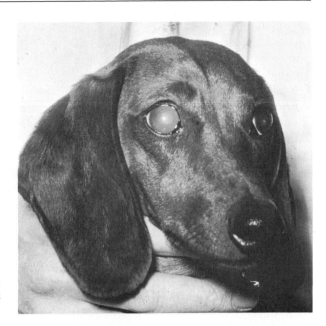

Figure 16–6. Blue-eye, a type III hypersensitivity reaction to canine adenovirus 1 (ICH), occurring in the cornea. (Courtesy of Dr. H. Reed.)

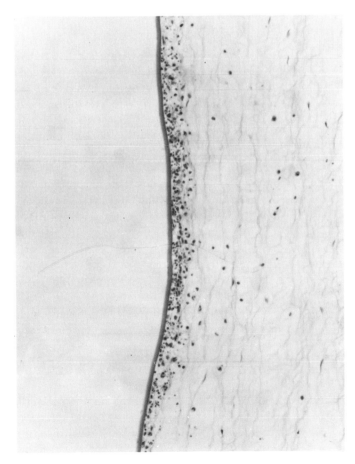

Figure 16–7. A section from the cornea of a dog suffering from blue-eye. Note the neutrophil infiltration of the posterior surface of the cornea as a result of virus-antibody complex deposition in this region. (From Carmichael LE. 1964. Pathol Vet 1 73–95. Used with permission.)

22), including glomerulonephritis and arteritis, and they show signs of autoimmunity by possessing autoantibodies to their own immunoglobulins (rheumatoid factors) and to DNA (antinuclear antibodies).

The immune complex-derived lesions of Aleutian disease include an arteritis in which IgG, C3 and viral antigen may be detected within vessel walls, and a glomerulonephritis in which "lumpy-bumpy" deposits of immune complexes containing virus and antibody may be identified. In addition, infected mink are anemic. Their erythrocytes can be shown to be coated with antibody which, when eluted, can be shown to be directed against the Aleutian disease virus. It is likely, therefore, that the erythrocytes of infected animals adsorb virus-antibody complexes from plasma. These coated erythrocytes are then rapidly removed from the circulation by mononuclear-phagocytic cells.

As might be predicted, the use of immunosuppressive agents such as cyclophosphamide or azathioprine in infected mink prevents the development of many of these lesions and so prolongs survival, whereas experimental vaccination with inactivated AD virus increases the severity of infections.

Feline Infectious Peritonitis (FIP)

FIP is a fatal disease of felids. It is caused by a coronavirus that is antigenically related to transmissible gastroenteritis virus of swine. FIP infects relatively young cats between 6 months and 5 years of age. The disease presents in two major forms: an effusive peritonitis (ascites) or pleuritis and a noneffusive form characterized by the development of multiple small granulomas on the surface of the major abdominal organs. Pleural lesions are uncommon in the noneffusive form of FIP. Some cats may show signs of central nervous system involvement and ocular lesions.

The pathogenesis of FIP differs between the two forms of the disease. After invading a cat, the virus first replicates in intestinal epithelium. It is then disseminated by blood-borne phagocytes and taken up by phagocytic cells in the target tissues. The course of the infection then depends upon the nature of the

immune response to the virus. In some cats, the immune response is almost entirely humoral. In these animals, antibody enhances virus uptake by phagocytic cells in which it then replicates. These antibodies also form immune complexes with the virus, and these immune complexes are deposited in the serosa to cause a pleuritis or peritonitis, and in glomeruli to cause glomerulonephritis. The vasculitis occurring in the serosa is responsible for the effusion of fibrin-rich fluid into the serosal cavities in cats with the "wet" form of the disease. This massive production of immune complexes may also be responsible for the occurrence of disseminated intravascular coagulation in these cats.

The immune mechanisms in the noneffusive form of FIP are less clear. The lesions probably arise as a result of a cell-mediated immune response against the virus since the granulomas are similar to those seen in diseases like tuberculosis and histoplasmosis.

Equine Infectious Anemia (EIA)

EIA is a persistent virus infection of horses, many of the lesions of which are attributable to the development of hypersensitivity reactions. The most obvious lesion is a hemolytic anemia in which the erythrocytes of infected horses adsorb circulating EIA virus onto their surfaces. Circulating antibody and complement then bind to the virus, as a result of which the erythrocytes are cleared from the circulation more rapidly than normal. In addition to the anemia, infected horses may also develop a glomerulonephritis as a result of immune complex deposition on glomerular basement membranes. Horses infected with EIA are immunosuppressed and have unusually low levels of IgG(T), although their circulating lymphocytes appear to be unaffected and respond normally to mitogens such as phytohemagglutinin.

Some Comments on Viral Vaccines

Because of the lack of chemotherapeutic antiviral agents, vaccination is the only effective method for the control of most viral diseases in the domestic animals. As a result, the development of viral vaccines is, in many ways, more advanced than that of their bacterial counterparts. It has, for example, proved relatively easy to attenuate many viruses so that effective vaccines containing modified live virus (MLV) derived from tissue culture are readily available.

As discussed in Chapter 14, MLV vaccines are usually good immunogens, but their use may involve certain risks. The most important problem encountered in the use of MLV vaccines is residual virulence. One serious example of this is the development of clinical rabies in some dogs following administration of low-egg-passage Flury-strain rabies vaccine and in cats following the use of SAD(ERA)-strain MLV rabies vaccine. Some strains of infectious bovine rhinotracheitis and equine herpesvirus vaccine may cause abortion when given to pregnant cows or mares, respectively, and MLV bluetongue vaccines may cause disease in fetal lambs if given to pregnant ewes (Chapter 13). More commonly, the residual virulence in these vaccines causes a relatively mild disease. Thus, intraocular or intranasal feline rhinotracheitis or calicivirus vaccine may cause a transient conjunctivitis or rhinitis, and some MLV canine distemper vaccines may cause transient thrombocytopenia. MLV infectious bursal disease vaccines, some canine parvovirus vaccines and some BVD vaccines can cause a mild immunosuppression.

Transient side effects like these, which may otherwise be regarded as inconsequential, can be of major significance in the broiler chicken industry, where even a minor slowing in growth can have major economic results. Thus, two strains of infectious bronchitis vaccine are available. The Massachusetts strain is mildly pathogenic but a good immunogen, whereas the Connecticut strain is nonpathogenic but a poor immunogen. It is common therefore, in order to minimize complications, to use the Connecticut strain for primary vaccination and, if boosters are required, to use the Massachusetts strain subsequently. Similarly, of the two major vaccine strains of Newcastle disease, the LaSota strain is a good immunogen but may provoke mild adverse reactions. In contrast, the B1 strain is considerably milder but is less immunogenic, especially if given in drinking water.

Because of problems of this nature, persistent attempts have been made to minimize residual virulence in vaccines. One method involves the use of temperature sensitive (ts) mutants. Ts strains of IBR virus that are now available will grow only at temperatures a few degrees lower than normal body temperature. As a result, when this organism is administered intranasally, it is able to colonize the relatively cool nasal mucosa but is unable to invade the rest of the body. Thus, the vaccine can stimulate a local immune response without incurring the risk of systemic invasion.

Another example of a genetically engineered vaccine is one against pseudorabies that uses a strain of virus from which the thymidine kinase gene has been deleted (Chapter 14).

Some strains of IBR vaccine may persist in vaccinated animals and give rise to a prolonged carrier state. Although this is a problem largely associated with herpesviruses, concerns have been expressed that the widespread use of MLV vaccines may serve to seed viruses into animal populations and that untoward consequences may develop in the future. This is a threat not to be taken lightly; indeed, it has been suggested that the sudden and widespread appearance of canine parvovirus in 1978 may have been facilitated by the use of MLV feline panleukopenia vaccines.

An alternative approach to overcoming the problems caused by MLV vaccines involves the increasing use of inactivated and subunit vaccines. Excellent inactivated vaccines are available against diseases such as foot-and-mouth disease, equine rhinopneumonitis, pseudorabies, feline panleukopenia, feline herpes (rhinotracheitis) and rabies. At their best, these vaccines confer immunity comparable in strength and duration to that induced by MLV vaccines, with the assurance that they are free of residual virulence. A general trend toward the use of more inactivated virus vaccines in the future is anticipated.

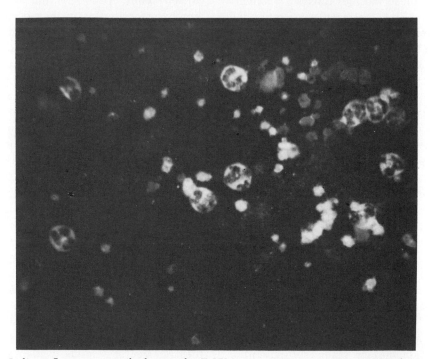

Figure 16–8. Indirect fluorescent antibody tests for FeLV in cats. *Top,* A negative reaction from a normal cat. *Bottom,* Cytoplasmic FeLV virion antigen in granulocytes, lymphocytes and platelets from a cat with naturally occurring lymphosarcoma. (From Hardy WD. 1974. Vet Clin North Am *4(1)* 141. Used with permission. Courtesy of Dr. Hardy.)

THE SERODIAGNOSIS OF VIRAL DISEASES

Tests Used to Detect and Identify Viruses

Among the simplest and most widely employed tests for the detection of viruses are the direct and indirect fluorescent antibody techniques. These may be used to identify virus in the tissues of infected animals (Fig. 16–8). If it is not possible to identify the virus in tissues, it is usually necessary to grow the virus in experimental animals, chick embryos or tissue cultures in order to provide sufficient antigen for testing. Once sufficient virus has accumulated, it may be identified by its reaction with specific antiserum. The tests commonly employed for this purpose are fluorescent antibody tests, ELISA, hemagglutination inhibition, virus neutralization, complement fixation and gel precipitation. The precise tests employed will depend on the nature of the unknown virus. Hemagglutination inhibition tests are technically simple and are preferred if the virus is a hemagglutinating one. They do, however, tend to be strain-specific. The complement fixation test and gel precipitation test, as a broad generalization, tend to be largely group-specific and thus lend themselves to attempts to identify the genus to which a virus belongs. In contrast, virus neutralization tests tend to be highly strain-specific, so much so that they are perhaps best employed in the classification of a virus into its subtypes rather than in identifying the specific genus of a particular organism. There are, of course, exceptions to these generalizations; for example, the New Jersey and Indiana strains of vesicular stomatitis virus do not cross-react in the complement fixation test.

Immunoelectron Microscopy

Specific antibodies may be employed to selectively enrich virus suspensions prior to electron microscopy. For example, a feces sample may be centrifuged, leaving a clear supernatant that contains a small number of many different viruses. After sonication to break up clumps, antibody specific for the virus of interest is added to the supernatant and, after a brief incubation, the fluid is centrifuged again. Virus particles clumped by antibody will be spun to the bottom, where they can be removed and examined by electron microscopy after negative staining (Fig. 16–9). The anti-

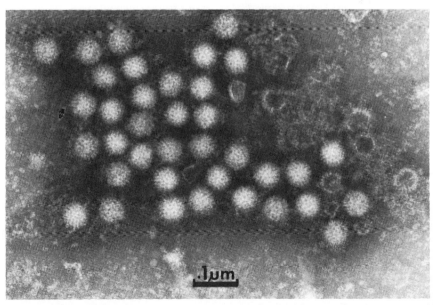

Figure 16–9. Immunoelectron microscopy of porcine rotavirus clumped by convalescent antiserum. × 130,500. (Courtesy of Dr. L. Saif.)

body, by clumping only the virus of interest, renders it much more visible in the electron microscope, and the presence of visible antibody within the virus-clumps provides direct confirmation of the identity of the virus.

Tests Used to Detect and Identify Antiviral Antibodies

In general, the most widely employed techniques for the identification of antibodies to viruses are hemagglutination inhibition, indirect ELISA, immunofluorescence, gel diffusion, complement fixation and virus neutralization. The first four of these are technically simple and are thus preferred. The complement fixation test and the virus neutralization tests are complex, thus restricting the circumstances in which they may be employed. The virus neutralization tests are also extremely specific, which, as discussed earlier, tends to reduce their value as screening tests.

ADDITIONAL SOURCES OF INFORMATION

Appel JMG, Mendelson SG and Hall WW. 1984. Macrophage Fc receptors control infectivity and neutralization of canine distemper virus-antibody complexes. J. Virol. *51* 643–649.

Appel JMG, Shek WR and Summers BA. 1982. Lymphocyte-mediated immune cytotoxicity in dogs infected with virulent canine distemper virus. Infect. Immun. *37* 592–600.

Gaudry D. 1983. Rabies vaccines: the Merieux experience. Vet. Med. (Small Anim. Clin.) *78* 525–530.

Gorman NT. 1983. The interaction of cells persistently infected with canine distemper virus with antiviral antibody and complement. Cell. Immunol. *77* 242–248.

Gresser I. 1977. On the varied biological effects of interferon. Cell. Immunol. *34* 406–415.

Hesse RA and Toth TE. 1983. Effects of bovine parainfluenza-3 virus on phagocytosis and phagosome-lysosome fusion of cultured bovine alveolar macrophages. Am. J. Vet. Res. *44* 1901–1907.

Horzinek MC and Osterhaus ADME. 1978. Feline infectious peritonitis: a coronavirus disease of cats. J. Small Anim. Pract. *19* 623–630.

Jacobse-Geels HEL, Daha MR and Horzinek MC. 1982. Antibody, immune complexes and complement fluctuations in kittens with experimentally induced feline infectious peritonitis. Am. J. Vet. Res. *43* 666–670.

Krakowa S, Higgins RJ and Koestner A. 1980. Canine distemper virus: review of structural and functional modulations in lymphoid tissues. Am. J. Vet. Res. *41* 284–292.

Lutz H, Petersen NC, Harris CW, et al. 1980. Detection of feline leukemia virus infections. Feline Pract. *10* 13–23.

Mathes LG, Olsen RG, Hebebrand LC, et al. 1978. Abrogation of lymphocyte blastogenesis by a feline leukemia virus protein. Nature *274* 687–689.

Mims CA (ed). 1985. Virus immunity and pathogenesis. Brit Med. Bull. *41* 1–102.

Mogensen SC. 1983. Interference of phagocytic functions by viruses. Clin. Immunol. Newslett. *4* 58–61.

Ohmann HB and Babiuk LA. 1986. Alteration of alveolar macrophage functions after aerosol infection with bovine herpesvirus type 1. Infect. Immun. *51* 344–347.

Palese P and Young JF. 1982. Variation of influenza A, B, and C viruses. Science *215* 1468–1474.

Pastoret PP, Babiuk LA, Misra V and Griebel P. 1980. Reactivation of temperature-sensitive and non–temperature-sensitive infectious bovine rhinotracheitis vaccine virus with dexamethasone. Infect. Immun. *129* 483–488.

Pedersen NC. 1983. Feline infectious peritonitis and feline enteric coronavirus infections. Part 2: Feline infectious peritonitis. Feline Pract. *13* 5–20.

Ringler SS and Krakowka S. 1985. Effect of canine distemper virus on natural killer cell activity in dogs. Am. J. Vet. Res. *46* 1781–1786.

Rojko JL and Olsen RG. 1984. The immunobiology of the feline leukemia virus. Vet. Immunol. Immunopathol. *6* 107–165.

Rouse BT and Babiuk LA. 1979. Mechanisms of viral immunopathology. Adv. Vet. Sci. Comp. Med. *23* 103–136.

Rouse BT, and Horohov DW. 1984. Cytotoxic T lymphocytes in herpesvirus infections. Vet. Immunol. Immunopathol. *6* 35–66.

Shively MA, Banks KL, Greenlee A and Klevjer-Anderson P. 1982. Antigenic stimulation of T lymphocytes in chronic nononcogenic retrovirus infection: equine infectious anemia. Infect. Immun. *36* 38–46.

17

Immunity to Parasites

The essence of successful parasitism is accommodation and survival; that is, the success of any parasite is measured not by the disturbances it imposes on a host but on its ability to adapt and integrate itself within a host's internal environment. From an immunological point of view, a parasite can be considered a success if it integrates itself into a host in such a way that it is not regarded as foreign.

These considerations apply not only to the protozoa and helminths that we conventionally consider parasites but also to other infectious agents, including bacteria and viruses. On this basis we may regard the intracellular bacteria and algae that serve as mitochondria and chloroplasts within animal and plant cells as the epitome of successful parasitism.

IMMUNITY TO PROTOZOA

Parasitic protozoa may be classified according to their degree of adaptation to a specific host. Some organisms such as the free-living amebae of the genus *Naegleria* are, apparently, totally unadapted to life in animal tissues. Because of this, their inadvertent invasion of the human nasal mucosa, which occurs as a result of swimming in contaminated water, leads to the development of hyperacute meningitis that is almost invariably fatal. Another example of an organism that is poorly adapted to its host is *Trypanosoma rhodesiense*. Although human trypanosomiasis caused by *Trypanosoma gambiense* has been known for hundreds of years and gives rise to a chronic disease usually lasting several years, disease due to *T. rhodesiense* is relatively recent, having been first recorded in 1908. It is not surprising, therefore, that the disease caused by this organism is rapidly progressive, with death occurring in some infected individuals within a few weeks. At the other extreme, *Toxoplasma gondii*, the causal agent of toxoplasmosis, is an organism that almost completely lacks species specificity in its tachyzoite stage, being capable of infecting any species of mammal and many species of birds.

Not surprisingly, *T. gondii*, being so adaptable, causes clinical disease in only a very small proportion of infected animals, and most carry the parasite throughout their lives without showing any ill effects.

Mechanisms of Resistance to Protozoa

Nonimmunological Defense Mechanisms

Although the nonimmunological mechanisms of resistance to protozoa have not been fully clarified, they appear, in general, to be qualitatively similar to those that operate in bacterial and viral diseases. Species influences are perhaps of most significance; for example, *Trypanosoma lewisi* is found only in the rat and *Trypanosoma musculi* in the mouse, where neither causes disease. *Trypanosoma brucei, Trypanosoma congolense* and *Trypanosoma vivax* appear not to cause disease in the wild ungulates of East Africa but are highly virulent for domestic cattle, presumably as a result of lack of mutual adaptation. Similarly, the coccidia are extremely host-specific; they include *T. gondii*, which in its tachyzoite stages can infect any species of mammal but in its coccidian stages will affect only felids (cats, tigers, etc.).

Presumably, these species' differences are but a reflection of somewhat more subtle genetic influences. Thus, some strains of African cattle, most notably N'Dama, show an increased resistance to infection by the pathogenic trypanosomes, which is probably based on a continuous selection of the most resistant animals over many years. Perhaps the best analyzed example of genetically determined resistance to a protozoan infection is sickle cell anemia and its role in resistance to malaria in humans. Individuals who inherit the sickle cell trait possess hemoglobin S (HbS) in which a residue of valine has replaced a residue of glutamic acid present in normal hemoglobin. The changes in the sequence of the hemoglobin molecule induced by this substitution cause deoxygenated hemoglobin molecules to precipitate when reduced, thus distorting the shape of the erythrocytes and resulting in increased erythrocyte fragility and clearance. Individuals who are homozygous for the sickle cell gene die when young from the results of severe anemia. Heterozygous individuals are also anemic, but in west central Africa the fact that hemoglobin S kills *Plasmodium falciparum* ensures that affected individuals are resistant to malaria. As a result of this, more of these individuals tend to survive to reproductive age than normal persons. The mutation is therefore maintained in the human population at a relatively high level.

Specific Immunity to Protozoa

The obvious inadequacies of the immune responses to many parasites led early investigators to conclude that successful parasites were, in general, poorly immunogenic. This is not the case; most parasites are fully antigenic, but in their adaptation to a parasitic existence they have developed mechanisms through which they may survive in the presence of an immune response. Therefore, like other antigenic particles, protozoa can stimulate both humoral and cell-mediated immune responses. In general, antibodies serve to control the level of parasites that exist free in the blood stream and tissue fluids, whereas cell-mediated immune responses are directed largely against intracellular parasites.

Serum antibodies directed against protozoan surface antigens may opsonize, agglutinate or immobilize them. Antibodies together with complement and cytotoxic cells may kill them, and some antibodies (called ablastins) may act to inhibit protozoan enzymes in such a way that their replication is prevented. In infections of the genital tract due to *Tritrichomonas fetus* and *Trichomonas vaginalis*, a local antibody response is stimulated in which, at least in humans, IgE production is prominent. The local type I hypersensitivity reaction that ensues provokes intense discomfort, but more importantly, by increasing vascular permeability, it permits IgG antibodies to reach the site of infection and immobilize and eliminate the organisms.

In babesiosis the infective stage of the organisms (sporozoites) invades red cells. This invasion apparently involves activation of the alternate complement pathway. Infected erythrocytes incorporate *Babesia* antigens into their membranes. These in turn induce antibodies that opsonize the red cells and lead to their removal by the mononuclear phagocytic system. In addition to the humoral response, infected red cells may also be destroyed by an antibody-dependent cell-mediated response. The *Babesia* antigen-opsonizing antibody complex on the surface of infected erythrocytes can be recognized by at least two effector cell types, a macrophage or a cytotoxic lymphocyte. Cytotoxic lymphocytes may be important early in infection when the number of infected erythrocytes is small.

Toxoplasma gondii is an obligate intracellular parasite whose tachyzoite stages replicate within cells (Fig. 17–1). When the number of intracellular organisms becomes excessive, the infected cell ruptures and the organisms released invade other cells. They penetrate these cells by means of a poorly understood mechanism that resembles phagocytosis. When *Toxoplasma* tachyzoites invade normal macrophages, however, they are not destroyed. In the normal process of phagocytosis, once a particle has been enclosed in a phagosome, it is usual for lysosomes to move through the cytoplasm and to empty their

hydrolytic enzymes into the space around the particle. This does not happen in cells that have phagocytosed toxoplasma. The lysosomes may move toward the phagosome, but they do not fuse with it. Thus *Toxoplasma* tachyzoites are able to replicate within the cell in an environment devoid of antibodies or lysosomal enzymes.

Normally, both antibody production and a cell-mediated immune response occur following infection with *Toxoplasma*. The antibodies acting in conjunction with complement can eliminate organisms found free in body fluids and thus reduce the spread of the organism between cells, but they will naturally have little or no influence on the intracellular forms of the parasite. These intracellular organisms are destroyed through a cell-mediated immune response similar to that described for *Listeria monocytogenes* and the mycobacteria (Fig. 17–2) (Chapter 7). Sensitized T lymphocytes release γ interferon in response to *Toxoplasma* ribonucleoproteins. This γ interferon can act on macrophages, first to make them resistant to the lethal effects of *Toxoplasma* and second to assist them in killing the intracellular organism by permitting lysosome-phagosome fusion. Some of these T cells may also release factors that interfere directly with

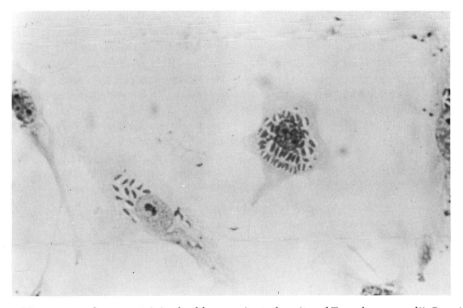

Figure 17–1. Mouse macrophages containing healthy, growing tachyzoites of *Toxoplasma gondii*. Once immunity develops, these cells acquire the ability to destroy ingested tachyzoites. (Courtesy of Dr. C. H. Lai.)

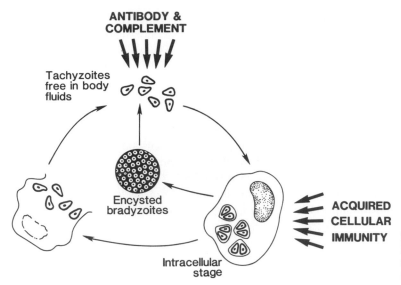

ANTIBODY & COMPLEMENT

Tachyzoites free in body fluids

Encysted bradyzoites

Intracellular stage

ACQUIRED CELLULAR IMMUNITY

Figure 17–2. The points in the life-cycle of *Toxoplasma gondii* at which the immune system can exert a controlling influence.

Toxoplasma replication. In addition, cytotoxic T cells can also destroy *Toxoplasma* tachyzoites and *Toxoplasma*-infected cells. In these ways, antibody-mediated and cell-mediated immune responses act together to ensure the elimination of the tachyzoite stage of this organism. However, *T. gondii* can exist in a cystic form. The cysts develop within cells during the course of infection. They appear to be nonimmunogenic and do not stimulate an inflammatory response. It is possible that this cyst stage is not recognized as foreign.

In *Theileria parva* infection (East Coast fever) of cattle, animals that have recovered from the disease are solidly immune. This immunity is T cell-mediated. The *Theileria* sporozoites preferentially invade lymphocytes, although binding to macrophages and monocytes can also occur. As the schizont stage of *Theileria* develops, these infected lymphocytes are transformed into enlarged cells (lymphoblasts). In cattle that recover from this infection, cytotoxic T lymphocytes are generated that can be shown to kill infected lymphoblasts from other cattle as long as they share the same class I MHC antigens. Thus this reaction is MHC-restricted and implies that the cytotoxic cell recognizes the surface epitopes induced by the parasite infection in association with class I antigens.

The evidence for cell-mediated immune mechanisms in other protozoan diseases is scanty, although in histomoniasis of turkeys, recovered birds show a short-lived resistance to reinfection that is not transferable by serum.

In some protozoan diseases, notably those due to coccidia, the mechanisms of protective immunity are unclear. For example, infection of chickens with some strains of the intestinal parasite *Eimeria maxima* leads to the development of a form of immunity that is capable of preventing reinfection. This immune response acts by inhibiting the growth of the trophozoite, the earliest invasive stage, within intestinal epithelial cells. This growth inhibition is reversible, since arrested stages may be transferred to normal animals and complete their development uneventfully. The mechanism of this resistance is unclear. Antibodies to *E. maxima* can be readily detected in the serum of immune chickens, and the phagocytic cells of these birds show an increased ability to ingest coccidian sporocysts. The results of attempts to detect a local immune response have been equivocal, although a slight measure of resistance can be provided by oral administration of IgA. In spite of all this, neither neonatal bursectomy, thymectomy nor the use of antilymphocyte serum significantly modifies the course of experimentally induced disease.

Immunity to intestinal coccidia is also observed in mammals. Infections by coccidia in lambs and by the coccidian stage of *T. gondii* in cats both effectively stimulate an immune response that is capable of inhibiting reinfection. In cats the shedding of *Toxoplasma* oocysts ceases abruptly about three weeks after infection, coincident with the appearance of serum antibodies. It is not entirely clear, however, whether it is these antibodies that effectively inhibit oocyst production. Bovine dialyzable leukocyte extract (Chapter 27) produced from sensitized calf lymphocytes can transfer delayed hypersensitivity reactions to *Eimeria bovis* as well as confer partial protection to recipient cattle. This implies that cell-mediated immunity may be of significance in this infection.

For many years it was thought that a common feature of many protozoan infections was premunition. Premunition is an old term (perhaps "co-infectious immunity" is better) used to describe resistance that is established after the primary infection has become chronic and is only effective if the parasite persists in the host. It was believed, for example, that only cattle actually infected with *Babesia* were resistant to clinical disease. If all organisms were removed from an animal, then resistance was considered to wane immediately. Further studies have shown that this is not entirely true. For example, cattle apparently cured of *Babesia* infection by chemotherapy have been shown to be resistant to challenge with the homologous strain of that organism for several years afterward. Nevertheless, the presence of infection does appear to be mandatory for protection against heterologous strains. Babesiosis is also of interest, since splenectomy of animals carrying the organisms will cause the development of clinical disease. Not only does the spleen serve as a source of antibodies in this disease, but it also removes infected erythrocytes. Cessation of these functions through splenectomy is apparently sufficient to allow the clinical disease to reappear.

Evasion of the Immune Response by Protozoa

Most important protozoan parasites have evolved mechanisms for evading the consequences of their hosts' immune responses. In general, these mechanisms resemble those evolved by other types of organisms. For example, live *Toxoplasma gondii* appears to be able to successfully avoid neutrophil attachment and phagocytosis. Many protozoa are immunosuppressive; for example, *Theileria parva* invades and destroys lymphocytes. Other protozoa such as the trypanosomes are also effectively immunosuppressive, but their mode of action is unclear. It has been suggested that trypanosomes may promote the development of suppressor cells. Other evidence suggests that they stimulate the B cell system to exhaustion, whereas some investigators believe that they release immunosuppressive factors.

Parasite-induced immunosuppression may be of great assistance to the parasite. For example, *Babesia bovis* is immunosuppressive for cattle. As a result, its host vector, the tick *Boophilus microplus*, is more able to survive on an infected animal. Consequently, infected cattle have more ticks than noninfected animals, and the efficiency of transmission of *B. bovis* is greatly enhanced. It must also be pointed out, however, that parasite-induced immunosuppression commonly leads to the death of host animals as a result of secondary infection, so it is not necessarily always beneficial to the parasite.

In addition to immunosuppression, protozoa have evolved two other extremely effective immunoevasive techniques. One involves becoming either hypo- or nonantigenic, and the other involves acquiring the ability to rapidly and repeatedly alter their surface antigens. An example of a hypoantigenic organism is the cyst stage of *T. gondii*, which, as mentioned previously, appears not to stimulate a host response. As an alternative to the evolution of nonimmunogenic stages, some protozoa can become functionally nonantigenic by masking themselves with host antigens. Examples of these include *Trypanosoma theileri* in cattle and *Trypanosoma lewisi* in rats. These are both nonpathogenic trypanosomes, which can survive in the blood stream of infected animals because they become covered with a layer of host serum proteins and so are not regarded as foreign. There is also some evidence to suggest that *T. brucei*, a pathogenic trypanosome of cattle, may adsorb either host serum

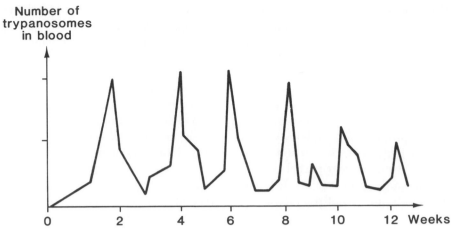

Figure 17–3. The time-course of *Trypanosoma congolense* parasitemia in an infected calf. Each parasitemic peak represents the development of a new, antigenically original population of organisms.

proteins or red cell antigens and so become functionally nonantigenic.

Although the absence of antigenicity may be considered the ultimate stage in the evasive process, many protozoa, especially the trypanosomes, have evolved the technique of antigenic variation to a high degree of sophistication. If cattle are infected with the pathogenic trypanosome *T. vivax*, *T. congolense* or *T. brucei* and the parasitemia is checked at regular intervals, it is found that the numbers of circulating organisms fluctuate greatly, with periods of high parasitemia alternating regularly with periods of low or undetectable parasitemia (Fig. 17–3). Serum taken from infected animals will react with trypanosomes isolated prior to the time of bleeding but not with those that develop later. Each peak period of high parasitemia corresponds to the development of a population of trypanosomes of a new antigenic type. The elimination of a population of one antigenic type leads to a fall in blood parasite levels. From the survivors, however, a proportion of parasites develop new surface antigens and a fresh population arises to produce yet another period of high parasitemia (Fig. 17–4). This cyclical fluctuation in parasite levels, with each peak reflect-

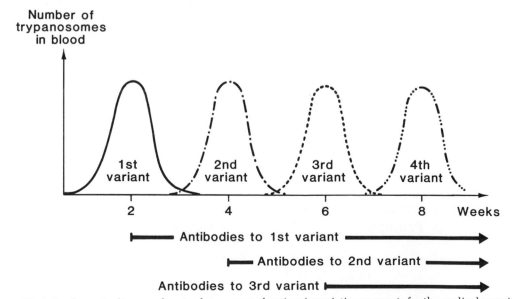

Figure 17–4. A schematic diagram showing how repeated antigenic variation accounts for the cyclical parasitemia observed in African trypanosomiasis. Each peak represents the growth of a new antigenic variant.

ing the appearance of a new antigenic variant population, can continue for a long time.

The variant antigens produced early in infection tend to develop in a fairly predictable sequence. As the infection progresses, however, the variant antigens become more random. Trypanosomes grown in tissue culture also show spontaneous antigenic variation, demonstrating that the variation is not necessarily induced by antibody. By means of electron microscopy, it can be shown that the variant antigen forms a thick coat over the surface of the trypanosome. When antigenic change occurs, the proteins in the old coat are shed and replaced by an antigenically different protein. Analysis of the genetics of this process indicates that the trypanosomes possess a large number of genes for coat protein and that antigenic variation occurs as a result of random gene rearrangement and selection.

Trypanosomiasis is not the only protozoan infection in which antigenic variation is seen. Minor antigenic variations have been recorded in babesiosis in which relapse strains appear to be antigenically different from the original strains. Antigenic variation is also seen in malaria, although the range of antigens and the differences between them are relatively small.

Since parasitic protozoa seek to evade the immune responses, it is not surprising that they also invade immunosuppressed individuals. Organisms that are normally maintained in a relatively quiescent state by the immune response, such as the cyst forms of *T. gondii* or *Cryptosporidium*, are capable of changing to a more active form and producing severe disease in immunosuppressed animals. For this reason, acute toxoplasmosis or cryptosporidiosis is not uncommonly seen in patients immunosuppressed for transplantation purposes, for cancer therapy or with AIDS.

Adverse Consequences of the Immune Response to Protozoa

As with the groups of organisms described earlier, the immune response against protozoa can give rise to each of the hypersensitivity types described in Chapter 19, and these may,

under some circumstances, contribute significantly to the pathogenesis of the disease process.

Type I hypersensitivity, as has been mentioned, is a feature of trichomoniasis and results in local irritation and inflammation in the genital tract. Type II cytotoxic reactions, which contribute to the development of anemia, are of significance in babesiosis and trypanosomiasis. In babesiosis, parasitized erythrocytes carry parasite-derived antigens on their surfaces and are thus recognized as foreign and eliminated by immune cytolysis and phagocytosis. In trypanosomiasis, either fragments of disrupted organisms or possibly preformed immune complexes bind to erythrocytes and provoke their immune elimination, thus contributing to the development of anemia. Immune complex formation on circulating erythrocytes is not the only problem of this type in trypanosomiasis. In many cases, systemic immune complex formation can also lead to the development of vasculitis and glomerulonephritis (type III hypersensitivity; Chapter 22). The actual cause, or causes, of death in trypanosomiasis is not clear, but it is likely that systemic immune complex deposition may contribute to the demise of infected animals.

It is probable that a type IV hypersensitivity reaction contributes to the inflammatory reaction that occurs when *Toxoplasma* cysts break down and release fresh tachyzoites. Extracts of *T. gondii* (toxoplasmin), if administered intradermally to infected animals, will result in the development of a delayed hypersensitivity response (Fig. 17–5), and this phenomenon has been used on occasion as a diagnostic test for this infection.

Vaccination Against Protozoan Infections

Successful vaccination against protozoan infections of domestic animals is currently limited to babesiosis and theileriosis. The *Babesia* species constitute a heterogeneous group of tick-borne organisms that parasitize erythrocytes and so cause anemia. A number of factors contribute to the resistance of animals against babesiosis, including genetic factors (Zebu cat-

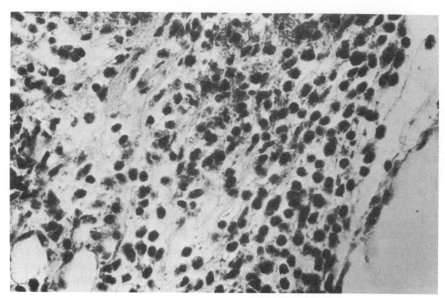

Figure 17–5. The characteristic mononuclear cell infiltration of a delayed hypersensitivity reaction in the skin of a mouse following an intradermal injection of an extract of *Toxoplasma gondii* called toxoplasmin. (Courtesy of Dr. C. H. Lai.)

tle are more resistant to disease than European cattle) and age (cattle show a significant resistance to babesiosis in the first six months of life). Animals that recover from acute babesiosis are resistant to further clinical disease, and this immunity has been considered to be a form of premunity (see page 237). It is possible to infect young calves deliberately so that they will acquire infection while they are still relatively insusceptible to disease, and thereafter be resistant to reinfection. The organisms employed for this procedure are first attenuated by repeated passage through splenectomized calves and then administered to recipient animals in whole blood. As might be anticipated, the side effects of this type of controlled infection may be relatively severe, and chemotherapy is commonly required to control them. The transfer of blood from one calf to another may also lead to sensitization and the production of isoantibodies against red cells. These antibodies complicate any attempts at blood transfusion in later life and may provoke hemolytic disease of the newborn in calves born from sensitized cows (Chapter 21). Cattle can be immunized against East Coast fever (*Theileria parva* infection) by in-

jecting them with sporozoites and treating them simultaneously with tetracycline.

Many attempts have been made to immunize poultry against coccidia, but it is clear that only infection with viable organisms can induce protective immunity. Thus, repeated dosing with small number of oocysts can provide some protection. Unfortunately, this technique may provoke severe reactions that require treatment with coccidiostats. Alternatively, oocysts may be attenuated by ionizing radiation. The results obtained by this method suggest that any protection obtained is due to infection and establishment of the few parasites whose life cycles have not been interrupted by the radiation.

In the case of a well-adapted organism such as *T. gondii*, not only does infection rarely lead to disease, but it also results in the development of strong life-long immunity to reinfection. Because of this, it would be difficult to produce a vaccine against this organism that would improve significantly on the natural infection. It may, however, be desirable to develop a vaccine for cats, which could inhibit oocyst production and thus break that segment of transmission cycle.

The Serodiagnosis of Protozoan Infections (Table 17–1)

In general, the tests used for the diagnosis of protozoan infections resemble those used in the other situations. Thus, the complement fixation test, immunofluorescence techniques and passive agglutination are used in the diagnosis of toxoplasmosis, babesiosis and trichomoniasis. There has been a distinct trend toward the use of primary binding tests, especially the ELISA and the indirect immunofluorescence tests.

IMMUNITY TO HELMINTHS

The immune system has not been conspicuously successful in producing absolute resistance to helminth infections in mammals. In a sense it has been detrimental, since the IgE-mediated immune reactions appear to have evolved largely for the control of these parasites. In Western society where parasites are largely controlled by hygienic measures, the problem of allergies is probably of much greater social significance than parasitism. On a worldwide basis, however, and in relation to domestic animals, helminth parasites remain of major significance.

It is not surprising that the immune system is relatively inefficient in controlling helminth parasites. After all, these organisms have adapted to an obligatory parasitic existence, and presumably this adaptation has involved confronting the immune system and either overcoming or evading it. Parasitic helminths are, therefore, not maladapted pathogenic organisms but fully adapted obligate parasites whose very survival depends on reaching some form of accommodation with the host. Consequently, if an organism of this type causes disease, it is likely to be expressed either very mildly or subclinically. Only when helminth parasites invade a host to which they are not fully adapted or in unusually large numbers does acute disease occur.

Mechanisms of Resistance to Helminths

Nonimmunological Defense Mechanisms

The factors that influence the course of helminth infections are many and complex. They include the influences not only of host-derived factors but also of factors derived from other helminths within the same host. For example, both intraspecies and interspecies competition are known to occur. In the former case, it is evident, particularly with respect to cestode infections, that the presence of adult worms in the intestine delays the further development of larval stages in the tissues. Consequently, for example, calves infected with *Cysticercus bovis* appear to be resistant to further infection by this organism. Similarly, lambs acquire resistance to *Echinococcus granulosus* to the extent that multiple dosing with ova does not result in the development of massive worm burdens. It is hypothesized that the original dose of eggs may stimulate "rejection" of subsequent doses. Interspecies competition between helminths for mutual habitats and nutrients serves to control the numbers and composition of an animal's helminth population.

Table 17–1 TESTS USED IN THE DIAGNOSIS OF SOME SELECTED PROTOZOAN INFECTIONS

Infection	Direct Agglutination	Passive Hemagglutination	Complement Fixation	Fluorescent Antibody Tests	Gel Diffusion	Skin Tests
Coccidiosis	−	−	−	−	−	−
Toxoplasmosis	−	+	+	+	−	+
Babesiosis	+	+	+	+	+	−
Trichomoniasis	+	+	+	+	−	+
Trypanosomiasis	+	+	+	−	−	−

The factors of host origin that influence helminth burdens include the age, breed and sex of the host. The influence of sex and age on helminth burdens appears to be largely hormonal. In animals whose sexual cycle is seasonal, parasites tend to synchronize their reproductive cycle with that of the host. For instance, ewes show a spring rise in fecal nematode ova, which coincides with lambing and the onset of lactation. Similarly, the development of helminth larvae ingested by cattle in autumn tends to be inhibited until spring. Perhaps the most evolved organisms in this respect are the nematodes of the genus *Toxocara*, the larvae of which may migrate from an infected bitch to the liver of the fetal pup, resulting in a congenital infection. Once born, the infected pups can reinfect their mother by the more conventional fecal-oral route.

A good example of genetically mediated resistance to helminths is the superior resistance of sheep with hemoglobin A to infestations with *Haemonchus contortus* and *Ostertagia circumcincta*, as compared to sheep with hemoglobin B. The reasons for this are unclear, but sheep with HbA mount a more effective self-cure reaction and a better immune response to many other antigens as well. Another example is the enhanced resistance of Zebu cattle to *Cooperia oncophora* compared to European cattle.

Specific Immunity to Helminths

Humoral Mechanisms. Helminths, in general, can be found in two situations in the body: in tissues as larval forms or within the gastrointestinal or respiratory tract as adults. Obviously, the form of the immune response that is most effective against each of these stages differs considerably.

Although conventional antibodies of the IgM, IgG and IgA isotypes are produced in response to helminth antigens, an increasing body of evidence suggests that the most significant immunoglobulin isotype involved in resistance to helminths is IgE. For example, IgE levels are usually extremely elevated in parasitized individuals. Many helminth infestations are associated with the characteristic signs of type I hypersensitivity, including eosinophilia, edema, asthma and urticarial dermatitis; and many helminth infections such as oesophagostomiasis, ancylostomiasis, strongyloidiasis, taeniasis and fascioliasis are accompanied by a positive passive cutaneous anaphylaxis (PCA) reaction to worm antigens (Chapter 20).

Many helminth antigens preferentially stimulate IgE production, so investigators who handle helminths regularly may become sensitized to worm antigens. These individuals then suffer from asthmatic attacks or cutaneous wheal-and-flare reactions (urticaria) on exposure to worms. In addition to being potent stimulators of IgE production against themselves, helminth antigens are also capable of acting as adjuvants, specific for IgE production against other, nonhelminth antigens.

Although IgE production and the allergies that result from it are considered by some to be only a nuisance, they appear to be of considerable benefit in controlling worm burdens. One of the best examples of this is the self-cure reaction seen in sheep infected with gastrointestinal nematodes, particularly *Haemonchus contortus*. These worms, which are embedded in the intestinal and abomasal mucosa, secrete antigens during their third ecdysis that act as allergens. As a result, the development of a worm burden provokes a local acute type I hypersensitivity reaction in the parasitized regions of the intestine. The combination of helminth antigens with mast cell–bound IgE leads to mast cell degranulation and the release of vasoactive amines. These compounds stimulate smooth muscle contraction and increase vascular permeability. Thus, in the self-cure reaction, violent contractions of the intestinal musculature and an increase in the permeability of intestinal capillaries occur, allowing an efflux of fluid into the intestinal lumen. This combination results in dislodgment and expulsion of the major portion of the animal's gastrointestinal worm burden (Fig. 17–6). In sheep that have just undergone self-cure, the PCA antibody titer is high (Chapter 20) and experimental administration of helminth antigens will result in acute anaphylaxis, confirming the role of type I hypersensitivity in this phenomenon.

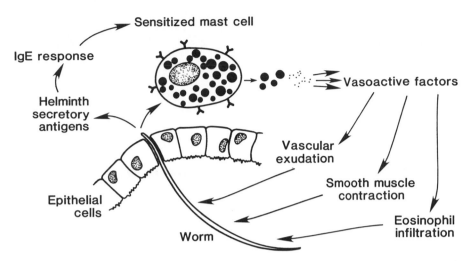

Figure 17–6. The mechanisms involved in the self-cure reaction against intestinal helminths.

A similar reaction is seen in fascioliasis in calves in which peak PCA titers coincide with expulsion of the parasite.

Macrophages, platelets and eosinophils also possess IgE Fc receptors. As a result, these cells can be sensitized by IgE and will bind to parasites. Once bound these cells are activated. For example, macrophages bound to helminth larvae through IgE show elevated lysosomal enzymes and increased release of reactive oxygen metabolites, interleukin 1, leukotrienes, prostaglandins and platelet activating factor (Chapter 20). The net effect of this is enhanced parasite destruction.

Eosinophils are attracted to sites of helminth invasion by ECF-A (eosinophil chemotactic factor of anaphylaxis) released by degranulating mast cells. In addition, this material mobilizes the body's eosinophil pool, resulting in the release of large numbers of eosinophils into the circulation. It is for this

reason that an eosinophilia is so characteristic of helminth infestations. Once they arrive at the site of helminth invasion, eosinophils attach to the parasites by means of IgE and IgG. They then degranulate, releasing their granule contents onto the helminth cuticle (Fig. 17–7). These granule contents include products of the respiratory burst, such as superoxides, hydrogen peroxide and other free radicals, and potent lytic enzymes such as lysophospholipase, and phospholipase D (Table 17–2). More importantly, however, the major basic

Table 17–2 THE CONTENTS OF EOSINOPHIL GRANULES

Major basic protein
Eosinophil cationic protein
Eosinophil peroxidase
Aryl sulfatase B
Phospholipase D
Lysophospholipase
Acid phosphatase
Collagenase
Histaminase
Kininase

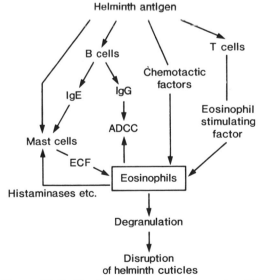

Figure 17–7. The interactions between eosinophils and other branches of the immune system that result in helminth destruction.

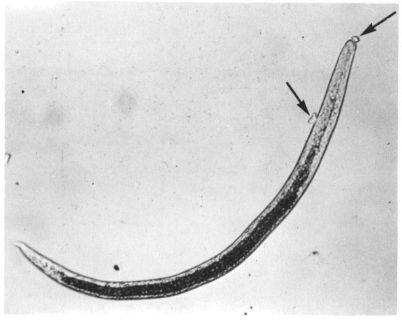

Figure 17–8. A *Toxocara canis* larva after incubation in specific antiserum. The immune precipitates at the oral and excretory pores are indicated by arrows. (Courtesy of Dr. D. H. DeSavigny.)

protein of the granules can cause direct damage to the cuticle and promote the adherence of additional eosinophils. The helminthicidal effects of eosinophils are enhanced by mast cell-derived factors such as histamine as well as by complement and by factors derived from T lymphocytes and macrophages.

While the IgE-dependent eosinophil-mediated antihelminth response is perhaps the most significant mechanism of resistance to helminths, antibodies of the other immunoglobulin isotypes also play a protective role. The mechanisms involved include antibody-mediated neutralization of the proteolytic enzymes used by larvae to penetrate tissues,

blocking of the anal and oral pores of these larvae by immune complexes as antibodies combine with their excretory and secretory products (Fig. 17–8) and prevention of ecdysis and inhibition of larval development by antibodies directed against exsheathing antigens. Other enzyme pathways may be blocked by antibodies acting against adult worms, causing possible arrest of egg production or even interference in the development of anatomical structures (Fig. 17–9). Thus, female *Ostertagia ostertagi* worms fail to develop vulvar flaps when grown in immune calves. Similarly, spicule morphology may be altered in *Cooperia* males derived from immune hosts. Larvae also

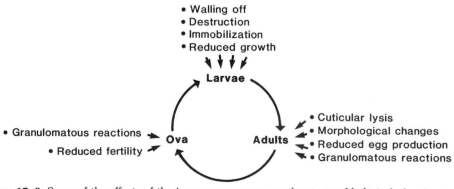

Figure 17–9. Some of the effects of the immune responses on the stages of helminth development.

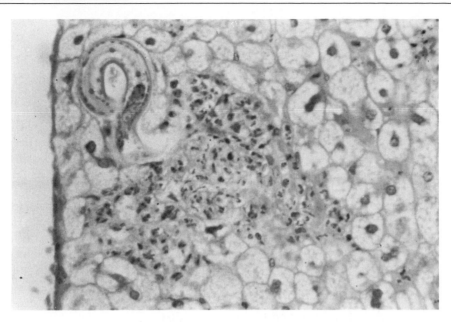

Figure 17–10. The cellular response to a helminth larva. This is a *T. canis* larva in the liver of a rabbit, 48 hours after administration of infective eggs. At this stage, most of the cells present are neutrophils. (Courtesy of Dr. J. P. Lautenslager.)

tend to cause tissue destruction and inflammation, attracting large numbers of neutrophils (Fig. 17–10).

Cell-Mediated Mechanisms. Many helminths, particularly those that undergo tissue migration, may be considered as functional xenografts. It is somewhat remarkable, therefore, that they are not precipitously rejected by the cell-mediated immune system. Their survival is a reflection of the success of their adaptation to existence within mammalian tissues. Nevertheless, there is evidence to suggest that sensitized T lymphocytes may successfully attack helminths that are either deeply embedded in the intestinal mucosa or undergoing prolonged tissue stages. For example, cell-mediated immune reactions have been shown to occur in *Trichinella spiralis* and *Trichostrongylus colubriformis* infections. In the former, immunity can be transferred to normal animals by lymphoid cells, and infected animals show delayed hypersensitivity reactions to intradermally inoculated worm antigens. *In vitro* tests for cell-mediated immunity such as MIF production and lymphocyte proliferation are also positive in these infections. (Trichinosis is also characterized by the occurrence of a massive eosinophilia. This appears to be associated with the presence of

T cells and may be due to the activity of an eosinophil-stimulating lymphokine.) In the case of *T. colubriformis*, immunity can be transferred to normal animals from immune ones by both cells and serum, and the site of worm attachment is subjected to a massive lymphocyte infiltration.

The cell-mediated immune responses participate in resistance against a number of other helminth infections. Thus, lymphocytes from sheep infected with *H. contortus* will release MIF and undergo blastogenesis in response to worm antigen, and it has been shown that immunity to this organism can be transferred to syngeneic sheep by using immune lymphocytes.

Sensitized T lymphocytes depress the activities of helminths by two mechanisms. First, the development of an inflammatory response of the delayed hypersensitivity type tends to attract mononuclear cells to the site of larval invasion and renders the local environment unsuitable for growth or migration. Second, cytotoxic lymphocytes may be capable of causing larval destruction. In connection with this, it has been shown that the treatment of experimental animals with BCG vaccine, a treatment that stimulates the T cell system (Chapter 27), inhibits the metastases of hydatid cysts

(*E. granulosus*); in these treated animals the space that surrounds the cysts may be filled with large lymphocytes. It is also not uncommon to observe large lymphocytes adhering firmly to migrating nematode larvae *in vivo*.

Evasion of the Immune Response by Helminths

Although the preceding discussion has noted a number of mechanisms whereby animals resist helminth infection, it is obvious, even to a casual observer, that these responses are not fully effective. The success of this adaptation is seen at its most marked extent in cestode infections in which cysticerci, in particular, appear to be able to survive indefinitely in the presence of a host response. Several mechanisms may be considered to play a role in this adaptation. They include mimicry of host antigens, absorption of host antigens, antigenic variation, shedding of the glycocalyx, blocking of antibodies and tolerance.

The first of these mechanisms introduces the concept that helminths may synthesize histocompatibility or blood group antigens to match those of their host. It is clear that a helminth cannot synthesize all antigens it could possibly require, since this would demand the existence of a genetic system similar in complexity to the antibody-producing system. Nevertheless, partial mimicry of host antigens is indeed possible, so that, for example, sheep respond to fewer antigens of *H. contortus* than do rabbits. This suggests that *H. contortus* possesses a closer antigenic similarity to sheep, its natural host, than to rabbits, which it does not normally infect. It has also been shown that many trematodes and cestodes are capable of synthesizing blood group antigens, which, if they happen to be identical to those of the host, also serve to reduce the effective antigenicity of the worm.

Second, there is a considerable amount of evidence that suggests that tissue helminths may be protected from the consequences of their host's immune response by the adsorption of host antigens onto their surface. An example of this is seen in adult *Taenia solium*

in pigs, which is coated with swine IgG. It is not clear whether this IgG is synthesized by the worm or if the worm synthesizes a receptor for IgG. Cysticerci can also adsorb histocompatibility antigens in this way.

A third mechanism of evasion of the immune response involves antigenic variation. Although helminths have not evolved a system as efficient as that seen in trypanosomiasis, gradual antigenic variation is recognized. Thus, the cuticular antigens of *T. spiralis* larvae show extensive changes following each molt. Even during their growth phase they show quantitative changes in the expression of surface protein antigens. This antigenic variation of the cuticular antigens may be accompanied by a shedding of the glycocalyx as is seen in *F. hepatica* exposed to specific antibodies.

Another response that may contribute to the survival of parasitic helminths is immunosuppression. For example, sheep infected with *H. contortus* may become specifically suppressed so that they are unreactive to *H. contortus* even though they remain responsive to unrelated antigens. The mechanisms involved in this response are unknown. *Oesophagostomum radiatum* secretes soluble factors that inhibit the responses of lymphocytes to mitogens. Other mechanisms may involve induction of specific suppressor cells, as has been demonstrated in filariasis or, alternatively, they may result from the production of soluble suppressor factors as has been demonstrated in fascioliasis. In other helminth infections, such as trichinosis, infected animals are nonspecifically immunosuppressed. This immunosuppression is reflected in a lowered resistance to other infections, a poor response to vaccination and a prolongation of skin graft survival.

It is theoretically possible that tolerance could occur in young animals that receive a high dose of parasite antigen either *in utero* as in toxocariasis or very soon after birth.

Vaccination Against Helminths

It is not surprising, considering the ineffectiveness of the host response to helminths, that vaccines are not widely available. Since vaccines consisting of dead organisms or extracts of organisms have been uniformly unsuccessful in conferring protection, studies have tended to concentrate on the use of irradiated material. Experimentally it has been shown, for instance, that irradiated metacercariae can reduce a *Fasciola hepatica* burden in calves, whereas irradiated ova of *Ascaridia galli* protect chickens against challenge by this helminth and UV-irradiated *Ascaris suum* eggs can confer protection on pigs. However, only very few of these preparations have been commercially produced with any success. Perhaps the most important of those that have is the vaccine that is used to protect calves against verminous pneumonia caused by the lungworm *Dictyocaulus viviparus*. In this vaccine, second-stage larvae hatched from ova in culture are exposed to 40,000 R x-irradiation, and two doses of these larvae are then fed to calves. The larvae succeed in penetrating the calf's intestine, but, since they are unable to develop to the third stage, they never reach the lung and for this reason are nonpathogenic. During their exsheathing process, however, they stimulate the development of antibodies that are then capable of blocking reinfection. The efficiency of this vaccine, like other vaccines, depends very much on timing and on the size of the challenge dose, since vaccinated calves may show mild pneumonic signs if placed on grossly infected pastures.

A similar type of vaccine has been used to protect puppies against the hookworm *Ancylostoma caninum*. In this case, irradiated larvae are administered three days after birth in order to provide immunity. Interestingly, passive immunity from the bitch does not appear to interfere with the development of resistance in the puppy.

The Serodiagnosis of Helminth Infections

Immunological tests have never been widely used in the diagnosis of helminth infestations. It has generally been much easier to arrive at a diagnosis by examining feces for ova. Nevertheless, there are three important helminth diseases—heartworm infestation, visceral larva migrans (*Toxocara canis*) and trichinosis—in which ova are not shed and in which serological diagnosis is almost essential. In all three cases ELISA tests have been found to be the most useful diagnostic techniques.

IMMUNITY TO ARTHROPODS

When arthropods bite an animal, they inject saliva. This saliva contains antigens and therefore induces immune responses. The immune responses induced by these antigens are of three types. Some salivary components are of low molecular weight, and as a result, they cannot function as normal antigens. They may, however, bind to skin proteins such as collagen and then function as haptens, stimulating a cell-mediated response. On subsequent exposure, these haptens will induce a delayed hypersensitivity reaction. Other salivary antigens may bind to epidermal Langerhans cells and induce cutaneous basophil hypersensitivity, a response associated with the production of IgG antibodies and a basophil infiltration. If the basophils are destroyed by antibasophil serum, then resistance to biting arthropods is reduced. The third type of response to arthropod saliva is an IgE response with an associated type I hypersensitivity. This response may induce a severe inflammatory response in the skin and as a result cause severe discomfort to the bitten animal. Each of these three types of response may modify the skin in such a way that the feeding of the offending arthropod is impaired and the animal may therefore be a less attractive source of food. (These hypersensitivities are discussed further in Chapter 23.)

Demodectic Mange

The mange mite *Demodex folliculorum* appears to be a normal symbiont commonly present in hair follicles and only occasionally causing disease. When demodectic mange does occur, the reaction around mites and mite fragments tends to be infiltrated by mononuclear cells together with a few plasma cells. Granuloma formation may occasionally occur. Although it has been suggested that this lesion is a type IV hypersensitivity reaction, perhaps a form of allergic contact dermatitis, it is more likely to be a foreign-body reaction. The absence of eosinophils and edema in the lesion suggests that type I hypersensitivity is relatively unimportant in this condition. It is of interest to note that immunosuppressive agents such as antilymphocyte serum, azathioprine and prolonged steroid therapy tend to predispose animals to the development of demodectic mange. Animals suffering from generalized demodecosis have normal neutrophil function and respond normally to vaccines or other foreign proteins. Nevertheless, their T cell response to plant mitogens such as phytohemagglutinin and concanavalin A is depressed. Serum from these animals is also able to suppress the reactivity of T cells from normal animals. However, if the T cells of a dog with demodecosis are washed free of serum, they regain their ability to respond to mitogens.

Flea Bite Dermatitis

Biting fleas secrete saliva into the skin wound. Some of the components of flea saliva are of relatively low molecular weight but can act as haptens by binding to dermal collagen. As a consequence of this, a local type IV hypersensitivity reaction characterized by a mononuclear cell infiltration occurs. In some sensitized animals, this type IV reaction is gradually replaced over a period of months by a type I reaction, and so the mononuclear cell infiltration gradually changes to an eosinophil infiltration.

Tick Infestation

It has been observed that ticks on nonimmune animals are larger than those on immune animals. Although the nature of this resistance is unclear, it has been suggested that local cell-mediated and immune complex hypersensitivities to tick saliva may act together to restrict the blood flow to the tick, thus reducing its food supply and stunting its growth. It is possible to immunize guinea pigs with tick homogenates and show that ticks feeding on these animals have reduced fertility and egg production.

ADDITIONAL SOURCES OF INFORMATION

Baker PE, Hagemo A, Knoblock K and Dubey JP. 1983. *Toxoplasma gondii:* Microassay to differentiate toxoplasma inhibiting factor and Interleukin 2. Exp. Parasitol. *55* 320–330.

Bloom BR. 1979. Games parasites play: how parasites evade immune surveillance. Nature *279* 21–26.

Butterworth AE and David JR. 1981. Current concepts: eosinophil function. N. Engl. J. Med. *304* 154–156.

Callow LL and Stewart NP. 1978. Immunosuppression by *Babesia bovis* against its tick vector *Boophilus microplus.* Nature *272* 818–819.

Capron A, Dessaint JP and Capron M. 1979. Immunoregulation of parasite infections. J. Allergy Clin. Immunol. *66* 91–96.

Coley SC and Leid RW. 1982. Effects of extracts of *Onchocerca cervicalis* from horses on the lytic activity of human, rat and equine complement. Clin. Immunol. Immunopathol. *23* 113–123.

Conception JE and Barriga OO. 1985. Transfer of infection-induced immune protection to *Toxocara canis* in a mouse model. Vet. Immunol. Immunopathol. *9* 371–382.

Gasbarre LC, Romanowski RD and Douvres FW. 1985. Suppression of antigen- and mitogen-induced proliferation of bovine lymphocytes by excretory-secretory products of *Oesophagostomum radiatum.* Infect. Immun. *48* 540–545.

Miller HRP. 1984. The protective mucosal response against gastrointestinal nematodes in ruminants and laboratory animals. Vet. Immunol. Immunopathol. *6* 167–259.

Miller TA. 1978. Immunology in intestinal parasitism. Vet. Clin. North Am. (Small Anim. Pract.) *8* 707–720.

Mitchell GF. 1979. Effector cells, molecules and mechanisms in host-protective immunity to parasites. Immunology *38* 209–223.

Nantulya VM, Musoke AJ, Rurangirwa FR et al. 1982. Immune depression in African trypanosomiasis: the role of antigenic competition. Clin. Exp. Immunol. *47* 234–242.

Oldham G and Williams L. 1985. Cell-mediated immunity to liver fluke antigens during experimental *Fasciola hepatica* infection of cattle. Parasite Immunol. *7* 503–516.

Rhodes MB, Keralis MB and Staudinger LA. 1982. Immune response of swine to oral inoculation with embryonated eggs of *Ascaris suum.* Am. J. Vet. Res. *43* 1604–1607.

Ribeiro JMC, Makoul GT, Levin T, Robinson DR and Spielman A. 1985. Antihemostatic, antiinflammatory and immunosuppressive properties of the saliva of the tick *Ixodes dammini*. J. Exp. Med. *161* 332–344.

Smith WD, Jackson F, Jackson E et al. 1984. Resistance to *Haemonchus contortus* transferred between genetically histocompatible sheep by immune lymphocytes. Res. Vet. Sci. *37* 199–204.

Spry CJF. 1985. Synthesis and secretion of eosinophil granule substances. Immunol. Today *6* 332–335.

Stear MJ, Newman MJ, Nicholas FW, Brown SC and Holroyd RG. 1984. Tick resistance and the major histocompatibility system. Aust. J. Exp. Biol. Med. Sci. *62* 47–52.

Townsend J and Duffus WPH. 1985. Antibody dependent cellular cytotoxicity of *Trypanosoma theileri* mediated by purified bovine isotypes and subisotypes. Parasite Immunol. *7* 175–179.

Urban JF and Tromba FG. 1982. Development of immune responsiveness to *Ascaris suum* antigens in pigs vaccinated with ultraviolet-attenuated eggs. Vet. Immunol. Immunopathol. *3* 399–410.

Urquhart GM. 1980. Application of immunity in the control of parasitic disease. Vet. Parasitol. *6* 217–239.

Zachary JF and Smith AR. 1985. Experimental porcine eperythrozoonosis: T-lymphocyte suppression and misdirected immune response. Am. J. Vet. Res. *46* 821–830.

18

Surveillance and Elimination of Foreign and Abnormal Cells

Although the immune responses first attracted the attention of scientists by virtue of the body's ability to recognize and eliminate invading microorganisms, the observation that animals also possess the ability to reject foreign tissue grafts has led to the development of a much broader view of the function of the immune system.

TERMINOLOGY

Genetically identical animals are said to be *syngeneic* or *allogeneic*. Genetically dissimilar animals of the same species are *allogeneic*. Animals of different species are *xenogeneic*.

A graft between two locations on the same animal is known as an *autograft*. A graft between two genetically identical animals is an *isograft*. A graft between two genetically dissimilar animals of the same species is an *allograft*. A graft between two animals of differing species is a *xenograft*.

THE ALLOGRAFT REACTION

If a kidney is surgically transplanted between unrelated mongrel dogs, it will survive for about a week (Table 18–1). The graft is eventually rejected as a result of disruption of its blood flow and tissue destruction leading to oliguria and eventually anuria. If a second kidney graft is made from the same donor, it will be rejected by the recipient within one

251

Table 18–1 SURVIVAL TIMES OF CANINE ALLOGRAFTS BETWEEN DLA-INCOMPATIBLE MONGREL DOGS*

Organ	Survival Time (Days)
Skin	12
Kidney	7
Liver	8
Pancreas	11
Lung	9
Small intestine	8
Heart	8
Tracheal cartilage	250
Parathyroids	<14

*Survival times are usually significantly longer in grafts between DLA-incompatible beagles or between DLA-compatible dogs.

to two days without ever becoming functional. This accelerated rejection of a second graft is known as a second-set reaction and is a form of secondary immune response. The second-set reaction is specific for a graft from the original donor or from a donor syngeneic with the first. Because the rejection process is directed against the histocompatibility antigens of the donor, it is not restricted to any particular site or to any specific organ, since histocompatibility antigens are present on all nucleated cells (Fig. 18–1).

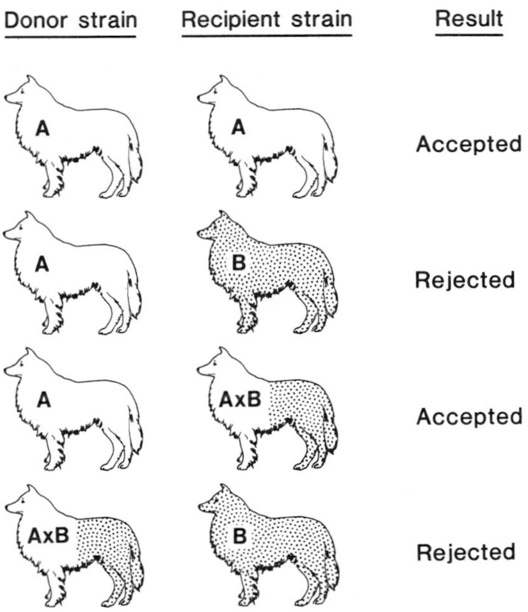

Donor strain	Recipient strain	Result
A	A	Accepted
A	B	Rejected
A	AxB	Accepted
AxB	B	Rejected

Figure 18–1. The laws of graft rejection. Grafts between histocompatible animals will be accepted. Grafts between incompatible animals will be rejected. An animal will accept a graft from one of its parents since it carries their histocompatibility antigens. A parent will not accept a graft from one of its offspring since the graft will carry foreign histocompatibility antigens.

Pathology of Allograft Rejection

The events that take place during graft rejection vary among different types of grafts. For example, if a skin graft is placed on an animal, it takes some time for vascular and lymphatic connections to be established between the graft and the host. Only when these connections are made can host cells penetrate the graft and commence the rejection process. The first indication of this is a transient neutrophil accumulation around the blood vessels at the base of the graft, and this is followed by an infiltration of mononuclear cells (lymphocytes and macrophages) that eventually extends throughout the grafted skin. The first signs of tissue damage are observed in the capillaries of the graft, whose endothelium is destroyed. As a result, thrombosis, vascular stasis and infarction follow rapidly. In renal grafts, the blood supply to the transplanted kidney is established at the time of transplantation. As a result, the whole organ gradually becomes infiltrated with mononuclear cells (Fig. 18–2), which damage the endothelium of small intertubular blood vessels. This vascular damage is progressive, and tubular destruction, infarction, hemorrhage and death of the grafted kidney follow thrombosis of these vessels.

In a second-set reaction, vascularization of skin grafts usually does not have time to occur, since an extensive and destructive mononuclear cell and neutrophil infiltration occurs in the graft bed. Similarly, the blood vessels of second kidney grafts become rapidly blocked as a result of thrombosis following destruction of vascular endothelium by serum antibodies and complement. Xenografts are usually rejected extremely promptly. For example, pig kidneys transplanted to dogs are irreversibly damaged in 10 to 20 minutes because of the presence of natural antibodies to pig antigens in dog serum.

Mechanisms of Allograft Rejection
(Fig. 18–3)

As described previously, the rejection of grafts is of two general types. In first-set reactions, grafts are rejected in a matter of days. In second-set reactions or xenografts, rejection

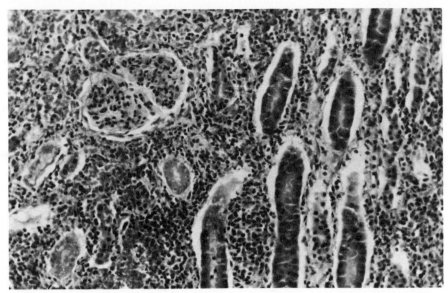

Figure 18–2. Section of a canine kidney that had been rejected after 14 days by an allogeneic canine recipient. Note the massive mononuclear cell infiltration. × 360. (From a specimen kindly provided by Dr. R. G. Thomson.)

may occur within hours. Both processes occur as a result of damage to vascular endothelium. The first-set reaction may be divided into two stages. First, information about the histocompatibility antigens of the graft must reach antigen-sensitive cells of the host. Second, effector cells from the host must invade the graft and mediate its destruction.

Sensitization of the Recipient

Information on graft antigens may reach the antigen-sensitive cells of the recipient by two routes. Either graft cells may release their histocompatibility antigens in soluble form, or, more importantly, circulating T cells may, on passing through the blood vessels of the graft, recognize foreign histocompatibility antigens on the endothelial cell surfaces. These T cells then pass from the graft in either the lymphatics or the blood vessels and eventually lodge in the draining lymph node as a consequence of local triggering of the lymphocyte "trap" (Chapter 5). It is probable, at least in skin grafts, that the lymphatic route is of most importance, since if a graft is prevented from

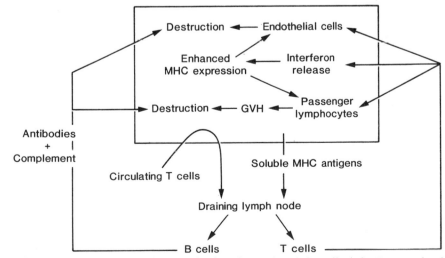

Figure 18–3. Some of the mechanisms involved in the rejection of an allograft. (See text for details.)

developing lymphatic connections with the host, then rejection is considerably delayed.

The cells that first recognize the foreign histocompatibility antigens of the graft divide and develop into cytotoxic T cells within the draining lymph node. The thymus-dependent paracortical regions of lymph nodes draining a graft contain increased numbers of cells, among which are clusters of large pyroninophilic cells. The numbers of these cells are greatest about six days after grafting and decline rapidly once the graft has been rejected. In addition to these signs of an active T cell-mediated immune response, it is also usual to observe some germinal center formation in the cortex and plasma cell accumulation in the medulla, suggesting that a humoral immune response also occurs.

Destruction of the Graft

As a result of the events that occur in the draining lymph node, cytotoxic T lymphocytes leave the node in the efferent lymph and reach the graft through the vascular system. When these T cells enter the graft they recognize that the histocompatibility antigens on the endothelial cells of the blood vessels are foreign. They therefore attach to and destroy the vascular endothelium by direct cytotoxicity. As a result of this endothelial damage, hemorrhage, platelet aggregation and thrombosis occur, and because of this failure in its blood supply, the grafted tissue dies.

Analysis of the rejection process shows that recipient animals mount immune responses against both class I and class II antigens in the graft. Antibodies to class I antigens are readily found in the serum after a graft has been rejected. However, their importance in the rejection process is probably less than that of the class II antigens. The intensity of the graft rejection process may be related to the number of foreign lymphocytes transplanted within the grafted tissue, and it has been suggested that a form of graft-versus-host response may contribute to the rejection process. If the grafted tissue contains a large number of "passenger" lymphocytes and macrophages then the rejection process is very severe. If, on the other hand, the graft contains few lymphocytes, then its survival is enhanced. Thus, thyroid cells and pancreatic islet cells have been experimentally transplanted to allogeneic hosts after prolonged tissue culture. This tissue culture permits the passenger lymphocytes and macrophages within the graft to die or lose their class II antigens. The recipient's T cells may also enhance the antigenicity of a graft by promoting the appearance of its class II antigens on endothelial cells through the release of interferon (Chapter 7).

Although sensitized T cells are most important in destroying foreign grafts, it is clear that antibodies also play a significant role in graft destruction (Table 18–2). This antibody-mediated destruction is brought about by antibodies, complement and neutrophils or through antibody-dependent cytotoxic cell activity (Chapter 6) and is especially important in second-set and xenograft reactions.

Cardiac Allografts

In humans and dogs that have received heart transplants, the pathology of the rejection process is uniquely different. The major lesion observed in rejected heart grafts is extensive endothelial cell proliferation in the walls of cardiac blood vessels (Fig. 18–4). The resulting obliteration of the blood vessel lumen eventually results in cardiac failure and death. A similar lesion is sometimes seen in renal allografts undergoing chronic rejection.

Table 18–2 MECHANISMS OF GRAFT DESTRUCTION

Mechanism	Pathway	Relative Importance
T cell-mediated cytotoxicity	Direct cytotoxicity	+++
	Lymphotoxins	+
Macrophage-mediated cytotoxicity	Direct cytotoxicity	+
ADCC	Several cell types using antibodies	++
Antibodies and complement	Direct cytolysis	+++

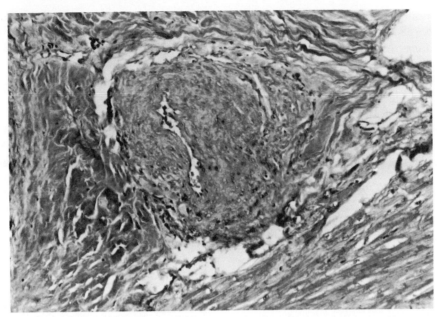

Figure 18–4. A section of coronary artery from a canine cardiac allograft, showing severe narrowing of the lumen as a result of endothelial proliferation. × 100. (From Penn, O. C. et al. 1976. Transplantation 22 313. The Williams & Wilkins Company, Baltimore. used with permission.)

Graft-Versus-Host (GVH) Disease

In Chapter 8 the normal lymphocyte transfer reaction, in which lymphocytes from a potential graft recipient are injected into a potential donor animal, was discussed. These transferred lymphocytes recognize that nearby cells carry "different" histocompatibility antigens and attack them, causing local inflammation. This reaction is particularly severe if the donor and recipient differ in class II antigens. In a normal lymphocyte transfer reaction, the results of this graft-versus-host disease are not usually serious, since the host is capable of destroying the foreign lymphocytes and thus terminating the attack. If, however, the host animal cannot, for some reason, destroy the grafted lymphocytes, then these cells may cause uncontrolled destruction of the host's tissues, and its eventual death. This type of GVH disease can occur if the recipient animal has been immunosuppressed or is immunodeficient. It has been observed in foals or puppies that receive bone marrow transplants in an attempt to cure congenital immunodeficiencies (Chapter 26). Animals suffering from a GVH disease develop lymphocytic infiltration of the intestine, skin and liver. This infiltration results in mucosal destruction and

diarrhea, ulcerative dermatitis and stomatitis, hepatic necrosis and jaundice. Eventually, there is cessation of growth (runting) and death. Although conventional immunosuppressive therapy may be used to prevent GVH disease, a superior approach is to selectively deplete the grafted marrow cells of cytotoxic T cell precursors by the use of specific monoclonal antibodies prior to transplantation.

Grafts That Are Not Rejected

Privileged Sites

Certain areas of the body, such as the anterior chamber of the eye, the cornea and the brain, lack effective lymphatic drainage. As a result, cytotoxic effector cells cannot reach grafts located in these tissues; therefore, these grafts survive relatively well (although antigen derived from these grafts may reach lymphoid tissue and sensitize the host). It is for this reason that corneal allografting is a successful procedure in human and canine surgery.

Pregnancy

The transfer of sperm from a male to an allogeneic female can be considered to be a natural allograft. While some cases of infertility may occur as a result of the female mounting an immune response against sperm antigens, this is an unusual event. One reason for the immunological acceptance of semen is that seminal plasma contains immunosuppressive factors such as uteroglobulin, transglutaminase, polyamines and prostaglandins. The immunosuppressive effect of semen is considered to be significant in the pathogenesis of AIDS.

Because the fetus and its placenta possess histocompatibility antigens derived from the male parent, the conceptus may be considered to be an allograft within the mother. Nevertheless, the fetus is successful in establishing and maintaining itself through pregnancy without suffering immunological damage. The reasons for this acceptance of the fetus and placenta are not completely understood. It is known that the uterus is not a privileged site, since other tissues, such as skin, grafted into the uterine wall are readily rejected. In fact, it is normal for the mother to recognize fetal antigens and undergo both humoral and cellular sensitization. One result of this is that the mother may make antibodies against fetal blood group antigens, and these may destroy fetal red cells in newborn animals following ingestion of colostrum (Chapter 21).

Several theories have been put forward to account for the lack of immunological attack on the fetus. One suggestion is that the fetus is protected from the mother's immune system by the trophoblast, which is that part of the placenta in closest contact with maternal tissue. Trophoblast cells have very low concentrations of histocompatibility antigens on their surface and are also covered by a layer of

nonimmunogenic sulfated mucoprotein. Nevertheless, mothers do develop antibodies against fetal MHC antigens, so the placenta must not prevent sensitization.

Second, the placenta is a source of immunosuppressive factors (Fig. 18–5). These include the hormones estradiol and progesterone and possibly also chorionic gonadotropin. In addition, a number of pregnancy-associated glycoproteins, including α_2-macroglobulin, uteroferrin and placental interferon, have immunosuppressive properties, and amniotic fluid is rich in immunosuppressive phospholipids.

Of much greater importance than the mechanisms described earlier is the production by the fetus of cells that can suppress the cytotoxic activities of maternal lymphocytes. Thus, lymphocytes in cord blood can suppress the activities of maternal T and B cells, and supernatants from cultures of these cells can suppress maternal B cell differentiation. One soluble suppressor factor that has been identified as coming from these fetal lymphocytes is prostaglandin E. Alpha-fetoprotein, the major protein in fetal serum, is immunosuppressive as a result of its ability to stimulate suppressor cell function.

A fourth important protective mechanism is mediated by "blocking antibody." The serum from multiparous animals can block the mixed lymphocyte reaction between fetal and maternal lymphocytes. The suppressive fraction consists of IgG antibody directed against paternal class II antigens. The blocking antibody coats placental cells, thus preventing their destruction by maternal T cells. This antibody can be eluted from the placenta and shown to

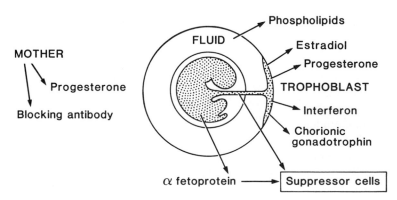

Figure 18–5. Some of the immunosuppressive factors that act to prevent the rejection of the fetus by the mother's immune system.

be capable of suppressing other cell-mediated immune reactions against paternal antigens, such as graft rejection. Absence of this blocking material has been shown to account for some cases of recurrent abortion in women.

It must not be assumed from the foregoing list of mechanisms that the pregnant female is grossly immunosuppressed. Pregnant animals have only minor deficiencies in cell-mediated immune reactivity to nonfetal antigens, showing, for example, a slight delay in the rejection of skin grafts, or transient unreactivity to the tuberculin skin test (Chapter 23). Nevertheless, this suppression may be significant in animals carrying parasites, in which the immune response can barely control the parasite. For example, normal adult sheep can usually prevent severe *Hemonchus contortus* infections. Nevertheless, severe infestations of *H. contortus* may develop in late pregnancy, perhaps as a result of periparturient immunosuppression. Similarly, this suppression may permit *Demodex* populations to rise in pregnant or lactating bitches and aid in the transmission of *Demodex* to their puppies. The intrauterine transmission of *Toxocara canis* to puppies may have a similar cause.

Cultured or Stored Organs

Because passenger lymphocytes contribute so significantly to the rejection process, graft survival is enhanced if these cells are removed from the graft before transplantation. One effective but rarely practical method is to treat the donor with immunosuppressive drugs prior to removal of the organ. An alternative method is to culture or freeze the organ for a period prior to grafting. For example, freeze-dried pig dermis is very useful in covering extensive wounds in horses and dogs without provoking rejection. Joints may be successfully transplanted in horses provided that they have been previously frozen. There have also been reports of successful aortic allografts in domestic animals after storage of the grafts in liquid nitrogen.

Immunologically Favored Organs

Pigs, rats and dogs that have received a liver allograft do not always mount an immune response against it. Although some animals destroy the grafted liver rapidly, in many, a response is mounted that is relatively weak and short-lived. As a result, the graft may survive for the normal lifespan of the animal. Because it is such a large organ, the grafted liver quickly traps most of the donor-reactive lymphocytes while at the same time releasing large quantities of soluble MHC antigens into the blood stream. The net effect of this is to rapidly eliminate any T cells reacting against the class I antigens of the graft. This process destroys the reactive cytotoxic T cells of the host but not helper T cells. The loss of cytotoxic T cells resulting from the presence of a liver graft of this type is able to prevent the rejection of other allografts (e.g., skin, heart or kidney) from the same donor. The presence of helper T cells permits the recipient to make antibodies against the graft and these may function as blocking antibodies and further enhance graft survival.

In some circumstances, such as in dogs that have maintained functioning renal allografts for several years, immunosuppressive therapy may be reduced gradually and eventually discontinued as graft acceptance becomes complete. It is probable that this is an example of high dose tolerance—that is, tolerance that results when the amount of antigen is in excess of the capacity of the antigen-sensitive cells to respond to it (Chapter 9). In the case of graft acceptance following immunosuppression, antigen-sensitive cells are gradually eliminated by the immunosuppressive drugs. Once their numbers are sufficiently low, the relatively large mass of grafted tissue may be sufficient to establish and maintain tolerance.

The Effect of Blood Transfusions

For many years, giving blood transfusions to potential renal allograft recipients was discouraged on the grounds that the foreign cells might sensitize the recipient and so hasten graft rejection. Experience has shown, however, that multiple transfusions given prior to transplantation greatly enhance graft survival not only in humans but also in pigs and dogs. The mechanisms involved are unclear, but the response may be due to the production of antibodies against T cell antigen receptors. Similar antibodies may be found in the blood of patients that have successfully retained renal allografts but not in those that have rejected grafts.

TUMORS AS ALLOGRAFTS

When organ transplantation became a common procedure in humans following the development of potent immunosuppressive agents, it was observed that immunosuppressed patients with prolonged graft survival were 80 to 100 times more likely to develop tumors than were nonimmunosuppressed individuals. It was therefore suggested that the immunocompetent cells suppressed by the antirejection therapy were also responsible for the prevention of neoplasia. It was from this suggestion that the concept of a surveillance function for the T cell system was developed, providing a stimulus for a growing interest in the role of the immune responses in preventing tumors.

Experimental evidence has shown that the concept of the T cells alone acting as a system to identify and destroy neoplastic cells is no longer tenable. Neoplasms are very heterogeneous, and it is unreasonable to assume, therefore, that a single branch of the immune system is responsible for protection against all tumors. In fact, different neoplasms may stimulate different forms of immune response, and it is probable that surveillance is mediated by T cells, natural killer (NK) cells, macrophages and antibodies, depending on the circumstances. For example, nude mice, which have no T cells, are no more susceptible to tumors, either natural or induced, than are normal mice. Their resistance to tumors is due not to T cells but to natural killer cells. It should also be pointed out that there is a great difference between the massive immune response triggered by allogeneic grafts and the host's responses to the very weak antigens associated with tumor cells. Although the original surveillance hypothesis has had to be greatly modified, there is good evidence to show that some tumor cells may be antigenic and that immunological techniques may be used to treat cancer. The increase in neoplasia seen in immunosuppressed individuals is probably a result of the destruction of several effector cell systems.

Tumor Antigens

Tumor cells may gain or lose antigens. For example, they may lose histocompatibility or blood group antigens, and some neoplasms of the intestine, such as colon carcinomas, may lose the ability to produce mucus. More commonly, tumor cells gain antigens, and some naturally occurring neoplasms of adult humans are characterized by the production of antigenic proteins normally found only in the fetus. For example, neoplasia of the gastrointestinal tract may produce a glycoprotein known as carcinoembryonic antigen (CEA), which is usually found only in the fetal intestine. The appearance of CEA in serum may indicate the presence of a colon or rectal adenocarcinoma. Other examples of the production of fetal antigens by tumor cells include the production of alpha-fetoprotein by hepatoma cells (alpha-fetoprotein is normally found only in the fetal liver), and squamous cell carcinoma cells of the horn may possess antigens also found in normal bovine fetal liver and skin.

Tumors induced by oncogenic viruses tend to gain new antigens characteristic of the inducing virus. These antigens, although coded for by the viral genome, are not part of the virus particle. Examples of this type of antigen include the FOCMA antigens found on the lymphoid cells of cats infected with feline leukemia virus (Chapter 26) and MATSA (Marek's tumor-specific antigens) found on Marek's disease virus-infected cells.

Chemically induced neoplasms are different from the virus-induced variety in that they carry surface antigens unique to the tumor and not to the inducing chemical. Tumors induced by a single chemical in different animals of the same species may be antigenically quite unrelated, and even within a single chemically induced tumor mass it is possible to demonstrate the existence of antigenically distinct sub-populations of cells.

IMMUNE RESPONSES TO TUMOR ANTIGENS

If tumor cells are sufficiently antigenically different from normal, they will be regarded as foreign and attacked. The major mechanisms of tumor cell destruction involve NK cells and cytotoxic T cells, although activated macrophages may also participate in this process.

Natural Killer Cells

Lymphocytes obtained from normal, nonimmune animals have a high level of spontaneous cytotoxic activity against a variety of tumor cells. These spontaneously cytotoxic cells are called natural killer (NK) cells (Fig. 18–6). Natural killer cells originate in bone marrow. They are found mainly in the secondary lymphoid organs, a smaller number are found in the bone marrow, and none are found in the thymus. They have been identified in mice, rats, humans, dogs, cats, swine, horses, cattle and chickens.

At first it was believed that NK cells functioned as an antitumor surveillance system. It was later shown, however, that they were active against a range of targets, including xenogeneic cells and virus-infected cells. NK cells are not adherent to glass and are not phagocytic. They are probably derived from the same stem cell pool as are T cells, since they carry low levels of Thy 1 on their surface, although they are not affected by anti-T cell serum. NK cells do not possess cell membrane-bound immunoglobulins but they do possess low avidity Fcγ receptors. They are present in nude (athymic) mice. NK cells destroy neoplasia and virus-infected cells by direct cytotoxicity and the release of perforins in the absence of prior antigenic stimulation (Fig. 18–7). Because NK cells possess Fc receptors they may participate in antibody-dependent cellular cytotoxicity (ADCC). There are probably several different types of NK cells. Thus "classical" NK cells lyse cells in suspension, for example, leukemia cells. In contrast, a subpopulation called natural cytotoxic (NC) cells will only destroy adherent cells. It is probable that subpopulations exist even within these different types.

Although NK cells are active in the nonimmunized animal, it can be shown that virus infections or administration of interferon inducers stimulates NK activity above normal levels. NK cells produce interferon upon encountering target cells. The interferon then acts to enhance NK activity by promoting the rapid differentiation of pre-NK cells. (Interferon also enhances T cell- and macrophage-mediated cytotoxicity.) The NK cell-interferon system probably plays a critical role in resis-

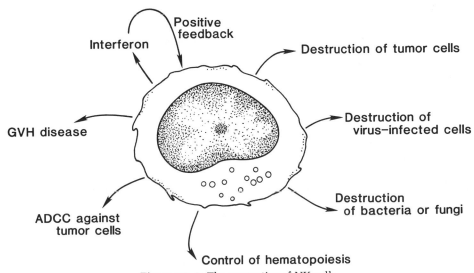

Figure 18–6. The properties of NK cells.

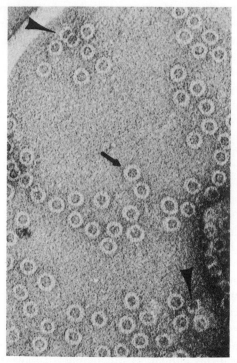

Figure 18–7. Polyperforins from human NK cells on the surface of a rabbit erythrocyte target. The arrowheads point to incomplete rings and double rings. (From Podack E. R. and Dennert G. 1983. Nature *307* 442. Used with permission.)

tance to neoplasia, and it may be shown that mice or humans deficient in NK cells (see the Chédiak-Higashi syndrome, Chapter 26) have an increased susceptibility to cancer. Neutralization of interferon by means of specific antisera enhances tumor growth in mice, presumably by depressing NK cell activity. Finally, preliminary studies suggest that interferon treatment may be useful in the therapy of some human and animal cancers.

T Cell-Mediated Immunity

It is occasionally possible to detect a cell-mediated response to tumor antigens either by skin testing or by an *in vitro* test such as macrophage migration inhibition. It is also possible to show that lymphocytes from some tumor-bearing animals may exert a cytotoxic effect on tumor cells cultured *in vitro*. Nevertheless, T cells are probably only significant in the control of virus-induced tumors.

Macrophage-Mediated Immunity

Macrophages have been credited with conferring immunity in several tumor systems. This may be a primary effect in which activated macrophages directly destroy the cancer cells. For example, bovine monocytes have been shown to be toxic for ocular squamous cell carcinoma cells. More commonly, stimulation of macrophages by bacteria or their products, for example, *Mycobacterium bovis* or *Propionobacterium acnes*, results in enhanced production of interleukin 1 and subsequent activation of helper T cell activity. Interleukin 1 has a cytostatic effect on some tumors.

Antibody-Mediated Immunity

Antibodies to tumor cells are commonly found in many tumor-bearing animals; for instance, about 50 per cent of sera from dogs with lymphosarcomas contain precipitating antitumor antibodies. These antibodies may be of some protective significance, since, in conjunction with complement, they may be capable of lysing free tumor cells. Antibodies do not appear to be effective in destroying the cells in solid neoplasia.

Immune Dysfunction in Tumor-Bearing Animals

Neoplasms are readily induced in experimental animals and are relatively common in domestic animals and in humans, suggesting that the immunological protective mechanisms are not very effective. Studies of tumor-bearing animals have demonstrated a number of mechanisms by which immune systems fail to reject neoplasia.

Immunosuppression

It is commonly observed that tumor-bearing animals are severely immunosuppressed. This suppression is most clearly seen in animals bearing lymphoid neoplasia; in these animals, tumors of B cells appear to suppress antibody formation, whereas T cell tumors generally suppress the cell-mediated immune responses (see Table 27–2). The suppression observed in leukemia virus infections is mainly due to the production of p15E, the potently immunosuppressive virus envelope protein. It may also be caused by the generalized disturbances in the lymphoid system brought about by these viruses. In some cases of melanoma the immunosuppression is a result of the neoplasm inhibiting the expression of class II histocompatibility antigens on macrophages and thus impairing antigen presentation. In contrast, immunosuppression observed in animals bearing chemically induced neoplasia appears to be due, at least in some cases, to the release of immunosuppressive factors such as prostaglandins from the tumor cells. Finally, it should be pointed out that the presence of actively growing tumor cells represents a severe protein drain on an animal. This protein loss may be reflected in an impaired immune response.

Although tumor cells may be antigenic and stimulate a protective cell-mediated immune response, the humoral immune response commonly has an opposite effect. Thus, the serum of a tumor-bearing animal when given to a second tumor-bearing animal may cause the neoplasm of the second animal to grow even faster—a phenomenon known as enhancement. Sera of this type may also inhibit the *in vitro* cytotoxicity of T cells for tumor cells. The nature of the factor(s) that causes tumor enhancement is not clear, but it may be either soluble antigen or antibody complexed to soluble tumor antigens. Many neoplasms release large quantities of cell surface antigen, and this may bind to cytotoxic T cells, saturating their antigen receptors and blocking their ability to bind to target cells. Of more importance is the production of blocking antibodies, non–complement-fixing antitumor antibodies that mask tumor antigens and thus protect the tumor cells from attack by cytotoxic T cells. In general, the presence or absence of these blocking factors correlates well with the state of progression or regression of a tumor.

Tumor Cell Selection

There are two mechanisms by which the biological activity of tumor cells might influence their survival. The first is "sneaking through," the process by which a neoplasm may not provide sufficient stimulus to induce an immune response until it has reached a size at which it cannot be controlled by the host. The second is tumor cell selection. Tumor cells that are very different from normal cells will be rapidly identified and eliminated without leading to disease. Tumor cells must, therefore, be selected for minimal antigenicity and for their ability to evade the host's immune system.

Some Specific Tumors

Transmissible Venereal Sarcoma

Transmissible venereal sarcoma of dogs is a neoplasm transmitted between animals by transplantation. In order to successfully colonize a new host, it must be able to establish itself in the face of gross histoincompatibility. It is not always successful, and after an initial growth phase the tumor often regresses. Nevertheless, lethal metastases do occasionally occur. Exposed dogs, whether or not they develop progressive neoplasia, develop antibodies to tumor cells, although the serum of dogs with regressive tumors is most effective in inhibiting tumor growth. If recipient dogs are immunosuppressed, the tendency to malignant growth is enhanced.

Warts

Warts are self-limiting neoplasms of epidermal cells induced by papilloma virus. The wart virus invades epidermal cells in the basal cell layer, but these cells do not express antigen. Since no viral antigen is expressed in this area where the blood supply is good, then the cells are not attacked by lymphocytes. As the infected cells move away from the basal layer toward the skin surface, they also move away from blood vessels, and the chances of immunological attack are minimized. Increasing amounts of virus are shed as the cells move toward the surface into a region devoid of antibodies or lymphocytes.

Equine Sarcoid

Equine sarcoid is a locally aggressive fibroblastic neoplasm of horse skin. It may be of virus origin. Two possible candidates are a retrovirus and bovine papilloma virus. Equine sarcoid is, however, unique in that it is remarkably amenable to immunotherapy. If BCG vaccine is infiltrated into the region between the tumor and normal skin, the tumor commonly regresses. The rate of regression will depend upon the size of the tumor (surgical extirpation is required to remove most of the tumor mass), and multiple treatments are usually necessary for a complete cure. Extracts of mycobacteria have also been used in treating this tumor. They possess the advantage of not rendering an animal tuberculin positive.

Ocular Squamous Cell Carcinoma

This is a common and economically important neoplasm of cattle, which responds to several forms of immunotherapy. One successful therapy involves inoculation of affected animals with a phenol saline extract of allogeneic carcinomas. This implies that these neoplasms possess characteristic tumor-associated antigens. Indeed, sera from affected cattle react with cancer cells (but not normal cells) obtained from the eyes of other cattle. It is also of interest to note that sera from some cattle with ocular squamous cell carcinoma also react with equine sarcoid and bovine papilloma cells.

TUMOR IMMUNOTHERAPY
(Table 18–3)

Two general approaches have been used in attempts to cure or modify tumor growth through immunotherapy. The simplest is to nonspecifically stimulate the immune system. Obviously, any improvement in an animal's immune capabilities will tend to enhance its resistance to neoplasia, although a cure may be expected only if the tumor mass is small or is surgically excised. The most widely used immune stimulant is the attenuated strain of

Table 18–3 TECHNIQUES IN TUMOR IMMUNOTHERAPY

Non-specific immune stimulation
  e.g., BCG, *Propionobacterium acnes*, interferons

Active immunization
  Immunization with chemically modified tumor cells, e.g., neuraminidase-treated
  Antiviral vaccination, e.g., Marek's disease, feline leukemia, warts

Passive immunization
  Cell-mediated immunity, e.g., dialyzable leukocyte extract
  Antibody-mediated immunity, e.g., immunotoxins

Mycobacterium bovis, bacille Calmette-Guerin (BCG). This organism has a nonspecific effect of cell-mediated immune reactivity. It may be given systemically, or, more effectively, it may be inoculated directly into the tumor mass. Techniques such as this have been employed with success in the treatment of equine sarcoid and ocular squamous cell carcinoma in cattle.

Other immunostimulants that have been employed, although generally with less success than BCG, include *Propionobacterium acnes*, thymus hormones, levamisole and various mixed bacterial vaccines. A related technique that has been used to treat dog skin tumors is to paint them with the contact allergen dinitrochlorobenzene. The local hypersensitivity reaction provoked by this compound appears to preferentially damage the tumor cells and cause tumor regression.

Specific immunotherapy, the second major approach, has also been attempted by many investigators. This may be achieved by active immunization, that is, vaccinating the animal with tumor cells or antigens. One such technique is to take tumor cells, emulsify them in Freund's complete adjuvant and inoculate the mixture into the host. This method has achieved some success in the treatment of canine lymphosarcoma. Lyophilized phenol-saline extracts of bovine ocular squamous cell carcinomas have produced encouraging remissions in cattle.

Because clinically obvious tumors must have evaded the animal's immune response already, it is essential to treat the tumor cells in an attempt to enhance their antigenicity. Thus, x-irradiated cells and neuraminidase- or glutaraldehyde-treated cells have been used in tumor vaccines with limited success.

Adoptive transfer of immune lymphocytes is, at least in theory, a logical method of conferring immunity against a neoplasm in an animal. In practice, however, this technique is not feasible, although some success has been achieved with dialyzable leukocyte extract obtained from these cells. Since this extract functions across species barriers, it is possible that it may be harvested from domestic animals and used therapeutically in humans (Chapter 27).

Passive immunization using serum from immune animals is generally considered undesirable because of the risk of tumor enhancement through transfer of blocking antibody. Nevertheless, as described earlier, serum from immune donors accelerates the regression of canine venereal sarcoma and normal cat serum causes rapid regression of FeLV-induced neoplasia. A related technique that shows promise of success is the use of immunotoxins. These are very specific antitumor antibodies (usually monoclonal antibodies) chemically conjugated to a potent cytotoxin. The antibody binds specifically to a tumor cell and so delivers its toxin directly to its target.

In contrast to the techniques described previously, most of which have met with only partial success, there are a number of successful techniques for vaccination against tumor viruses. The most important of these is the vaccine against Marek's disease, a T cell neoplasm of chickens caused by a herpesvirus. The immune response evoked by this vaccine has two components. First, humoral and cell-mediated responses act directly on the virus to reduce the quantity available to infect cells. Second, there is a cell-mediated immune response against antigens generated by the virus on the surface of the tumor cells. These antigens, known as MATSA (Marek's tumor-specific antigens), provoke successful antitumor immunity. Both the antiviral and antitumor immune responses act synergistically to protect the birds.

More recently a vaccine has been developed against feline leukemia. This consists of the supernatant fluid derived from a culture of persistently infected cat cells. It contains all the major viral antigens in soluble form (see Chapter 16). Success has also been achieved with formalized wart vaccines in cattle. In view of this, it is perhaps possible to predict that future successes are more likely to result from the development of vaccines against oncogenic viruses such as these rather than from more esoteric immunological approaches directed toward the destruction of the tumor cells.

ADDITIONAL SOURCES OF INFORMATION

Abruzzo LV and Rowley DA. 1983. Homeostasis of the antibody response: immunoregulation by NK cells. Science 222 581–585.

Adams DO and Nathan CF. 1983. Molecular mechanisms in tumor-cell killing by activated macrophages. Immunol. Today 4 166–170.

Al-Yaman F and Willenberg DO. 1984. Immune reactivity to autochthonous ocular squamous cell carcinoma. Vet. Immunol. Immunopathol. 7 153–168.

Baldwin RW. 1982. Manipulation of host resistance in cancer therapy. Springer Semin. Immunopathol. 5 113–125.

Beer AE and Billingham RE. 1978. Immunoregulatory aspects of pregnancy. Fed. Proc. 37 2374–2378.

Bloom BL. 1982. Natural killers to rescue immune surveillance? Nature 300 214–215.

Bloomberg MS, Goring RL and Born F. 1984. Frozen diaphyseal bone allografts combined with external and internal pin splintage in small animal orthopedic surgery. JAVMA 20 393–402.

Broder S and Waldmann TA. 1978. The suppressor-cell network in cancer. N. Engl. J. Med. 299 1281–1284.

Chism SE, Burton RC and Warner NL. 1978. Immunogenicity of oncofetal antigens: a review. Clin. Immunol. Immunopathol. 11 346–373.

Essex M and Grant CK. 1979. Tumor immunology in domestic animals. Adv. Vet. Sci. Comp. Med. 23 183–228.

Finco DR, Rawlings CA, Barsanti JA and Crowell WA. 1985. Kidney graft survival in transfused and nontransfused Beagle dogs. Am. J. Vet. Res. 46 2327–2331.

Herberman RB and Ortaldo JR. 1981. Natural killer cells: their role in defenses against disease. Science 214 24–30.

Hill DL, Yang TJ and Wachtel A. 1984. Canine transmissible venereal sarcoma: tumor cell and infiltrating leukocyte ultrastructure at differing growth stages. Vet. Pathol. 21 39–45.

Jacoby DR, Olding LB and Oldstone MBA. 1984. Immunologic regulation of fetal-maternal balance. Adv. Immunol. 35 157–208.

James K and Hargreave TB. 1984. Immunosuppression by seminal plasma and its possible clinical significance. Immunol. Today 5 357–363.

Kamada N. 1985. Transplantation tolerance and immunosuppression follow liver grafting in rats. Immunol. Today 6 336–342.

Kelly GE. 1977. Current prospects for renal transplantation in veterinary practice. Aust. Vet. J. 53 53–60.

Kolb M, Sale GE, Lerner KG et al. 1979. Pathology of acute graft-versus-host disease in the dog. Am. J. Pathol. 96 581–594.

Kuchroo VK and Spradbrow PB. 1985. Tumor-associated antigens in bovine ocular squamous cell carcinoma: Studies with sera from tumor bearing animals. Vet. Immunol. Immunopathol. 9 23–36.

Marx JL. 1980. Natural killer cells help defend the body. Science 210 624–626.

Perryman LE and Liu IKM. 1980. Graft-versus-host reactions in foals with combined immunodeficiency. Am. J. Vet. Res. 41 187–192.

Ringler SS and Krakowka S. 1985. Cell surface markers of the canine natural killer (NK) cell. Vet. Immunol. Immunopathol. 9 1–12.

Robins RA and Baldwin RW. 1985. T cell subsets in tumor rejection responses. Immunol. Today 6 55–58.

Russell PS and Cosimi AB. 1979. Transplantation. N. Engl. J. Med. 301 470–479.

Segal-Eiras A, Robins RA, Hannaout D et al. 1982. Circulatory immune complexes in dogs with osteosarcoma. Brit. J. Cancer 46 444–447.

Tompkins MB, Huber K and Tompkins WAF. 1983. Natural cell-mediated cytotoxicity in the domestic cat: properties and specificity of effector cells. Am. J. Vet. Res. 44 1525–1529.

Tompkins MB and Tompkins WAF. 1985. Stimulation of a cell-mediated cytotoxic response to FeLV-induced T cell lymphomas in the cat. J. Immunol. 135 2817–2823.

Vitetta ES, Krolick KA, Miyama-Inaba M, Cushley W and Uhr JW. 1983. Immunotoxins, a new approach to cancer therapy. Science 219 644–650.

IV

HYPERSENSITIVITY AND INFLAMMATION

19

Inflammation

Inflammation is the response of tissues to irritation or injury. It is a vital protective mechanism since it provides a means by which defensive factors, such as immunoglobulins, complement and phagocytic cells, which are normally confined to the blood stream, can gain direct access to sites of microbial invasion or tissue damage. Immunoglobulins and complement components occur in tissue fluids at a much lower concentration than in the blood. In addition, large molecules such as IgM cannot leave normal blood vessels. Inflammation may therefore be considered a method by which immunological protective mechanisms are focused at a localized region of tissue.

CLASSIFICATION OF INFLAMMATION

Inflammation is classified according to its severity and duration, so recent inflammation or acute inflammation has very different characteristics from the reactions seen in prolonged or chronic inflammation.

ACUTE INFLAMMATION

Acute inflammation develops within a few hours after a tissue is damaged or infected. In its classic form, acute inflammation has five cardinal signs: heat, redness, swelling, pain and loss of function. All these signs are a direct result of changes in the behavior of local blood vessels (Fig. 19–1). Immediately following injury, there is a transient constriction of local arterioles followed shortly thereafter by dilatation of all the small blood vessels in the area. As a result, the blood flow to the area increases significantly for several hours. Eventually the flow diminishes and gradually returns to normal. While the blood vessels are

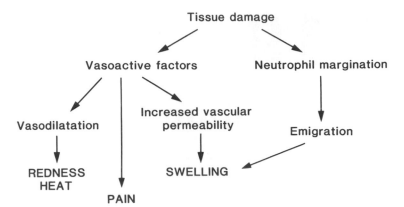

Figure 19–1. The characteristics of the acute inflammatory response.

dilated there is also an increase in their permeability, and protein-rich plasma exudes into the tissues where it causes local edema and swelling.

Within a few hours of the onset of these vascular changes, leukocytes (neutrophils, eosinophils and monocytes) adhere to the vascular endothelium in a process called pavementing. If the blood vessels are also damaged, then platelets may also bind to the vessel walls and release both vasoactive and clotting factors.

After adhering to the vessel walls, the leukocytes migrate into the surrounding tissues through the gaps between endothelial cells (Fig. 19–2). Since neutrophils and eosinophils are the most mobile of all the blood leukocytes, these cells will be the first to arrive in the inflamed tissues. Blood monocytes move more slowly and hence arrive later. Once within tissues, the cells are attracted by chemotactic factors to sites of bacterial growth and tissue damage. There they proceed to phagocytose and destroy any foreign material and, in the case of monocytes, remove dead and dying tissue.

Changes in Vascular Permeability

Vascular permeability in acute inflammation increases in two stages. First, there is an immediate increase mediated by vasoactive factors released by damaged tissues. The second phase of increased vascular permeability occurs several hours after the onset of inflammation, at the time when the leukocytes are commencing to emigrate. This escape of fluid

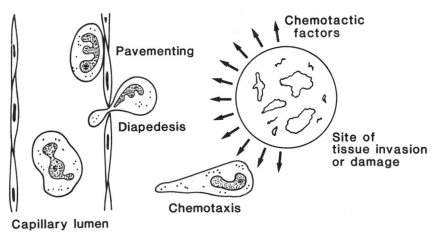

Figure 19–2. The basic features of acute inflammation. The release of chemotactic factors from damaged tissues results in the emigration of cells from nearby capillaries.

is due to contraction of the endothelial and perivascular cells, as a result of which the endothelial cells are pulled apart and so permit the escape of fluid through the intercellular spaces.

The Coagulation System

When fluid exudes from the blood stream into the tissues, three enzyme cascades are activated: the complement system, the coagulation system and the fibrinolytic system. The coagulation system is an enzyme cascade that is triggered following activation of the first component, Hageman factor (Factor XII) (Fig. 19–3). Hageman factor is activated as a result of vascular endothelial damage. This endothelial damage, in turn, leads to a series of enzyme reactions as a result of which large quantities of thrombin, the main clotting enzyme, are formed. Thrombin acts on the fibrinogen in tissue fluid and plasma to produce insoluble strands of fibrin. This fibrin is laid down in inflamed tissues and capillaries and forms an effective barrier to the spread of infection.

Activated Hageman factor, in addition to starting the coagulation cascade, also initiates the fibrinolytic system. This leads to activation of plasminogen activator, which in turn generates plasmin, a potent fibrinolytic enzyme. In destroying fibrin, plasmin releases peptide fragments that are chemotactic for neutrophils.

Hageman factor, plasmin and some neutrophil and macrophage enzymes act on another pre-enzyme to generate the enzyme kallikrein. Kallikrein acts on plasma α globulins (kininogens) to cleave off small peptides called kinins. Kinins are very potent vasodilators and increase vascular permeability.

Vasoactive Factors (Table 19–1)

Histamine

Histamine is an amine formed by the decarboxylation of the amino acid histidine and stored, preformed, within granules in mast cells. Once mast cell granules are exposed to the extracellular fluid by tissue damage, histamine is released through exchange with sodium ions. Histamine possesses biological activities that affect blood vessels, smooth muscle and exocrine glands. For example, it dilates most micro blood vessels (e.g., capillaries and venules) but contracts certain specific vessels, including the pulmonary vessels of herbivores and the hepatic veins of dogs. It also causes increased permeability of microvessels so that intradermal inoculation of histamine gives a "wheal and flare" reaction. Histamine causes smooth muscle contraction, particularly of the bronchi, gastrointestinal tract, uterus and bladder. Finally, it is a potent stimulator of exocrine secretions, stimulating bronchial mucus secretion, lacrimation and salivation. Dogs with mast cell tumors occa-

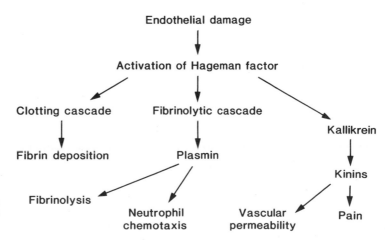

Figure 19–3. The role of Hageman factor in the development of acute inflammation.

Table 19–1 INFLAMMATORY MEDIATORS

Mediator	Major Source	Function
Histamine	Mast cells, Basophils	Increased vascular permeability, pain
Serotonin	Platelets, Mast cells	Increased vascular permeability
Kinins	Serum kininogens	Vasodilation, increased vascular permeability, pain
Prostaglandins	Arachidonic acid	Vasodilation
Leukotriene B_4	Arachidonic acid	Neutrophil chemotaxis, increased vascular permeability
Leukotrienes C_4, D_4, E_4	Arachidonic acid	Smooth muscle contraction, increased vascular permeability
Platelet activating factor	Phagocytic cells	Platelet secretion, neutrophil secretion, increased vascular permeability
Fibrinogen breakdown products	Blood clot	Smooth muscle contraction, neutrophil chemotaxis, increased vascular permeability
C3a and C5a	Complement	Mast cell degranulation, smooth muscle contraction, neutrophil chemotaxis (C5a)
Interleukin 1	Macrophages	Fever, amino acid mobilization, fibroblast proliferation, lethargy, immune stimulation, neutrophilia, induction of acute-phase proteins

sionally present with gastric ulcers due to the histamine-mediated stimulation of gastric secretion.

In small quantities, histamine is chemotactic for eosinophils, which, possessing large quantities of histaminases, can readily break it down. Other enzymes that can inactivate histamine include diamine oxidase (histaminase), coenzyme A, which can acetylate histamine, and imidazole N-methyl transferase, which can methylate it.

Serotonin (5–Hydroxytryptamine)

Serotonin, a derivative of the amino acid tryptophan, is released from the mast cells of some species of rodents and the large domestic herbivores. It also exists preformed in platelets, in central nervous tissue and in the argentophil cells of the intestine. It is released from platelets through the activity of a number of factors including platelet activating factor (Chapter 20). Serotonin normally causes a vasoconstriction that results in a rise in blood pressure (except in cattle in which it is a vasodilator). It appears to have little effect on

vascular permeability, except in rats and mice in which serotonin readily induces wheal and flare reactions.

Factors Derived from Arachidonic Acid

When tissues are damaged or stimulated, cell membrane phospholipases can act on the phospholipids in cell walls to release fatty acids. The most important of these fatty acids is an unsaturated long-chain fatty acid called arachidonic acid. Arachidonic acid is metabolized by two alternative pathways (Fig. 19–4). Under the influence of enzymes known as lipoxygenases, it first gives rise to hydroperoxyeicasotetraenoic acids (HPETEs). These in turn give rise to hydroxyeicasotetraenoic acids (HETEs) and to leukotrienes. Under the influence of enzymes known as cyclooxygenases, arachidonic acid yields prostaglandins, prostacyclin and thromboxane.

Leukotrienes. Four major groups of leukotrienes play a central role in the inflammatory response. Leukotriene B_4 acts to stimulate neutrophil and eosinophil chemotaxis and random motility and enhances their expression of

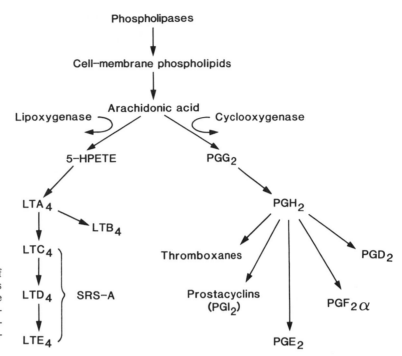

Figure 19–4. The production of leukotrienes and prostaglandins by the actions of lipoxygenase and cyclooxygenase on arachidonic acid. (Leukotrienes are abbreviated to LT and prostaglandins are abbreviated to PG.)

C3b receptors. The other major leukotrienes, leukotrienes C_4, D_4 and E_4, collectively represent what was formerly known as slow-reacting substance of anaphylaxis (SRS-A); they provoke a slow contraction of smooth muscle. Leukotrienes C_4 and D_4 are up to 20,000 times more potent than histamine in contracting the smooth muscle of bronchioles in certain species and are potent stimulators of increased vascular permeability.

Prostaglandins. Prostaglandins are a family of complex lipids with a wide range of activities. They consist of four groups of compounds: the PGE series, the PGF series, the thromboxanes (TxA_2) and the prostacyclins (PGI_2). The enzymes that generate the prostacyclins are found in vascular endothelial cells, the thromboxanes are found in platelets, and the other prostaglandins can be generated by most nucleated cells. The biological activities of the prostaglandins vary widely, and since many different prostaglandins are released in inflamed tissues, the net effect may be very complex. For example, $PGF_{2\alpha}$ and thromboxane (TxA_2) cause smooth muscle to contract and provoke vasoconstriction. Other prostaglandins such as PGE_1, PGE_2 and prostacyclin (PGI_1) cause smooth muscle relaxation and vasodilation. PGI_2, PGE_1, and $PGF_{2\alpha}$ inhibit platelet aggregation, PGE_2 and TxA_2 promote platelet aggregation and the release of platelet mediators such as serotonin, whereas $PGF_{2\alpha}$ promotes mast cell-mediator release.

Vasoactive Polypeptides

Several polypeptides have either potent vasoactive or chemotactic properties. The most important of these are the kinins and the anaphylatoxins. Kinins are basic polypeptides, the most important of which is bradykinin. They are derived from two serum proteins (kininogens) by the activity of proteolytic enzymes called kallikreins. Kallikreins may be produced directly from mast cells and basophils or indirectly from activated platelets. They may also be produced in plasma by the action of Hageman factor (factor XII) on inert prekallikrein (kallikreininogen). Kinins increase vascular permeability and stimulate smooth muscle contraction at least partly through the stimulation of release of leukotrienes and prostaglandins. They also stimulate pain receptors.

The anaphylatoxins are derived from the cleavage of the alpha chains of two complement components C3 and C5 and are known as C3a and C5a, respectively (Chapter 10). They both act indirectly on blood vessel permeability by promoting histamine release from mast cells. In addition, C5a is a very potent chemoattractant for neutrophils.

An important vasoactive peptide called PF/dil (permeability factor in diluted serum) is a fragment of the blood clotting protein Hageman factor. PF/dil activates prekallikreins, the proteolytic enzymes responsible for the generation of kinins. It is generated by damage to vascular endothelium.

Neutrophil-Derived Factors

Upon phagocytosis of particles by neutrophils, the primary granules fuse with the phagosomes to form phagolysosomes. Since this fusion may occur before the particle is completely ingested, many lysosomal enzymes may be released into the tissues. These enzymes include the kallikreins and enzymes of the respiratory burst such as superoxide dismutase as well as reactive oxidizing products of the respiratory burst.

Platelet-Derived Factors

If vascular endothelium is damaged, it provides a stimulus for local clumping of platelets.

When platelets clump they are stimulated to release many potent vasoactive agents, especially serotonin and thromboxanes.

Migration of Leukocytes

Emigration of leukocytes is an active process that takes place independently of the increased vascular permeability of acute inflammation. The leukocytes adhere to the vascular epithelium, insert their pseudopodia into the interendothelial junctions and migrate between the endothelial cells and the basement membrane. Subsequently the leukocytes move through the basement membrane into the tissue spaces under the influence of chemotactic factors (Fig. 19–5).

The most important chemotactic factor produced during acute inflammation is known as C5a. This peptide not only attracts neutrophils to sites of complement activation, but also triggers their adherence to endothelial cells. C5a is relatively unstable and readily looses its terminal arginine to form C5a des arg. C5a des arg has lost its ability to increase vascular permeability, but remains potently chemotactic in the presence of serum (Chapter 10.)

When vascular damage activates Hageman factor, both kallikrein and plasminogen activator are generated and are chemotactic for

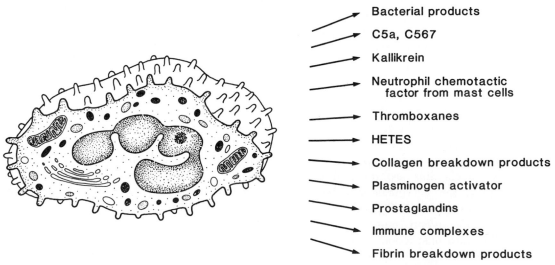

Bacterial products

C5a, C567

Kallikrein

Neutrophil chemotactic factor from mast cells

Thromboxanes

HETES

Collagen breakdown products

Plasminogen activator

Prostaglandins

Immune complexes

Fibrin breakdown products

Figure 19–5. Some of the factors that are chemotactic for neutrophils.

neutrophils. Other neutrophil chemotactic factors include collagen, chemotactic lymphokines and chemotactic factors derived from macrophages, fibroblasts, and mast cells as well as factors released from neutrophils themselves. For example, leukoegressin is a chemotactic peptide derived from cleavage of IgG by neutrophil proteolytic enzymes. Bacterial products are also chemotactic and thus attract neutrophils to sites of bacterial invasion. The most potent chemotactic factor known is leukotriene B_4, which has detectable activity at a concentration of 10^{-4} M.

Once neutrophils have reached the site of tissue damage or invasion they ingest and destroy foreign material as described in Chapter 2. Most neutrophils die soon after this, but those that survive eventually become unresponsive to chemotactic agents, enabling them to move away once their task is complete.

Control of Acute Inflammation

Since acute inflammation has the potential to cause severe tissue damage, it must be carefully controlled. Plasma contains several factors that either inactivate inflammatory mediators directly or inhibit the enzymes that generate the mediators. Thus α_1-antitrypsin and α_2-macroglobulin block the proteases released from neutrophil granules, as well as thrombin, plasmin and C1 esterase. Eosinophils probably play an important role in influencing the inflammatory response mediated by mast cell factors (Chapter 20).

INFLAMMATION AS A CONSEQUENCE OF IMMUNE REACTIONS

Inflammatory responses of immunological origin are known as hypersensitivity reactions and may be classified into four basic types (Figs. 19–6 and 19–7) as suggested by Gell and Coombs.

Type I or Immediate Hypersensitivity (Chapter 20)

IgE and some IgG subisotypes can attach to mast cells or basophils through sites on their Fc region. If antigen binds to this cell-fixed antibody, then the mast cell or basophil will respond by releasing the vasoactive factors, especially histamine, contained within its granules. These factors cause local acute inflammation within a few minutes.

Type II or Cytotoxic Hypersensitivity (Chapter 21)

Antibodies may participate in the destruction of cells either by activating complement or through the activities of cytotoxic cells. Cells such as neutrophils, macrophages and some lymphocytes possess receptors for the Fc portion of immunoglobulin. These cells may kill target cells coated with immune complexes by antibody-dependent cellular cytotoxicity (ADCC) (Chapter 7). Cells destroyed either in this way or through complement-mediated lysis may initiate an acute inflammatory reaction because of the release of biologically active cell breakdown products. This form of inflammation may be observed in graft rejection (Chapter 18).

Type III or Immune Complex Hypersensitivity (Chapter 22)

Immune complexes may activate complement even if deposited in tissues. Activation of complement in this way will attract neutrophils through the production of C5a, and the neutrophils will attempt to ingest the immune complexes. Unfortunately, under these circumstances neutrophils may release the proteolytic enzymes from their granules, resulting in tissue destruction (see Fig. 22–1). Neutrophil-activated plasmin may in turn activate the complement system; platelet aggregation may result in the release of more vasoactive factors; and mast cell degranulation may be mediated by anaphylatoxins. The total effect is therefore

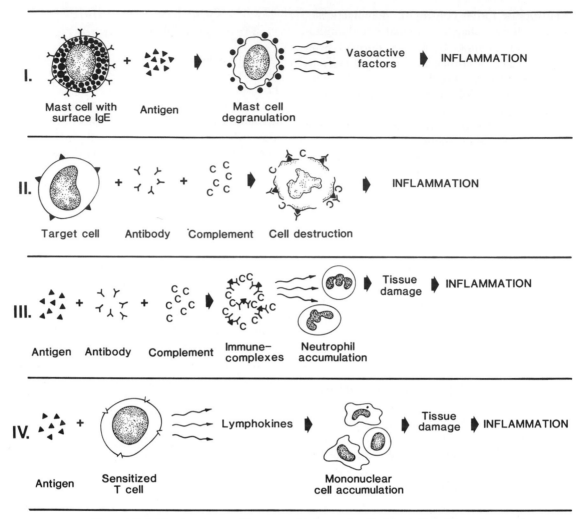

Figure 19–6. The four types of hypersensitivity as classified by Gell and Coombs.

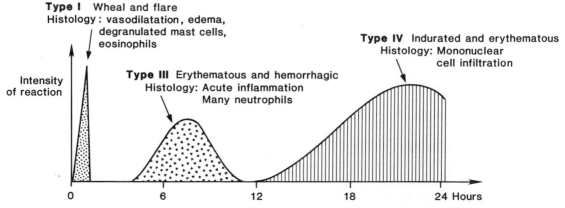

Figure 19–7. The time-course, character and histology of inflammatory skin reactions resulting from intradermal injection of antigen and caused by hypersensitivity types I, III and IV.

one of acute inflammation and tissue destruction.

Type IV or Delayed Hypersensitivity (Chapter 23)

Cell-mediated immune reactions may also participate in acute inflammatory reactions. Thus, if antigen is injected into an animal possessing appropriately sensitized T cells, then a local inflammatory reaction may occur. This form of reaction is known as delayed hypersensitivity, since it generally takes at least 24 hours after administration of antigen for the response to reach maximal intensity. The inflammatory response is caused by the release of vasoactive factors from mast cells and basophils and of chemotactic and vasoactive lymphokines by sensitized T cells (see Fig. 23–2). This type of reaction occurs in response to many bacterial antigens as well as in response to virus-infected cells and in graft rejection.

CHRONIC INFLAMMATION

Several hours after neutrophils have arrived at an inflammatory focus, the monocytes begin to arrive. These monocytes are attracted by many of the factors that attract neutrophils, as well as by collagen-breakdown products and by factors released by lymphocytes. Once they reach the tissues the monocytes (now called macrophages) not only will eliminate any invading bacteria, but will also phagocytose and destroy damaged cells and tissues, including neutrophils and fibrin deposits. By releasing fibronectin and interleukin 1 (IL-1), macrophages attract fibroblasts. Interleukin 1 promotes fibroblast proliferation, and these cells then begin to synthesize the collagen required to repair any tissue damage. The collagen tends to be deposited throughout the lesion and is then gradually remodeled over several weeks or months as the area gradually returns to normal.

The final result of this healing process depends to a large extent on the effectiveness of the preceding acute inflammation. If the cause of the inflammation is rapidly and completely removed then healing will follow uneventfully. If, however, the offending material or organism cannot be destroyed because it is not susceptible to destruction by the enzymes of macrophages or neutrophils, then the chronic inflammatory process may persist. Thus, prolonged chronic inflammation results from the presence of bacteria such as *Mycobacterium tuberculosis*, fungi such as *Cryptococcus*, parasite eggs such as those derived from schistosomes, or inorganic material such as asbestos crystals. In these cases, the prolonged, continuous chemotactic stimulus results in the continuous arrival of new macrophages and fibroblasts and the excessive deposition of collagen around the irritant focus. The lesion that develops in this way is known as a granuloma.

If the persistent irritant is nonantigenic, for example, silica, talc or mineral oil, then few neutrophils or lymphocytes will be attracted to the lesion. Epithelioid and giant cells, however, are formed in an attempt to destroy the offending material. If the material is toxic for macrophages, as is asbestos, macrophage enzymes may be released, leading to excessive tissue damage and eventually to fibrosis and scarring.

If the foreign material is immunogenic, then the initial inflammatory response may be similar to that seen in a delayed hypersensitivity reaction (Chapter 23). As a result of the release of lymphokines and of persistent immune stimulation, this type of granuloma will contain lymphocytes as well as macrophages and fibroblasts and probably some neutrophils, eosinophils and basophils also. Macrophages within these granulomas may form giant cells. These chronically stimulated macrophages will also release interleukin 1, which can stimulate collagen deposition by fibroblasts and thus eventually "wall-off" the lesion from the rest of the body. Antigens that provoke this form of granulomatous hypersensitivity include bacteria such as the Mycobacteria and *Brucella abortus* and parasites such as filariae and schistosomes. Occasionally an animal may develop a granuloma characterized by an excessive infiltration with eosinophils. The cause of this is unknown.

These chronic granulomatous reactions whether caused by immunological or foreign body reactions are of importance, since they may enlarge and eventually involve normal tissues. Thus, in asbestosis, for example, death eventually occurs as a result of the gradual replacement of normal lung tissues by granulomatous tissue.

INTERLEUKIN 1 AND THE SYSTEMIC RESPONSE TO INFLAMMATION

When an animal suffers from microbial invasion and undergoes tissue injury and inflammation, a generalized set of systemic responses consistently occurs. This includes the development of a fever, a neutrophilia (elevated blood neutrophils), lethargy, and eventual muscle wasting. This general response is mediated by interleukin 1 (Fig. 19–8).

Interleukin 1 is a protein occurring in two forms, with molecular weights of 15,000 and 35,000 daltons. Both have identical biological activities. Interleukin 1 (IL-1) is made by Langerhans cells and by some epithelial cells such as keratocytes and corneal cells, but the major source of IL-1 is from macrophages. Macrophages release IL-1 following exposure to the stimulus of invading microorganisms, foreign antigens, microbial products or damaged or inflamed tissue.

Interleukin 1 causes a great variety of biological activities, all of which promote elimination of microbial invaders and repair of damaged tissue. The biological activities of endotoxins—fever, neutrophilia, immune stimulation and complement activation—can all be mimicked by interleukin 1. It seems reasonable to suggest, therefore, that endotoxins act *in vivo* by promoting the release of interleukin 1 from macrophages.

IL-1-Induced Fever

Interleukin 1 acts on the thermoregulatory center in the anterior hypothalamus to induce increased prostaglandin synthesis. This causes the thermostatic set-point to rise. In response to this rise, there is increased heat conservation by vasoconstriction and heat production by shivering. The body temperature therefore rises until it reaches the new set-point, and a fever occurs. This fever promotes T cell proliferation and enhances the production of cytotoxic T cells and immunoglobulin synthesis. The alternate complement pathway also functions optimally at temperatures around 39°C. The febrile response may also reduce the proliferation of some bacteria and viruses. Interleukin 1 can also cause sleep by promoting the release of sleep-inducing factors in the

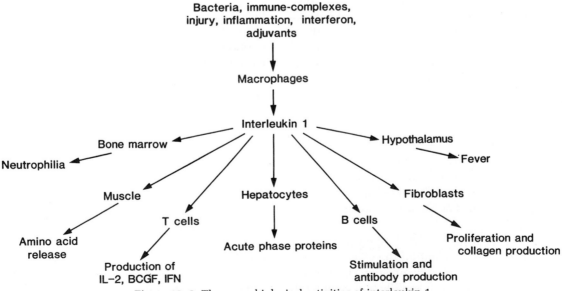

Figure 19–8. The many biological activities of interleukin 1.

brain. Increased lethargy is commonly associated with a fever and may, by reducing the energy demands of an animal, enhance the efficiency of defense and repair mechanisms.

Hibernation

Some mammals, most notably bears, some rodents and bats, are able to hibernate. At this time their temperature may fall to very low levels. If bats, for example, are cooled to around 8°C they cease antibody production, but rewarming permits rapid resumption of antibody synthesis. The cessation of immune responses in hibernating bats may be of importance for the ability of the bat to act as a carrier of viral pathogens such as rabies.

IL-1-Induced Immune Stimulation

Interleukin 1 acts on T cells to provoke their release of interleukin 2 and B cell growth factor (Chapter 6). It is thus necessary for T helper cell activity and the successful initiation of the immune response.

IL-1-Induced Metabolic Changes

In addition to its effects on the nervous and immune systems, interleukin 1 has profound metabolic effects. It acts on skeletal muscle to enhance protein catabolism and thus mobilizes a pool of available amino acids. This eventually results in muscle wastage. The newly available amino acids are available for increased immunoglobulin synthesis by B cells and for enhanced protein synthesis by hepatocytes.

IL-1-Induction of Acute-Phase Proteins

Under the influence of interleukin 1, hepatocytes show increased synthesis of a large number of proteins. Because this synthesis is associated with acute infections and inflammation, those proteins whose concentrations rise so rapidly are known as acute-phase proteins.

One group of proteins increase their concentrations two or three fold (Fig. 19–9). Many of these act by minimizing tissue damage. These include protease inhibitors such as α_1-antitrypsin, α_1-antichymotrypsin and α_2-macroglobulin. All of these can inhibit the damage caused by the release of neutrophil proteases in sites of acute inflammation. Ceruloplasmin is an acute-phase protein that may reduce tissue injury by scavenging free oxide radicals such as the superoxide anions released during the respiratory burst.

Other acute-phase proteins synthesized by hepatocytes include haptoglobin and transferrin. As described in Chapter 15, these proteins adsorb iron molecules, making them unavailable to invading bacteria. In this way they inhibit bacterial proliferation and invasion. These proteins also reduce iron availability for red cell production so that anemia is commonly associated with severe or chronic infections. A rise in the third component of complement may also enhance antimicrobial resistance.

Two of the acute-phase proteins may rise a thousandfold following invasion and tissue damage. These are C-reactive protein (CRP) and serum amyloid A (SAA). CRP was first identified and named for its ability to bind and precipitate the C-polysaccharide of *Streptococcus pneumoniae*. Its structure and amino acid sequence show that it is a member of the

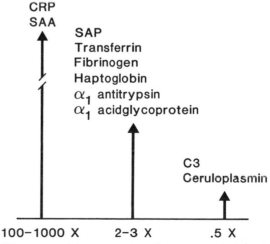

Figure 19–9. The major acute-phase proteins released by the actions of interleukin 1, showing the magnitude of their increase.

immunoglobulin superfamily, with features akin to an isolated immunoglobulin domain. As a result, it can activate the classical complement pathway (Chapter 10) and function as an opsonin by binding to phagocyte Fc receptors. CRP is synthesized by hepatocytes and is released into the circulation under the influence of IL-1. It can bind to activated lymphocytes, to invading organisms and to damaged tissues, where it activates complement. It promotes the phagocytosis and removal of damaged, dying or dead cells and organisms. CRP may therefore promote tissue healing by enhancing the repair of damaged tissue.

SAA, in contrast, is closely related to the major protein of reactive amyloidosis. (Reactive amyloidosis is a disease that results from very prolonged inflammation. It is discussed in detail in a following section.) SAA binds to cell membranes but is immunosuppressive, inhibiting both B cell and macrophage function. It has been suggested, therefore, that SAA may exert a negative feedback on interleukin 1 production by macrophages.

IL-1-Induced Neutrophilia

Interleukin 1 acts directly on bone marrow to stimulate the release of neutrophils into the circulation, causing a neutrophilia. Interleukin 1 is also chemotactic for neutrophils and thus attracts them to sites of bacterial invasion where interleukin 1 is being released. Interleukin 1 may also enhance the bactericidal activity of these cells by stimulating their oxidative metabolism.

In conclusion, therefore, interleukin 1 may account for many of the clinical features of acute infection. In doing so, it is probable that it plays a significant protective role. For this reason, it seems reasonable to question the strenuous efforts we make to reduce some of these clinical features such as fever through the use of anti-inflammatory drugs.

Amyloidosis

Amyloid is the name given to an amorphous, eosinophilic, hyaline, extracellular substance that infiltrates tissues in certain pathological conditions. It is found in all domestic animals, particularly cattle, horses and dogs. It may be classified as either "immunocytic," if it is associated with a myeloma or other lymphoid tumor, or "reactive," if it is associated with chronic suppurative conditions such as mastitis, osteomyelitis, abscesses, traumatic pericarditis or tuberculosis (Fig. 19–10). Reactive amyloidosis is a major cause of death in animals repeatedly immunized for commercial antiserum production. It is also commonly associated with autoimmune disorders. Several other well-defined forms of amyloidosis are seen in domestic animals; for example, old dogs may suffer from vascular amyloidosis in which amyloid is deposited in the media of leptomeningeal and cortical arteries. An inherited form of amyloid has been described in Abyssinian cats. Tumor-like amyloid nodules and subcutaneous amyloid have been reported in horses, but in general, amyloid deposits are usually found in the liver, spleen and kidneys, particularly within glomeruli. Amyloidosis may be produced in laboratory mice by feeding them a diet rich in casein or by injecting

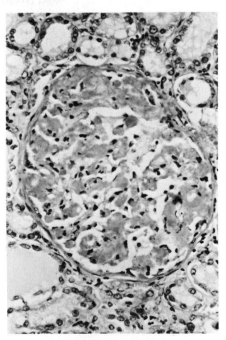

Figure 19–10. Secondary amyloid deposited in the glomerulus of a dog. ×250. (Courtesy of Dr. L. G. Adams.)

large or repeated doses of bacterial endotoxin or Freund's complete adjuvant.

On electron microscopy all forms of amyloid can be shown to consist of a felt-like mass of protein fibrils. By x-ray crystallography it can be further shown that all amyloid proteins have their polypeptide chains arranged in the form known as β-pleated sheets. This is a uniquely stable molecular conformation that renders the fibrils both extremely insoluble and almost totally resistant to normal proteolytic enzymes. Consequently, once deposited in tissues, they are almost impossible to remove. The accumulation of amyloid in tissues is essentially irreversible, leading to gradual cell loss and tissue destruction.

The β-pleated sheet configuration of amyloid also gives it unique staining properties; it stains metachromatically with toluidine blue and binds specifically to congo red.

Although all amyloid proteins have the β-pleated sheet configuration, biochemical analysis has shown that most are composed of one of two basic proteins (Fig. 19–11). In immunogenic amyloid and a few cases of reactive amyloid, this protein is known as AL. AL protein is a proteolytic digestion product of immunoglobulin light chains. In animals with myelomas, light chains are usually generated in excess, and limited proteolytic digestion of these permits the V_L region to assume a β-pleated sheet configuration. It has been suggested that immunogenic amyloid deposits

consist of light chains modified by proteolytic enzymes from cells such as macrophages and deposited in tissues in excessive amounts.

The major protein component of reactive amyloid is known as AA. AA is not immunoglobulin-derived, but may be deposited in close association with plasma cells. It is derived by partial proteolytic digestion of serum amyloid A (SAA). SAA is found in high concentrations in the serum of humans and animals with experimental or natural amyloidosis and in the serum of patients undergoing chronic antigenic stimulation, as in tuberculosis or rheumatoid arthritis. It is found in low levels in normal serum and is produced by hepatocytes and fibroblasts in response to IL-1. Since SAA has been shown to be strongly immunosuppressive in mice, it has been suggested that SAA normally serves to control the immune response and that, under conditions of chronic antigenic stimulation, excessive production of SAA and its subsequent digestion can lead to the deposition of AA as amyloid in tissues. The major protein in familial amyloid of Abyssinian cats is also AA.

Reactive amyloid also contains, in addition to AA, a small quantity of a protein known as amyloid P (AP). Serum amyloid P is another acute-phase protein whose concentration rises 10 to 40 fold in infected animals. This is assumed to be a protective response, since AP enhances the bactericidal activity of macrophages. Although AL and AA are associated with the two major forms of amyloid, it must be emphasized that any protein that can form extensive β-pleated sheets will give rise to amyloid if deposited in tissues. Many of the less common manifestations of amyloidosis may, therefore, be caused by proteins distinct from AL or AA. It has been suggested that a more appropriate collective term for the amyloidoses is β fibrilloses, since the β-pleated conformational structure is the common feature of all these conditions.

ADDITIONAL SOURCES OF INFORMATION

Boyce JT, DiBartola SP, Chew DJ and Gasper PW. 1984. Familial renal amyloidosis in Abyssinian Cats. Vet. Pathol. *21* 33–38.

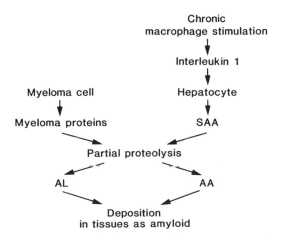

Figure 19–11. The pathogenesis of immunogenic and reactive amyloid.

Caspi D, Baltz ML, Snel F et al. 1984. Isolation and characterization of C-reactive protein from a dog. Immunology 53 307–313.

Dinarello CA. 1984. Interleukin 1 and the pathogenesis of the acute-phase response. N. Engl. J. Med. 311 1413–1418.

Glenner GG. 1980. Amyloid deposits and amyloidosis: the β fibrilloses. N. Engl. J. Med. 302 1283–1292 and 1333–1343.

Higgins AJ and Lees P. 1984. The acute inflammatory process, arachidonic acid metabolism and the mode of action of antiinflammatory drugs. Equine Vet. J. 16 163–175.

Jampel HD, Duff GW, Gershon RK et al. 1983. Fever and immunoregulation. III. Hyperthermia augments the primary in vitro humoral immune response. J. Exp. Med. 157 1229–1238.

Kushner I, Gewurz H and Benson MD. 1981. C-reactive protein and the acute-phase response. J. Lab. Clin. Med. 97 739–749.

Liggit HD, Leid RW and Huston L. 1984. Aggregation of bovine platelets by acetyl glyceryl ether phosphorylcholine (platelet activating factor). Vet. Immunol. Immunopathol. 7 81–88.

Ryan GB and Majno G. 1977. Acute inflammation. Am. J. Pathol. 86 183–276.

Samuelsson B. 1983. Leukotrienes: Mediators of immediate hypersensitivity reactions and inflammation. Science 220 568–575.

Weissmann G, Smolen JE and Korchak HM. 1980. Release of inflammatory mediators from stimulated neutrophils. N. Engl. J. Med. 303 27–34.

20

Type I Hypersensitivity: Allergies and Anaphylaxis

Type I hypersensitivities are inflammatory reactions mediated by certain immunoglobulin isotypes, especially IgE, bound to mast cells and basophils; the reactions result from the release of pharmacologically active factors by these cells (Fig. 20–1).

Of all the adverse consequences of the immune response, the most dramatic are those of type I hypersensitivity. These reactions are variously termed immediate hypersensitivity, allergies or anaphylaxis. Because they cause so much discomfort and distress, any beneficial effects are not immediately obvious; nevertheless, certain features of this type of hypersensitivity do give us indications of a beneficial biological function. First, it is probable that the localized acute inflammatory response that occurs in this condition plays a significant role in antigen elimination. Second,

this type of hypersensitivity is commonly associated with helminth antigens and appears to play an important role in resistance to these parasites (Chapter 17). Third, statistical evidence suggests that individuals who suffer from allergies are less likely than unaffected people to die from cancer. The mechanism and significance of this phenomenon are unknown.

INDUCTION OF TYPE I HYPERSENSITIVITY

Type I hypersensitivity is mediated by antibodies of the IgE isotype. The conditions under which IgE rather than IgG antibodies are produced are not entirely clear. The antigens that induce IgE antibodies have no dis-

TERMINOLOGY

Before the antibodies that mediate type I hypersensitivity were characterized as IgE, they were known as reagins, or reaginic antibodies. Because they bind to cells, they are also cytotropic or cytophilic. If they can bind only to cells of their own species, they are said to be homocytotropic. IgE is not, strictly speaking, homocytotropic, since it may bind to cells from several different species of mammals. IgE mediates an immediate hypersensitivity reaction, so called because of its rapid development following exposure to antigen. This type of hypersensitivity reaction is also known as allergy. Antigens that stimulate allergies may be termed allergens. However, many clinicians and laymen use the term allergy to describe any unpleasant reaction to foreign material. If an immediate hypersensitivity reaction is systemic and severe, it is termed anaphylaxis. Sometimes an animal suffers from a reaction similar to anaphylaxis but which may not be immunologically mediated. This type of reaction is described as anaphylactoid. In this chapter, the term "type I hypersensitivity" is employed since it has an etiological connotation that many of the other terms now lack.

some proteins in insect venoms. Freund's complete adjuvant or killed *Bordetella pertussis* organisms may act to preferentially stimulate IgE production in some animals.

In many species, including dogs and humans, the ability to respond to antigen by production of IgE antibodies is largely inherited; therefore, some individuals have a higher than normal tendency to mount an IgE response. These individuals are said to be atopic, and about 1 to 2 per cent of the dog population in North America is affected in this way. If both parents are atopic, then most of their progeny will be atopic also and will suffer from type I hypersensitivities. If only one parent is atopic, then the percentage of atopic offspring varies. There also appears to be a breed predisposition to atopy. Atopic dermatitis is most commonly observed in terriers (Cairn, West Highland White, Scottish), Dalmatians and Irish setters. It is rarely seen in Cocker spaniels.

Immunoglobulin E

IgE is a heat-labile immunoglobulin of conventional four-chain structure. Because of the addition of an extra constant domain near the hinge, its heavy chain contains four C_H regions and one V_H region. IgE thus has a molecular

cernible unique biochemical features. Certain antigens are, however, potent stimulators of this type of response. These include proteins of pollen grains, some helminth antigens and

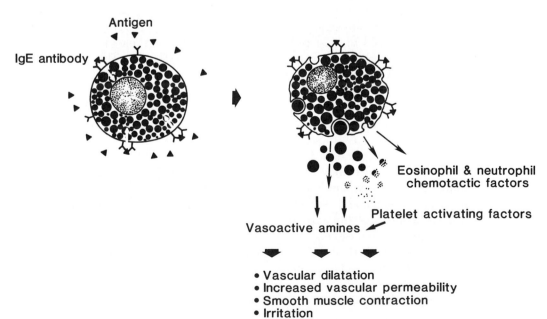

Figure 20–1. The mechanism of type I hypersensitivity.

weight of 196,000 daltons, which is somewhat greater than that of IgG. IgE is produced by plasma cells, most of which are located near epithelial surfaces. It is found in serum in exquisitely small quantities (9 to 700 μg/ml in dogs). Much of the IgE is normally bound through its C_H3 and C_H4 regions to mast cells and basophils. When attached to these cells it has a half-life of 11 to 12 days. When free in serum its half-life is only about two days. The precise level of IgE in serum appears to be related to the parasite burden of the animal.

Some IgG subisotypes may also bind to mast cells and participate in type I hypersensitivity reactions. However, the affinity of these subisotypes for mast cell receptors is considerably lower than that of IgE, and they may be considered to be of much less practical importance.

Mast Cells and Basophils

Mast cells are large, round cells (15 to 20 μm diameter) distributed throughout the body in connective tissue (Figs. 20–2 and 20–3). Their most characteristic feature is a cytoplasm packed with large granules that stain metachromatically with dyes such as toluidine blue. The granules usually mask the relatively large, bean-shaped nucleus.

Mast cells, at least in rodents and humans, fall into two populations differentiated on the basis of their origins and functions (Table 20–1). Ordinary connective tissue mast cells arise from precursors in fetal liver and bone marrow. Their numbers increase slowly in tissues, although irritation may cause local proliferation. Connective tissue mast cells contain many uniform granules and are rich in histamine and heparin. Their life span is at least six months.

Mucosal mast cells differ from the mast cells located in connective tissue elsewhere in several respects. For example, they tend to have few, variable-sized granules. The granules of these mast cells contain, not heparin, but chondroitin sulfate E. As a result they have different staining properties. They contain little histamine and produce different prostaglandins and leukotrienes as well as platelet activating factor. While connective tissue mast cells remain at relatively constant levels, mucosal mast cells proliferate in response to interleukin 3. Thus T cell-deficient animals are also deficient in mucosal mast cells. It has been suggested that these mucosal mast cells respond specifically to nematode antigens.

The Response of Mast Cells to Antigen

Mast cells possess Fc receptors specific for IgE and hence are able to bind free IgE molecules. When IgE binds to mast cell receptors no visible change occurs in the structure of the mast cells. When antigen binds to mast cell IgE and cross-links two IgE mole-

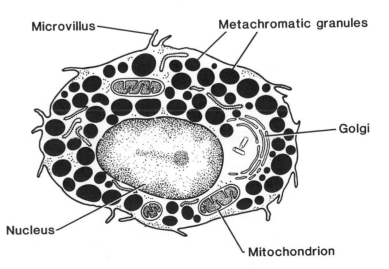

Figure 20–2. The structural features of a connective tissue mast cell.

Microvillus — Metachromatic granules — Golgi — Nucleus — Mitochondrion

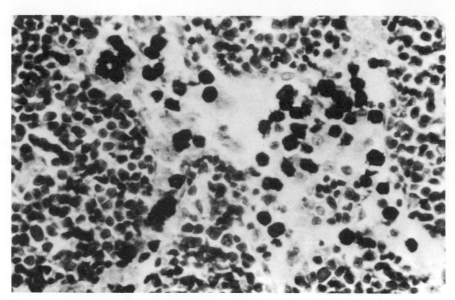

Figure 20–3. A section of human mesenteric lymph node stained to show mast cells. The mast cells stain intensely because of the heparin in their cytoplasmic granules.

cules, a series of reactions are triggered that cause the mast cell granules to migrate to the cell surface, fuse with the cell membrane and be extruded from the cell, releasing their granule contents into the surrounding tissues. The cell membrane metabolism of arachidonic acid is also stimulated. These mast cell responses are extremely rapid, occurring only a few seconds after antigen binds to antibody on the cell surface (Fig. 20–4). Degranulated mast cells do not die, but they are difficult to identify because of an absence of characteristic morphological features. Degranulated mucosal mast cells are known as globule leukocytes. These cells are prominent in the intestinal wall of animals after elimination of helminth infections as a result of the process of "self-cure" (Chapter 17).

Strictly speaking, peripheral blood basophils should not be considered simply as circulating mast cells. They may, however, be passively sensitized with IgE, and they will respond to antigen in a manner apparently similar to that of mast cells.

Agents that initiate mast cell degranulation by nonimmunological mechanisms include drugs such as the antibiotic polymyxin B, morphine, and tubocurarine and the anaphylatoxins C3a and C5a.

Biologically Active Agents Released in Type I Hypersensitivity

Once exposed to extracellular fluid, mast cell granules release their vasoactive agents. In addition, the combination of IgE with antigen on the surface of these cells provokes the

Table 20–1 THE DIFFERENCES BETWEEN CONNECTIVE TISSUE AND MUCOSAL MAST CELLS

Property	Connective Tissue Mast Cells	Mucosal Mast Cells
Granules	Many, uniform size	Few, variable size
Size	~20 μm	~10 μm
IL-3 dependent	No	Yes
Proteoglycan	Heparin	Chondroitin sulfate E
Histamine content	~15 pg/cell	~ 1.5 pg/cell
Life span	>6 mo.	<40 days

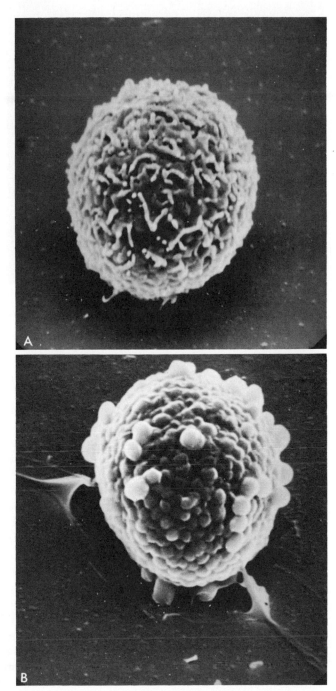

Figure 20–4. Scanning electron micrographs of a normal rat mast cell (*A*), a sensitized mast cell fixed five seconds after exposure to antigon (*B*).

Illustration continued on following page

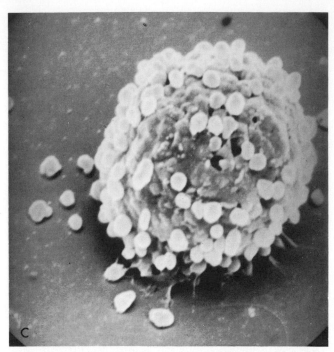

Figure 20–4 *Continued* A sensitized mast cell fixed 60 seconds after exposure to antigen (*C*). × 3000. (From Tizard I. R. and Holmes W. L. 1974. Int Arch Allergy Appl Immunol 46 867–879. Used with permission from the publisher, S. Karger, Basel.)

formation of other vasoactive substances. It is these agents, both those released preformed from granules and those newly synthesized, that generate the characteristic inflammatory lesions of type I hypersensitivity (Table 20–2).

Mast cell granules contain high concentrations of histamine and (in some species) serotonin. While these two compounds are very

Table 20–2 THE MAJOR MEDIATORS OF TYPE I HYPERSENSITIVITY

Agent	Stored	Newly Formed
Vasoactive factors		
Histamine	+	
Serotonin	+	
Leukotrienes C_4 and D_4		+
Prostaglandins		+
Activators		
Platelet activating factor		+
Tryptase	+	
Kallikreins (kinins)		+
Chemoattractants		
ECF-A*	+	
NCF†	+	
Leukotriene B_4		+
Anticoagulants		
Heparin	+	
Chondroitin sulfate E	+	

*Eosinophil chemotactic factor of anaphylaxis
†Neutrophil chemotactic factor

important mediators of inflammation, they are only part of the total spectrum of inflammatory mediators released following mast cell degranulation. More than half the protein in the mast cell granules consists of trypsin or chymotrypsin-like neutral proteases. These proteases can destroy nearby cells and activate the complement components C3 and C5 to generate anaphylatoxins. Mast cell granules also contain kallikreins (Chapter 19) and so act on kininogens to generate kinins such as bradykinin. Both the kinins and the anaphylatoxins are powerful vasoactive agents.

Platelet activating factor (PAF) is a phospholipid acether closely related to lecithin. It is synthesized by mast cells following exposure to antigen or to anaphylatoxins. It is also synthesized by platelets. PAF is a potent aggregator of platelets and makes them release their vasoactive factors, especially serotonin, and synthesize thromboxanes. It also causes a thrombocytopenia. PAF acts on neutrophils in a similar fashion. Thus, it promotes neutrophil aggregation, degranulation, chemotaxis, the release of oxygen radicals and a neutropenia. PAF at very low concentrations causes smooth muscle contraction. It is inactivated by the enzyme phospholipase D found in eosinophils.

Activation of cell membrane phospholipases

is also provoked by antigen binding to IgE on the mast cell surface. This leads to the release of arachidonic acid from cell membrane phospholipids. Arachidonic acid is the substrate for cyclooxygenase and for lipoxygenase. The products of the cyclooxygenase pathway are the prostaglandins, prostacyclins and thromboxanes; the products of the lipoxygenase pathway are leukotrienes (see Chapter 19). All of these have major effects on vascular tone and permeability. It is possible that different subclasses of mast cells give rise to different products from these pathways.

Mast cell granules also release two peptides that are chemotactic for eosinophils (eosinophil chemotactic factors of anaphylaxis, ECF-A). Both are tetrapeptides that exist preformed within mast cell granules. These factors account, at least in part, for the eosinophilia so characteristic of type I hypersensitivity reactions, including helminth infestations.

Other factors that are found in mast cell granules and are released on degranulation include a neutrophil chemotactic factor (NCFA) and a neutrophil immobilization factor. The latter factor, as its name suggests, stops the emigration of neutrophils once they have been attracted to the area by the chemotactic factor. It does not interfere with the phagocytic activities of the cells.

Proteoglycans such as heparin from connective tissue mast cells and chondroitin sulfate E from mucosal mast cells are also released on mast cell degranulation. Heparin is largely responsible for the metachromatic staining properties of connective tissue mast cells. It is released from the granules independently of histamine. Because of the anticoagulant properties of heparin, blood from animals suffering from anaphylaxis and from dogs with mast cell tumors may fail to coagulate.

Control of Type I Hypersensitivity

Regulation of the IgE Response

It is well recognized that not all individuals are equally able to mount an IgE response. The reasons for this are primarily genetic. The ability to mount an IgE response is regulated by several different immune response genes.

From studies of the immune system of atopic individuals, it is clear that some individuals have a deficiency of suppressor cells, as a result of which their IgE-producing B cells can function at a higher rate than normal. It has proved possible to remedy this by the use of "desensitizing" injections of antigen. The original rationale for administering antigen to atopic individuals was to stimulate the production of IgG-blocking antibodies. It was anticipated that these would compete with IgE for antigen and hence prevent the antigen from reaching the mast cells. It is now believed that desensitizing injections also promote suppressor cell activity and in some way directly reduce the sensitivity of mast cells to antigen.

The role of blocking antibodies was first shown in beekeepers who, in spite of being stung frequently and of having high levels of IgE in their serum, usually suffered minimal discomfort. Analysis of their serum showed that they had very high levels of IgG against bee venom. If venom-allergic individuals were passively immunized with serum from these beekeepers they could be made temporarily "immune" to allergic reactions to venom. In addition, this hyperimmune serum effectively prevented degranulation and histamine release from sensitized mast cells *in vitro*.

In hyposensitization therapy, antigen is administered in a form designed to stimulate the immune response while reducing, as far as possible, the risks of anaphylactic shock. Thus, antigen may be administered in a suspension with alum or in a water-in-oil emulsion to form a depot. Generally, aqueous allergens are rapidly absorbed but require frequent injections. The alum- or oil-adjuvanted allergens are slowly absorbed and require fewer injections. The first injections contain only a very small quantity of allergen. Over a number of weeks, the dosage is gradually increased. If an animal's allergy is of the seasonal type, the course of injections should be timed to reach completion just prior to the anticipated antigen exposure.

A newer approach to the selective stimulation of suppressor cells in atopic individuals is to modify the allergen by attaching it to a nonimmunogenic polymer such as polyethylene glycol. This molecule can, when bound to an allergen, promote specific suppression of the IgE response.

Regulation of Mast Cell Degranulation

The release of vasoactive agents from mast cells is modulated by intracellular cyclic nucleotides. Elevation of cyclic AMP or depression of cyclic GMP inhibits mast cell degranulation, whereas depression of cyclic AMP or elevation of cyclic GMP enhances degranulation. The precise relationship between these two compounds is complex, and the final response may depend on the cyclic AMP-to-cyclic GMP ratio.

On the surface of mast cells there are two types of receptors for adrenergic agents (adrenoceptors), named α and β receptors. Compounds that stimulate the α receptor enhance mast cell degranulation because they depress intracellular cyclic AMP (Table 20–3). Compounds that stimulate the β receptor have the reverse effect and thus depress mast cell degranulation. Drugs that either stimulate the α receptor, such as norepinephrine and phenylephrine, or block the β receptor, such as propranolol, therefore enhance mast cell degranulation. Drugs that stimulate the β receptor, thus raising cyclic AMP levels and inhibiting mast cell degranulation, include isoproterenol, epinephrine and salbutamol. Recently, it has become clear that β-receptor impairment can also contribute to the atopic state. For example, the effects of β-receptor activation can be inhibited by certain respiratory tract pathogens such as *Bordetella pertussis* or *Hemophilus influenzae* or by auto-antibodies directed against the β receptor. Because of this impairment, affected individuals are more susceptible to hypersensitivity conditions such as chronic asthma. It is also of interest to note that histamine itself tends

to suppress mast cell degranulation by binding to mast cell H2 receptors and so elevating intracellular cyclic AMP.

Regulation of the Response to Mast Cell-Derived Mediators

The α and β adrenoceptors are found not only on mast cells but also on secretory and smooth muscle cells throughout the body. Stimulators of α adrenoceptors mediate vasoconstriction (see Table 20–3). Consequently, α adrenergic agents may be of use in the treatment of anaphylaxis, reducing edema and raising blood pressure. Stimulators of β adrenoceptors mediate smooth muscle relaxation and may therefore be useful in modulating the severity of smooth muscle contraction.

Pure α and β receptor stimulants are of only limited use in the treatment of anaphylaxis because each alone is insufficient to counteract all the effects of mast cell-derived factors. Epinephrine, on the other hand, has both α and β adrenergic activity and therefore, in addition to causing vasoconstriction in skin and viscera, its β effects cause smooth muscle to relax. This combination of effects is well suited to combat the vasodilation and smooth muscle contraction produced by histamine. Ideally, epinephrine solution should be available whenever potential allergens are administered to animals.

The Role of Eosinophils

Eosinophils are attracted to the site of mast cell degranulation by ECF-A, by leukotriene B$_4$ and by histamine and its breakdown products. Their function, once they arrive, is a matter of debate. For many years it was believed that eosinophils served to suppress inflammation by destroying the factors released by mast cells (Fig. 20–5). It is now clear, however, that the pro-inflammatory factors

Table 20–3 EFFECTS OF STIMULATING α AND β ADRENOCEPTORS

System	Stimulation of α Adrenoceptor	Stimulation of β Adrenoceptor
Cyclic nucleotides	Lowers cAMP Raises cGMP	Raises cAMP Lowers cGMP
Mast cell degranulation	Enhances	Depresses
Smooth muscle	Contracts	Relaxes
Blood vessels	Constricts	Dilates

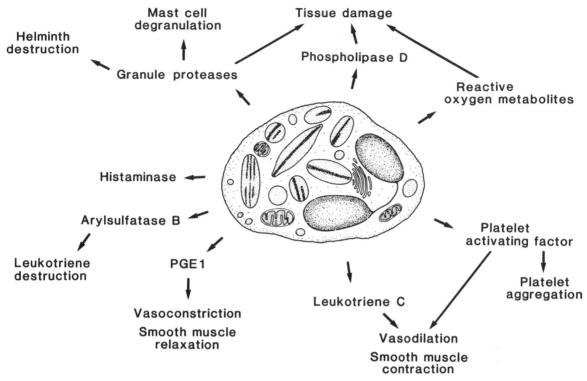

Figure 20–5. The functions of eosinophils.

released by eosinophils greatly outweigh the effects of the anti-inflammatory factors. Thus although eosinophils release diamine oxidase, which acts as a histaminase, arylsulfatase B, which may destroy leukotrienes, and PGE_1, which has vasoconstrictor and smooth muscle relaxant effects, they also release leukotriene C, PAF, phospholipase D, toxic granule proteins and reactive oxygen metabolites. In addition, the eosinophil granule enzymes may promote mast cell degranulation. It is also of interest to note that eosinophils and basophils share eosinophil basic protein and lysophospholipase and are therefore probably closely related. It may be that mast cells, basophils and eosinophils constitute a family of cells whose function is to enhance the inflammatory responses.

Measurement of Type I Hypersensitivity

The term hypersensitivity is used to denote a severe reaction that occurs in response to normally harmless material. For example, normal animals do not react to antigens injected intradermally. If, however, IgE antibodies are produced against an antigen and if these antibodies bind to skin mast cells, then intradermal inoculation of antigen, even in very dilute solution, will provoke a local inflammatory reaction. Because of the nature of the mast cell response, vasoactive agents are released within minutes to produce erythema as a result of capillary dilatation and circumscribed edema (a wheal) due to increased vascular permeability. The reaction may also involve an erythematous "flare" due to arteriolar dilatation brought about by a local axon reflex. This type of response to antigen reaches maximal intensity within 30 minutes and then fades and disappears within a few hours.

Direct skin testing of this type has been widely used for the identification of specific allergens in atopic dogs. The results obtained can vary widely for several reasons. One important factor is the concentration of antigen in commercial skin testing products. For example, dogs may be up to 10 times less sensitive to intradermal allergens such as pollens, fungi or danders than humans, and males are less sensitive than females. Other problems may arise because of the presence of preservatives in the allergen solutions. The precise set of allergens used for testing varies between different parts of the country; however, they commonly include an assortment of allergens from trees, grasses, fungi, ragweed, danders, house dust and insects.

Two other skin testing techniques may be used to detect reaginic antibodies to specific antigens. One, named the Prausnitz-Kustner or P-K test, is a skin test in which serum from a test animal is injected intradermally into a normal animal. After a period of 24 to 48 hours, which allows antibodies to bind to skin mast cells, the antigen is injected at the same site. In a positive reaction, a wheal and flare response occurs within one to two minutes. An alternative method is called the passive cutaneous anaphylaxis (PCA) test. In this test, increasing dilutions of serum are injected at different sites in the skin of a normal animal. After waiting for 24 to 48 hours, the antigen solution is administered intravenously. In a positive reaction, each injection site shows an immediate inflammatory response. The injected antibodies may remain fixed in the skin for a very long period. In the case of the calf, this may be up to eight weeks. In the PCA test it is sometimes difficult to detect very mild inflammatory responses. One way to render them more visible is to inject the test animal intravenously with Evans blue dye. The dye binds to serum albumin and does not normally leave the blood stream. At sites of acute inflammation in which vascular permeability is increased, the dye-labeled albumin enters the tissue fluid and forms a striking blue patch. The size of this patch may be used as a measure of the intensity of the inflammatory reaction (Fig. 20–6).

An *in vitro* experimental test of immediate hypersensitivity is the Schultz-Dale technique. In this test, a strip of smooth muscle such as intestine is removed from a sensitized animal, washed and suspended in physiological saline. If this tissue is then exposed to specific antigen, degranulation of the mast cells within it will cause it to contract violently. This test may be modified by preincubating the smooth muscle from a normal animal in serum derived from a sensitized one. This passively sensitized muscle will then contract on exposure to specific antigen. Other smooth muscle-containing tissues, such as the uterus, bronchus or trachea and certain blood vessels, may also be employed to demonstrate Schultz-Dale reactions.

If it is necessary to measure the level of specific IgE in the serum of an allergic animal, then the serological test of choice is the radioallergosorbent test (RAST) (Chapter 11).

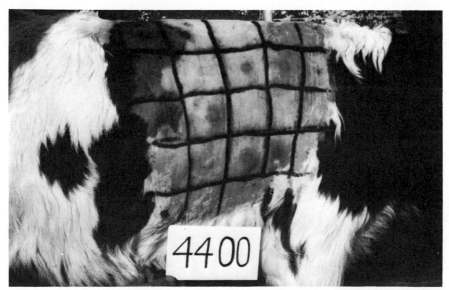

Figure 20–6. Passive cutaneous anaphylaxis (PCA) reactions in a calf. Several different sera were tested for PCA activity on the flank of a normal calf. (Courtesy of Dr. P. Eyre.)

Table 20-4 COMPARISON OF ANAPHYLAXIS IN VARIOUS SPECIES*

Species	Main Shock Organ	Symptoms	Pathology	Major Pharmacological Mediators
Cattle and sheep	Respiratory tract	Cough, dyspnea, collapse	Lung edema, emphysema, hemorrage	Leukotrienes, kinins, histamine
Horse	Respiratory tract, intestine	Cough, dyspnea, diarrhea	Emphysema, intestinal hemorrhage	Histamine, serotonin, kinins
Swine	Respiratory tract, intestine	Cyanosis, itch, staggering, collapse	Systemic hypotension	Histamine (uncertain)
Cat	Respiratory tract, intestine	Itch, vomiting, dyspnea, diarrhea	Lung edema, intestinal edema	Histamine, leukotrienes
Dog	Hepatic veins	Vomiting, diarrhea, dyspnea, collapse	Hepatic engorgement, visceral hemorrhage	Histamine, leukotrienes
Chicken	Respiratory tract	Dyspnea, convulsions, collapse	Lung edema	Histamine, serotonin, leukotrienes
Man	Respiratory tract	Urticaria, dyspnea	Lung edema, emphysema	Histamine, leukotrienes

*Modified from Eyre P. 1972. The biochemical pharmacology of allergic reactions in domestic animals. Vet Rev 23 3–16. Used with permission.

CLINICAL MANIFESTATIONS OF TYPE I HYPERSENSITIVITY

All the clinical signs of type I hypersensitivity relate to the release of vasoactive substances from mast cells and basophils. The severity and location of these reactions depends on the number and location of the mast cells stimulated, and this, in turn, is dependent on the amount of antigen and its route of administration. In its most extreme form, antigen administered rapidly and intravenously will cause generalized mast cell degranulation. If the rate of release of vasoactive agents from these mast cells is in excess of the body's ability to respond to the rapid changes in its vascular system, the animal will suffer from anaphylactic shock and may die. If, on the other hand, antigen is administered either locally in small quantities or slowly, then the clinical signs of hypersensitivity will be much less severe, since the animal will have had an opportunity to compensate for the vascular changes provoked by the mast cell-derived factors.

Acute Systemic Anaphylaxis
(Table 20–4)

In cattle, acute anaphylaxis is characterized by profound systemic hypotension and pulmo-nary hypertension. The major organ involved in the reaction is the lung. The pulmonary hypertension occurs as a result of constriction of the pulmonary vein and leads to severe dyspnea with pulmonary edema. Other events that take place include contraction of the smooth muscle of the bladder and intestine, resulting in urination, defecation and bloating. It seems likely that the main mediators of anaphylaxis in the bovine are serotonin, kinins and the leukotrienes. Histamine is of much less importance. Dopamine also functions in bovine anaphylaxis by enhancing histamine and leukotriene release from the lung, thus exerting a form of positive feedback. Cattle are also of interest since, in contrast to the other species, drugs that stimulate the β adrenoceptor, such as isoproterenol, potentiate histamine release from leukocytes, whereas drugs that stimulate the α receptor, such as norepinephrine, inhibit histamine release. In addition, epinephrine potentiates histamine release in the bovine. The significance of these anomalous effects is unclear.

In sheep, too, pulmonary signs predominate in acute anaphylaxis as a result of constriction of the bronchi and pulmonary vessels. Smooth muscle contraction also occurs in the bladder and intestine with predictable results. The major mediators of type I hypersensitivity in sheep are histamine, serotonin, leukotrienes and kinins.

The major shock organs of horses are the lungs and the intestine. Bronchial and bronchiolar constriction in anaphylaxis leads to coughing, dyspnea and eventually apnea. On necropsy, severe pulmonary emphysema and peribronchiolar edema are commonly seen. In addition to the lung lesions, edematous hemorrhagic enterocolitis may occur, resulting in severe diarrhea. Pathologically, the intestinal lesion resembles that of colitis X, a disease associated with salmonellosis. It is tempting to suggest that an anaphylactic reaction may play a role in colitis X. The major mediators in horses are probably histamine and serotonin.

In pigs, acute systemic anaphylaxis is largely the result of systemic and pulmonary hypertension, leading to dyspnea and death. In some pigs the intestine shows signs of involvement, whereas in others no gross lesions are observed. The most significant mediator so far identified in this species is histamine.

Dogs differ from the other domestic animals in that the major organ involved in acute anaphylaxis is not the lung but the liver, specifically the hepatic veins. Dogs undergoing anaphylaxis show initial excitement followed by vomiting, defecation and urination. As the anaphylactic reaction progresses, the dog collapses with muscular weakness and depressed respiration, becomes comatose, convulses and dies within an hour. On necropsy, the liver and intestine are massively engorged, perhaps holding up to 60 per cent of the animal's total blood volume. All these signs are a result of occlusion of the hepatic vein, which results in portal hypertension and visceral pooling. The mechanism of this is probably a combination of smooth muscle contraction in the vessel walls and of occlusion secondary to hepatic swelling.

In cats, the shock organ is the lung. Cats undergoing anaphylaxis will show vigorous scratching around the face and head as histamine is released into the skin, followed by dyspnea, salivation, vomiting, incoordination and collapse. On necropsy, there are bronchoconstriction, emphysema, pulmonary hemorrhage and edema of the glottis. The relative importance of the major pharmacological mediators in this species is not known.

The signs of acute anaphylaxis in chickens are similar to those in mammals. They show increased salivation, defecation, ruffling of feathers, dyspnea, convulsions, cyanosis, collapse and death. The major target organ is probably the lung, and death is due to pulmonary arterial hypotension, right heart dilatation and cardiac arrest. The pharmacological agents involved include histamine, serotonin, the kinins and the leukotrienes.

Specific Allergic Conditions

Although acute systemic anaphylaxis is the most dramatic of the type I hypersensitivity reactions, it is more common to observe local allergic reactions, the sites of which are referable to the route of administration of antigens. For example, inhaled antigens (allergens) provoke an initial response in the upper respiratory tract, trachea and bronchi, resulting in fluid exudation from the nasal mucosa (hay fever) and tracheobronchial constriction (asthma). Aerosolized antigen will also contact the eyes and provoke conjunctivitis and intense lacrimation. Ingested antigens may provoke diarrhea and colic as the intestinal smooth muscle contracts violently, and if sufficiently severe the resulting diarrhea may be hemorrhagic. Antigen reaching the skin will cause a local hypersensitivity reaction similar to that described following a skin test. The reaction is erythematous and edematous and is said to be of an urticarial type (*urtica* is Latin for "stinging nettle"). Urticarial lesions are extremely irritating because of the histamine released; consequently, the true nature of the lesion may be masked by scratching (Fig. 20–7).

Milk Allergy

Jersey cattle may become allergic to the α casein of their own milk. Normally, this material is synthesized in the udder, and, provided that the animals are milked regularly, nothing untoward occurs. If the milking is delayed, however, then the increased intramammary pressure forces milk proteins back into the blood stream. In allergic cattle, the

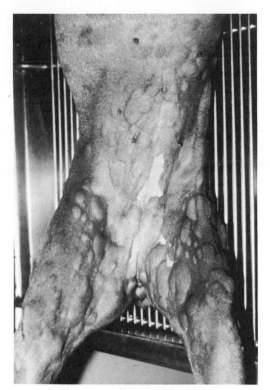

Figure 20–7. Severe urticaria in a boxer stung by three wasps. (Courtesy of Dr. G. Elissalde.)

times hemorrhagic diarrhea occurring soon after feeding. About half the dogs suffer from skin disease. The skin reactions are usually urticarial and erythematous and may involve the feet, eyes, ears, axillae or perianal area. The lesion itself is highly pruritic and is thus commonly masked by self-inflicted trauma. This pruritus tends to respond poorly to steroids. In chronic cases the skin may be hyperpigmented, lichenified and secondarily infected. The foods involved vary but are usually protein-rich, e.g., cow's milk, wheat meal, fish, chicken, beef or eggs. In pigs, fishmeal and alfalfa have been incriminated, and in horses, wild oats, white clover and alfalfa have been recognized as allergens. Diagnosis of suspected food allergies is made by removing all potential allergens and then testing using a trial diet, since skin tests are of little help. Mutton and brown rice are usually hypoallergenic for dogs since mutton is not commonly employed in commercial dog foods. This diet may be supplemented by various foods until the allergen is identified by a recurrence of clinical signs.

result of this may range from mild discomfort with urticarial skin lesions to acute systemic anaphylaxis and death. The condition can be readily treated by prompt milking, although some seriously affected animals may have to go for several lactations without drying off because of the severe reactions that occur on cessation of milking.

Food Allergy

It has been claimed that up to 30 per cent of skin diseases seen in dogs are due to allergic dermatitis and that responses to ingested allergens may account for 1 per cent of cutaneous disease in dogs and cats. The clinical signs of food allergies are observed both in the digestive tract and on the skin.

About 10 to 15 per cent of the dogs suffering from food allergy have gastrointestinal problems. The intestinal reaction may be mild, perhaps showing only as an irregularity in the consistency of the feces, or it may be severe, with vomiting, cramps, and violent, some-

Basenji dogs appear to suffer from type I hypersensitivities to an unusual degree. Thus their airways are unusually sensitive, and they suffer from a condition similar to that seen in human asthmatics. Basenjis also suffer from immunoproliferative small intestinal disease. This condition is characterized by chronic diarrhea, anorexia, gastritis, hypergammaglobulinemia and a lymphocytic-plasmacytic infiltration of the intestinal lamina propria. The cause of this disease is unknown, but the association of degranulated mast cells with the cellular infiltration suggests that it may be due in part to a hypersensitivity reaction.

Allergies to Inhaled Antigens

The most significant allergies of humans are hay fever and asthma. Both of these allergies are caused by exposure to antigenic particles suspended in inhaled air. Hay fever is generally due to pollens, whereas asthma is etiologically complex, involving both pharmacological and psychological factors as well as allergy. Asthma can be provoked by many allergens, including fungal spores and mites present in house dust, and may also occur as a result of food allergies.

In dogs and cats, inhalant allergy most commonly leads to an atopic dermatitis manifested primarily as pruritus. Many affected animals have a history of foot licking, face rubbing or axillary pruritus. The specific lesions vary greatly, ranging from acute erythema and edema to more chronic secondary changes including crusting, scaling, hyperpigmentation and pyoderma. Some animals may suffer from otitis externa and conjunctivitis. The major allergens implicated include molds; tree, weed and grass pollens; house dusts; animal danders; and fabrics such as kapok or wool. Most animals develop multiple sensitivities. Diagnosis is based primarily on history and identification of the offending antigens by direct skin testing. Canine atopy may be treated by the use of corticosteroids or by hyposensitization therapy. Antihistamines and non-steroidal anti-inflammatory drugs seem to be of little help.

Nasolacrimal urticaria (hay fever) is an uncommon manifestation of respiratory allergy in dogs and cats. Pollens usually provoke a rhinitis and conjunctivitis characterized by a profuse watery nasal discharge and excessive lacrimation. If the offending allergenic particles are sufficiently small, they may reach the bronchi or bronchioles (see Fig. 12–1), where the resulting local reaction can cause bronchoconstriction, wheezing and recurrent asthma-like paroxysmal dyspnea.

In Australia, a form of nasal granuloma occurs in cattle, which consists of numerous polypoid nodules, 1 to 4 mm in diameter, situated in the anterior nasal mucosa. The nodules contain large numbers of mast cells, eosinophils and plasma cells and probably arise as a result of repeated exposure to an unidentified inhaled antigen. These lesions are intensely pruritic and cause great distress to affected animals.

Chronic obstructive pulmonary disease (COPD) (as in asthma in humans or heaves in horses) may be due in part to bronchopulmonary hypersensitivity to inhaled allergens. Horses suffering from COPD may show posi-tive skin reactions to many fungal extracts (such as *Aspergillus* spp., *Alternaria* spp. and *Cladosporium* spp.) and always have large numbers of eosinophils and high titers of antibody to equine influenza in their bronchial secretions. The significance of the latter finding is not yet clear. There is no correlation between the severity of COPD and circulating levels of mast cell-derived mediators. Removal of clinically affected horses to air-conditioned stalls permits improvement of the disease, but this is reversed if the horses are returned to dusty stables.

Allergies to Vaccines and Drugs

The induction of an IgE response is a potential hazard that may arise from the administration of any antigen, including vaccines, and this factor must be considered in undertaking any vaccination process. In practice, severe problems have been associated with the use of killed foot-and-mouth disease vaccines, rabies vaccines and contagious bovine pleuropneumonia vaccines in cattle.

It is not uncommon for an IgE response to occur following administration of drugs. Most drug molecules are too small to be antigenic, but many can bind to host proteins and then act as haptens. Penicillin allergy, for example, may be produced in animals either through therapeutic exposure or by ingestion of penicillin-contaminated milk. The penicillin molecule is degraded *in vivo* to several compounds, the most important of which contains a penicilloyl epitope. This penicilloyl group can bind to proteins and stimulate the immune system (see Fig. 3–2). In animals sensitized in this way, parenteral administration of penicillin may lead to acute systemic anaphylaxis or milder forms of allergy, whereas feeding of penicillin-contaminated milk to these animals can lead to severe diarrhea.

Allergies to many other drugs, especially antibiotics and hormones, have been reported in the domestic animals. Even substances contained in leather preservatives used in harnesses, in catgut sutures or in compounds such as methyl cellulose or carboxymethylcellulose used as stabilizers in vaccines may provoke local allergic responses.

Allergies to Parasites

The role of the IgE-mast cell-vasoactive amine system in immunity to helminths was first observed in the self-cure phenomenon (Chapter 17). In general, helminths appear to stimulate IgE responses preferentially, and helminth infestations are commonly associated with many of the signs of allergy and anaphylaxis; for example, animals with tapeworms may exhibit signs of respiratory distress or urticaria. Rupture of a hydatid cyst during surgery or transfusion of blood from a dog infected with *Dirofilaria immitis* to a sensitized animal may provoke anaphylaxis.

Allergies are also commonly associated with the response of animals to arthropod parasites. Insect stings account for a significant number of human deaths each year as a result of acute anaphylaxis following sensitization by venom. Anaphylaxis can also occur in cattle infested with the warble fly (*Hypoderma bovis*). The pupae of this fly develop under the skin on the back of cattle after the larvae have migrated through the tissues from the site of egg deposition on the hind leg. Because the pupae are so obvious, it is tempting to remove them manually. Unfortunately, if they rupture during this process, the release of coelomic fluid into the sensitized animal may provoke an anaphylaxis-like response and even kill the animal. The precise role of anaphylaxis in this condition is unclear.

In horses and cattle, hypersensitivity to insect bites may cause an allergic dermatitis known as Queensland itch, Gulf Coast itch or "sweet itch." The flies involved include the midges (*Culicoides* spp.) and the black flies (*Simulium* spp.). If animals are allergic to antigens in the saliva of these insects, biting results in the development of urticaria accompanied by intense itching. The itching may provoke severe self-mutilation with subsequent secondary infection that may mask the original allergic nature of the lesion.

In mange due to *Sarcoptes scabiei* in dogs and to *Octodectes cyanotis* in cats, a type I hypersensitivity may contribute to the development of the lesions. The infested dermis is infiltrated with mast cells, lymphocytes and plasma cells, and an intradermal injection of mite antigen leads to an immediate wheal and flare response. Infested animals may also possess precipitins to mite antigens, and it is possible that immune complexes may also contribute to the development of the lesion.

IgE antibodies may be produced in some animals in response to bee, wasp and hornet stings so that a second sting in a sensitized animal may provoke acute systemic anaphylaxis. The offending allergens include phospholipases, hyaluronidase and several peptides (see Fig. 20–7).

The response of animals to arthropod allergens is not inevitably a type I hypersensitivity. Thus, the reactions to *Demodex* mites and to components of flea saliva are largely mediated by cells (type IV hypersensitivity, Chapter 23).

Laminitis

Laminitis is a syndrome seen in all the hoofed animals. It is etiologically complex and is associated with a wide variety of predisposing causes, but one of the factors that may play a role in some cases of laminitis is type I hypersensitivity. The condition occurs as a result of engorgement of the vascular bed of the laminae of the hoof. This engorgement, occurring in a tissue where there is no room for swelling to occur, leads to intense pain and discomfort. A condition resembling laminitis may be produced in some animals by intravenous histamine, and in affected calves, blood histamine levels may be raised. However, the source of this histamine is not known. It may be derived directly from food or, alternatively, may represent a product of food allergy. In rare cases, antihistamines may be of assistance in treatment.

PREVENTION AND TREATMENT OF TYPE I HYPERSENSITIVITY

In order to prevent type I hypersensitivity reactions, it is essential that the allergen(s) be identified and removed. This may be extremely difficult and tedious. Intradermal skin testing using dilute solutions of a variety of potential antigens may be of assistance. Alternatively (or additionally) in food allergies a change of diet and the readdition of individual components on a test basis may enable the investigator to identify a specific antigen or, more commonly, a group of antigens.

When elimination of the offending allergen is not possible, as, for example, in allergies to pollens, desensitization therapy performed as described previously (see page 287) may prove effective.

Treatment of type I hypersensitivity reactions may be accomplished by means of a number of different drugs. One group comprises the sympathomimetic agents, which act as β adrenoceptor stimulants. These include epinephrine and isoprenaline. Salbutamol is a more selective β stimulant that causes bronchodilation. Sympathomimetics that act as α adrenoceptor inhibitors include methoxamine and phenylephrine. All have been used extensively in humans and are available for use in animals.

Another group of drugs widely employed in the treatment of type I hypersensitivity reactions are the specific pharmacological inhibitors. These drugs, by mimicking the structure of the active mediators, competitively block specific receptors. Thus, antihistamines such as pyrilamine, promethazine and diphenhydramine can effectively inhibit the activities of histamine. However, since histamine is but one of a large number of mast cell-derived mediators, antihistamines possess limited effectiveness in controlling hypersensitivity diseases. The tryptamine antagonist cyproheptadine can block receptors for both serotonin and histamine and may be of assistance in some situations.

Nonsteroidal anti-inflammatory drugs (NSAIDs) such as acetylsalicylic acid and phenylbutazone are antagonists of the leukotrienes and kinins and are widely used in veterinary medicine as anti-inflammatory agents. They may also be useful in the treatment of acute hypersensitivities.

As an alternative to the specific pharmacological agents described above, considerable use is made of corticosteroids as anti-inflammatory drugs. The corticosteroids can suppress all aspects of inflammation by inhibiting cell membrane phospholipases, so blocking the production of prostaglandins and leukotrienes. Corticosteroids have a considerable palliative effect on chronic type I hypersensi-

tivities, but it must be borne in mind that these drugs are immunosuppressive and increase an animal's susceptibility to infection (Chapter 27).

Two other drugs that may be of assistance in the treatment of type I hypersensitivity are disodium cromoglycate, which interferes with the release of histamine and leukotrienes from mast cells, and diethylcarbamazine citrate, an anthelmintic with similar pharmacological properties.

ADDITIONAL SOURCES OF INFORMATION

August JR. 1982. The intradermal test as a diagnostic aid for canine atopic disease. JAVMA 18 164–171.

Austin KF. 1984. The heterogeneity of mast cell populations and products. Hosp. Pract. 19 135–146.

Befus AD, Bienenstock J and Denburg JA. 1985. Mast cell differentiation and heterogeneity. Immunol. Today 6 281–284.

Davis LE. 1984. Hypersensitivity reactions induced by antimicrobial drugs. JAVMA 185 1131–1136.

Eyre P. 1980. Pharmacological aspects of hypersensitivity in domestic animals: a review. Vet. Res. Comm. 4 83–98.

Frick OL and Brooks DL. 1983. Immunoglobulin E antibodies to pollens augmented in dogs by virus vaccines. Am. J. Vet. Res. 44 440–445.

Huntley JF, Newlands G and Miller HRP. 1984. The isolation and characterization of globule leukocytes: their deriviation from mucosal mast cells in parasitized sheep. Parasite Immunol. 6 371–390.

Ishizaka K. 1981. Regulation of the IgE antibody response. Int. Arch. Allergy Appl. Immunol. 66 (suppl 1) 1–7.

Jarrett EE and Haig DM. 1984. Mucosal mast cells in vivo and in vitro. Immunol. Today 5 115–118

Jarrett EE, MacKenzie S and Bennich H. 1980. Parasite-induced "nonspecific" IgE does not protect against allergic reactions. Nature 283 302–303.

Kay AB. 1985. Eosinophils as effector cells in immunity and hypersensitivity disorders. Clin. Exp. Immunol. 62 1–12.

Kuehl FA and Egan RW. 1980. Prostaglandins, arachidonic acid and inflammation. Science 210 978–984.

Marsh DG, Meyers DA and Bias WB. 1981. The epidemiology and genetics of atopic allergy. N. Engl. J. Med. 305 155–159.

Ochoa R, Breitschwerdt EB and Lincoln KL. 1984. Immunoproliferative small intestinal disease in Basenji dogs. Am. J. Vet. Res. 45 482–490.

Peters JE, Hirshman CA and Malley A. 1982. The Basenji-greyhound dog model of asthma: leukocyte histamine release, serum IgE and airway response to inhaled antigen. J. Immunol. 129 1245–1249.

Scott DW. 1981. Observations on canine atopy. J. Amer. Anim. Hosp. Assoc. 17 91–100.

Willemse A, Noordzij A, Rutten PMG and Bernadina WE. 1985. Induction of non-IgE anaphylactic antibodies in dogs. Clin. Exp. Immunol. 59 351–358.

21

Erythrocyte Antigens and Type II Hypersensitivity

Erythrocytes, like nucleated cells, possess characteristic cell-surface antigens. Unlike the histocompatibility antigens, however, erythrocyte surface antigens are not intimately linked to an animal's ability to mount an immune response, although they do influence graft rejection. (Grafts incompatible in the major blood groups are rapidly rejected.)

Except in the case of the M and C antigens of sheep erythrocytes, which are associated with the membrane potassium pump and amino acid transport, respectively, the exact functions of these antigens are unknown. Most erythrocyte surface antigens are either carbohydrate or glycolipid in nature and are integral components of the cell membrane. Exceptions are those antigens that are found free in serum, saliva and other body fluids and are passively adsorbed onto erythrocyte surfaces. Examples of such antigens include the J antigens of cattle, the R antigens of sheep, the A and O antigens of pigs and the Tr antigens of dogs.

If normal erythrocytes are administered to an allogeneic recipient, their surface antigens will stimulate an immune response. This response results in the rapid elimination of the transfused erythrocytes through intravascular hemolysis mediated by antibody and complement and through extravascular destruction occurring as a result of opsonization and clearance by the cells of the mononuclear-phagocytic system. Cell destruction mediated by antibodies in this way is classified as a type II hypersensitivity reaction.

BLOOD GROUPS

The antigens found on the surface of erythrocytes are termed blood group antigens. There are many different blood group antigens on the surface of an animal's red cells, and they vary in their antigenicity, some being more potent and therefore of greater importance than others. Blood group antigens are secondary gene products. The primary gene products are enzymes that act as sugar transferases. It is these enzymes that determine the structure of the blood group antigens. The expression of blood group antigens is therefore genetically controlled. In each blood group system there exists a variable number of alternative alleles or phenogroups. (A phenogroup is a set of alleles inherited in a group of two or more.) As a result, the complexity of the erythrocyte blood group systems may vary greatly. They range from simple systems like the L system of cattle, which consists of two alleles controlling a single alloantigen system, to the highly complex B system. The B system of cattle contains several hundred alleles or phenogroups that, together with the other cattle blood groups, may yield millions of unique blood group combinations.

In addition to possessing blood group antigens on their cells, animals may also possess serum antibodies directed against foreign blood group factors. For example, J-negative cattle commonly carry antibodies to the J factor in their serum, while A-negative pigs can possess anti-A antibodies. These "natural alloantibodies" are thought to be derived not from prior contact with foreign red cells but as a result of exposure to similar or identical epitopes (heterophile antigens) that commonly occur in nature. Many blood group antigens, for example, are common structural components of a wide range of organisms including plants, bacteria, protozoa and helminths. The presence of these natural alloantibodies is not, however, a uniform phenomenon, and not all blood group factors are accompanied by the production of natural alloantibodies to their alternative alleles.

Blood Transfusion and the Consequences of Incompatible Transfusions

Red cells can be readily transfused from one animal to another. If the donor's erythrocytes carry antigens identical to those found on the recipient's erythrocytes, no immune response will result. If, however, the recipient possesses natural alloantibodies to antigens on donor erythrocytes, they will be subject to immediate attack. Natural alloantibodies are usually (but not always) of the IgM isotype. When these antibodies combine with foreign erythrocyte antigens, they may cause agglutination, immune hemolysis, opsonization and phagocytosis of the transfused cells. In the absence of naturally occurring antibodies, allogeneic erythrocytes stimulate an immune response in the recipient. The transfused cells then circulate for a period of time before antibody production takes place and immune elimination occurs. A second transfusion with identical allogeneic cells results in their immediate destruction.

Although the body is able to eliminate small numbers of aged red cells on a continuing basis, the rapid destruction of large numbers of foreign red cells following an incompatible transfusion can lead to the development of severe pathological reactions. The signs of this destructive process are, in general, referable to massive hemolysis. They include tremors, paresis and convulsions, disseminated intravascular coagulation, fever and hemoglobinuria. In some animals dyspnea, coughing and diarrhea may also be observed. Treatment of these transfusion reactions consists of stopping the transfusion and maintaining urine flow with a diuretic, since accumulation of hemoglobin within the kidney may result in renal tubular destruction. Recovery occurs following elimination of all the foreign erythrocytes.

The occurrence of transfusion reactions may be prevented by prior testing of the recipient's serum for antibodies against donor red cells. The test for compatibility is known as crossmatching and is performed by mixing recipient serum with donor erythrocytes. It is usual to obtain serum and washed erythrocytes from both donor and recipient. Donor erythrocytes are mixed with recipient serum, and recipient erythrocytes are mixed with the donor serum and then incubated at 37°C for 30 minutes. If the donor's erythrocytes are lysed or agglutinated by the recipient's serum, then no transfusion should be attempted with those cells. It is occasionally found that the donor's serum may be capable of reacting with the recipient's red cells. This is not of major clinical significance, since donor antibodies given intravenously are rapidly diluted within the recipient. Nevertheless, blood giving such a reaction is best avoided.

HEMOLYTIC DISEASE OF THE NEWBORN

Female animals may become sensitized to allogeneic red cells not only through incompatible blood transfusions given for clinical reasons but also through leakage of fetal erythrocytes into the maternal blood stream by way of the placenta. In animals sensitized by either of these routes, antibodies to the allogeneic erythrocytes are concentrated in colostrum. On ingestion by the newborn animal, these colostral antibodies are absorbed through the intestinal wall and so reach the circulation. If the absorbed antibodies are directed against antigens present on the erythrocytes of the newborn animal, then these erythrocytes will be rapidly destroyed. The disease arising from this massive erythrocyte destruction occurs in many of the domestic animal species as well as in humans and is known as hemolytic disease of the newborn.

Blood Groups, Blood Transfusion and Hemolytic Disease in the Domestic Animals (Table 21–1)

Cattle

Cattle possess eleven blood group systems: A, B, C, F, J, L, M, S, T, Z and R', of which two (B and J) are of the greatest importance.

The B blood group system of cattle is one of the most complex systems known; it is estimated to contain more than sixty different antigens. Blocks of these antigens tend to be inherited together as phenogroups. Because of this complexity, it is generally impossible to obtain bovine blood from a donor animal that is absolutely identical to that of the recipient. Indeed, it has been suggested that the complexity of the B system is such that there exist sufficient different antigenic combinations to provide a unique identifying character for each bovine in the world. Naturally, such a system provides an ideal method for the accurate identification of individual animals, and many breed societies utilize blood grouping as a check on the identity of registered animals.

The J antigen is a lipid that is found free in body fluids and is passively adsorbed onto erythrocytes. Therefore, it is not a true red cell antigen. It is absent from the erythrocytes of newborn calves but is acquired within the first six months of life. J-positive cattle are of two types. Some possess J antigen in high concentration, and this may be detected both on their erythrocytes and in serum. Other J-positive animals possess low levels of this antigen, which is only with great difficulty detected on erythrocytes. J-negative cattle, lacking the J antigen completely, may possess natural anti-J antibodies, although the level of these antibodies shows a marked seasonal variation, being highest in the summer and fall. Because of the presence of these antibodies, transfusion of J-positive erythrocytes into J-negative recipients may result in a transfusion reaction even in the absence of known prior sensitization.

Hemolytic disease of newborn calves is rare

Table 21–1 DOMESTIC ANIMAL BLOOD GROUPS

Species	Blood Group Systems	Serology
Bovine	A, B, C, F, J,* L, M, R', S, T, Z	Hemolytic
Sheep	A, B, C, D, M, R,* X	Hemolytic, Agglutinating (D only)
Pig	A,* B, C, D, E, F, G, H, I, J, K, L, M, N, O	Agglutinating, Hemolytic, Antiglobulin
Horse	A, C, D, K, P, Q, U	Agglutinating, Hemolytic
Dog	A, B, C, D, F, J, K, L, M, N, Tr*	Agglutinating, Hemolytic, Antiglobulin
Cat	AB	Agglutinating, Hemolytic

*Soluble blood group substances.

but may occur as a result of vaccinating calves against anaplasmosis or babesiosis. These vaccines consist of blood derived from infected calves. In the case of anaplasma vaccines, the blood from a large number of donor animals is pooled, freeze-dried and then mixed with adjuvant before being administered to cattle. The vaccine against babesiosis consists of relatively fresh, infected calf blood. Both vaccines result in infection and, consequently, the development of premunity (Chapter 17) in the recipient animals. They also cause the production of anti-erythrocyte alloantibodies directed primarily against antigens of the A and F systems. Cows sensitized to erythrocyte antigens by these vaccines and then mated with bulls carrying the same blood groups can transmit colostral alloantibodies to their calves, which may then develop a hemolytic disease.

The clinical signs of hemolytic disease in calves vary with the amount of colostrum ingested. Calves are usually healthy at birth but commence to show symptoms from 12 hours to five days afterward. In acute cases, death may occur within 24 hours after birth, with the animals developing respiratory distress and hemoglobinuria. On necropsy they are found to have severe pulmonary edema, splenomegaly and dark kidneys. Less severely affected animals develop anemia and jaundice and may die during the first week of life. The erythrocytes of affected calves are antiglobulin-positive and may sometimes be lysed by the addition of hemolytic complement (fresh, normal rabbit serum). Death is due to disseminated intravascular coagulation (DIC) as a result of activation of the clotting system by erythrocyte ghosts.

Serological Testing. Bovine blood groups are detected by a hemolytic test. The red cells are incubated in specific antisera and rabbit serum is used as a source of complement.

Sheep

The blood groups of sheep resemble those of cattle. Sheep have seven blood groups: A, B, C, D, M, R and X. The ovine equivalent of the bovine B system is also termed B and, like the bovine system, is relatively complex,

containing at least 52 different alleles. Sheep also possess an equivalent of the bovine J system, which is known as the R system. Two blood group antigens are found in this system, R and O, coded for by alleles R and r. The production of R and O substances is controlled by a gene called I and its recessive allele i. If a sheep is homozygous for i, it will possess neither R nor O antigens. This interaction between the I/i genes and the RO system is known as an epistatic effect (Fig. 21–1). A similar effect is seen in the A-O system of pigs (Example 1). R and O antigens are soluble substances found free in the serum of II or Ii sheep and are passively adsorbed to erythrocytes. Erythrocytes from ii sheep may acquire R or O by incubation in appropriate serum. Natural anti-R antibodies may be found in R-negative sheep. Sheep fall into two groups, according to whether their red cells have high or low potassium levels. This is regulated by the M blood group system.

Sheep erythrocytes are commonly used as a tool in immunological research, since they are a very economical source of antigen. Antibodies against these cells produced in species other than sheep tend to be directed mainly against sheep-specific antigens. Some of these species antigens are also heterophile, that is, they are found in a wide variety of different organisms, particularly bacteria. Consequently, "natural" antibodies to sheep erythrocytes are found in the serum of many normal animals. These heterophile antigens include the M antigen and the Forssman antigen. Antibodies against the M antigen are elevated in the viral infection of humans known as infectious mononucleosis. The Forssman antigen is a glycolipid common to the erythrocytes of many mammals, including horses, dogs, cats and mice; it is absent in humans, cattle, pigs, rabbits and rats.

Serological Testing. Ovine blood groups are detected by hemolytic tests. The only exception to this rule is the D system, which is detected by agglutination.

Pigs

Fifteen pig blood group systems have been identified. They are identified by the letters

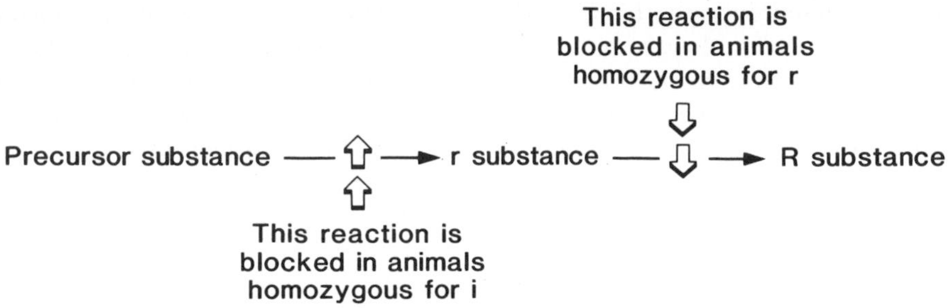

This reaction is blocked in animals homozygous for r

⇩

Precursor substance —— ⇧ ——▶ r substance —— ⇧/⇩ ——▶ R substance

⇧

This reaction is blocked in animals homozygous for i

Figure 21–1. The regulation of the expression of R blood group antigens in sheep. Animals homozygous for i will have neither R nor O blood group antigens. Animals homozygous for r will possess blood group O. Only animals that possess both I and R genes will possess blood group R.

from A to O. Of these, the most important is the A system. The A system contains two factors A and O. Their expression is controlled by a gene called S (secretor). In the homozygous recessive state (ss) this gene can prevent the production of the A and O substances. As a result, the amount of these antigens bound to red cells in these animals is reduced to an undetectable level (see Example 1). A and O,

like J in cattle and R and O in sheep, are soluble antigens found in serum and passively adsorbed onto red cells after birth. Natural anti-A antibodies may occur in A-negative pigs, and transfusion of A-positive blood into such an animal may cause transient collapse and hemoglobinuria.

Hemolytic disease of the newborn in piglets used to occur as a result of the use of hog

---

Example 1. The Inheritance of the A Blood Group System in Pigs

In pigs, the expression of the A blood groups is under the control of two loci. One, the A locus, contains two alleles, A and O, of which A is dominant. The other, the S locus, also contains two alleles, S and its recessive allele s. The S locus controls the expression of the A system so that A or O blood group factors will only be expressed if the animal carries at least one S gene.

Possible genotypes are therefore

AA   AO   OO   and SS, Ss and ss

These may be combined thus

Animals that are   AASS ⎫
                  AASs ⎪
                  AOSS ⎬ will all have A red cells
                  AOSs ⎭

Animals that are   OOSS ⎫ will all have O red cells
        or   OOSs ⎭

Animals that are   AAss ⎫
                  AOss ⎬ will have neither A nor O red cells i.e., − red cells
                  OOss ⎭

If we cross an animal of blood group O whose genotype is OOSs with an animal of blood group − whose genotype is AOss, then the offspring may be either

AOSs   with blood group A
OOSs   with blood group O
AOss ⎫
OOss ⎭ with blood group −

cholera vaccine containing pig blood. This vaccine consisted of pooled blood from viremic pigs inactivated with the dye crystal violet. Sensitization of sows by means of this vaccine led to the occasional occurrence of hemolytic disease of their offspring. There appeared to be a breed predisposition to this disease, which was most commonly seen in the offspring of Essex and Wessex sows. Affected piglets did not necessarily show clinical disease, although their red cells were shown to be sensitized by antibody. Other piglets showed rapidly progressive weakness and pallor of mucous membranes preceding death, and those animals that survived longest showed hemoglobinuria and jaundice. The severity of the reaction did not appear to be directly related to the anti-erythrocyte antibody titer in the piglet serum. Since the withdrawal of all live hog cholera virus vaccines, the problems associated with their use have disappeared.

True alloimmunization of pregnancy has also been recorded in the pig. The alloantibodies responsible are usually directed against antigens of the E system. In addition to the development of hemolytic anemia in newborn piglets, the presence of antibodies to platelet antigens may result in the development of thrombocytopenia, reflected clinically as a bleeding problem on tail docking and a tendency to bruise easily (neonatal purpura). On blood smears, the platelets may be clumped, and an antiglobulin test on them will be positive. Deprivation of colostrum in an attempt to prevent piglets from absorbing antierythrocyte antibodies may lead to difficulties because the newborn colostrum-deprived animals lack resistance to infection.

Serological Testing. Pig blood groups are detected by agglutination, hemolytic and antiglobulin tests. Each type of test is characteristic of certain blood groups.

Horses

Horses possess seven internationally recognized blood group systems: A, C, D, K, P, Q and U. There are other systems that are not officially recognized. The major clinical significance of equine blood groups lies in the fact that hemolytic disease of the newborn foal is not uncommon. In mules, in which the antigenic differences between dam and sire are great, about 8 to 10 per cent of foals may be affected. In thoroughbreds the prevalence is considerably less, ranging from 0.05 to 1 per cent of foals. This is in spite of the fact that in up to 25 per cent of pregnancies the mare and the stallion are incompatible.

The mechanism of alloimmunization is unclear, but fetal erythrocytes are assumed to gain access to the maternal circulation throughout pregnancy (Fig. 21–2). Mares have been shown to respond to fetal erythrocytes as early as day 56 postconception. The greatest leakage probably occurs during the last month of pregnancy and during parturition, as a result of breakdown of placental blood vessels. Necrotic foci are found in many equine placentas after birth.

The major sensitizing blood group antigen is Aa, followed (in decreasing order of importance) by Qa, R and S. (Factors R and S belong to the Q system.) The degree of maternal sensitization is usually relatively weak following a first pregnancy. However, if repeated pregnancies result in exposure to the same erythrocyte antigens, then the mare's response will be stimulated considerably. Hemolytic disease is therefore usually only a problem in mares that have had several foals.

The antibodies produced by the mare do not cross the placenta; instead, they reach the foal by way of the colostrum. Affected foals are, therefore, born healthy but begin to sicken several hours after birth. The most potent antibodies formed are those directed against Aa, and disease due to these antibodies may develop within 12 hours. Anti-Qa antibodies produce a less severe disease of slower onset, and disease due to anti-R or anti-S antibodies is milder still. The earliest signs are those of weakness and depression. The mucous membranes of affected foals may be pale and may eventually show a distinct jaundice, and hemoglobinuria may be present. Some foals sicken and die so rapidly that they do not have time to develop jaundice.

Hemolytic disease is readily diagnosed by clinical signs alone. Hematological examination is of little diagnostic use but may be of assistance in assessing appropriate treatment. Definitive diagnosis requires that immunoglobulin be demonstrated on the surface of the red cells of the foal. In the case of anti-Aa or anti-Qa antibodies, addition of a source of complement (fresh, normal rabbit serum) will cause rapid hemolysis. Since factors R and S are not as antigenic as Aa and Qa, antibodies to them can be detected *in vivo* only by means of a direct antiglobulin test involving an anti-equine globulin serum (Chapter 11). If hemolytic disease is anticipated, it is possible to test the serum of a pregnant mare for antibodies by means of an indirect antiglobulin test. By using erythrocytes from a horse with a major sensitizing blood group it is possible to show that the antibody titer may increase significantly in the month prior to parturition if sensitization is occurring. Testing of the foal's erythrocytes against the mare's colostrum is of limited usefulness because of the tendency of colostrum to induce rouleaux formation, which mimics agglutination.

The prognosis of hemolytic disease is good provided the condition is diagnosed sufficiently early and the appropriate treatment instituted rapidly. In acute cases, blood transfusion is necessary. Although exchange transfusion is efficient, it requires a donor capable of providing at least 5 liters of blood as well as a double intravenous catheter and an anesthetized foal. A much simpler technique is to transfuse washed cells from the mare. About 3 to 4 liters of blood are collected in sodium citrate and centrifuged, and the plasma is discarded. The red cells are washed once in saline and transfused slowly into the foal. The blood is usually given in divided doses about six hours apart. Milder cases of hemolytic disease may require only careful nursing.

If hemolytic disease is anticipated as a result of either a rising antibody titer or the previous birth of a hemolytic foal, it may be prevented by stripping off the mare's colostrum and giving the foal colostrum from another mare. The foal should not be allowed to suckle its mare for 24 to 36 hours. Once suckling is permitted, the foal should only be allowed to take small quantities at first and should be observed carefully for any adverse side effects.

Serological Testing. Horse blood groups may be identified by means of agglutination, hemolytic and antiglobulin tests. As in the pig, each blood group system has a preferred test system. The complement used in the hemolytic test comes from rabbits but it must be absorbed before use in order to remove any anti-horse antibodies.

Dogs

In dogs at least eleven blood group systems exist: A, Tr, B, C, D, F, J, K, L, M and N. Only one of these, the A system, is sufficiently

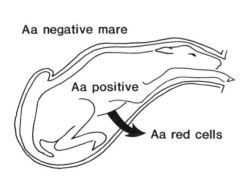

Aa negative mare

Aa positive

Aa red cells

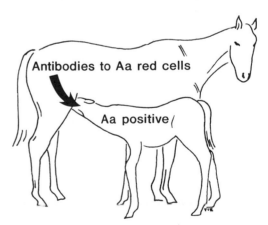

Antibodies to Aa red cells

Aa positive

Erythrocyte destruction following colostrum consumption

Figure 21–2. The pathogenesis of hemolytic disease of the newborn in foals. In the first stage, fetal lymphocytes leak into the maternal circulation and sensitize her. In the second stage, these antibodies are concentrated in colostrum and are then ingested by the suckling foal. These ingested antibodies enter the foal's circulation and cause erythrocyte destruction.

strong to be of clinical significance. About 60 per cent of dogs are A-positive; the remainder are A-negative. Naturally occurring antibodies to A occur in about 10 per cent of A-negative dogs, but these are usually of low titer and not of clinical significance. Therefore, unmatched first transfusions in the dog are usually safe. If, however, an A-negative dog is sensitized by transfusion of A-positive blood, high titered anti-A antibodies may be produced. Subsequent transfusion of A-positive blood into such an animal could lead to a severe reaction. Similarly, if a bitch is sensitized by incompatible transfusions, hemolytic disease may occur in her pups if she is mated to an A-positive dog. Natural hemolytic disease of the newborn in dogs is extremely rare. The Tr system is a soluble antigen system similar to the sheep R and pig O systems. Its expression is controlled by an epistatic gene.

Serological Testing. Agglutination at 4°C, and hemolytic and antiglobulin tests have all been used for the detection of canine blood groups. The source of complement can be either fresh dog serum or fresh rabbit serum.

Cats

In cats only one major blood group system, the AB system, has been reported. Cats may be either A, B or AB. About 75 to 95 per cent of cats are A-positive, about 5 to 25 per cent are B-positive and less than 1 per cent are AB. Severe transfusion reactions have been described in group B cats that received only very small quantities of group A blood, since most B cats possess anti-A antibodies. (Interestingly, very few A cats possess anti-B antibodies.) Thus a group B cat given as little as 1 ml of group A blood will go into shock hypotension, apnea and AV block within a few minutes. Cross-matching, therefore, is essential in this species. The A antigen is found on cat lymphocytes, but the B antigen is not. Hemolytic disease of the newborn has been recorded in cats but is very rare. Affected kittens suffered from severe anemia and intravascular hemolysis, and antibodies to the sire's red cells were present in the queen's serum.

Serological Testing. Agglutination and hemolytic tests are used for feline blood typing.

Chickens

Chickens are similar to mammals with respect to possessing blood group systems. They have at least twelve different blood group systems with multiple alleles. The erythrocyte B system is also the major histocompatibility system in the chicken. A hemolytic disease may be artificially produced in chicken embryos by vaccinating the hen with cock erythrocytes.

Hemolytic Disease of the Newborn in Man

In humans, hemolytic disease of the newborn is due almost entirely to alloimmunization against the antigens of the Rhesus (Rh) system. The condition is, or should be, of historical interest only, since a very simple but effective technique is available for its prevention.

The prevention of hemolytic disease in humans depends on preventing an Rh-negative mother from reacting to the Rh-positive fetal red cells that escape from the placenta into her circulation at parturition. Strong human anti-Rh globulin is obtained from male volunteers and given to mothers at risk soon after birth. It acts, just as other systems of passive immunization do, by specifically inhibiting the immune response to that antigen. Routine use of this material will therefore prevent maternal sensitization, antibody production and hemolytic disease.

Detection of Freemartins

In about 90 per cent of dizygotic bovine twins, anastomosis of placental blood vessels occurs *in utero*, and, as a result, the erythrocytes of these animals become indiscriminately mixed. Mixing of hematopoietic stem cells also occurs, and, consequently, each calf will carry erythrocytes of its twin's phenotype for the rest of its life. A calf carrying this cell mixture is known as a chimera (Chapter 13). Although no adverse consequences arise from this cell mixing and subsequent tolerance, problems may occur if the calves are of different sexes. In particular, the transfusion of male hormones to the female calf *in utero* may result in dysgenesis of the female reproductive tract. Externally, some of these female calves appear to be quite normal; however, on reaching reproductive age they are found to be infertile and are known as freemartins. It is obviously desirable for a farmer to be able to identify a freemartin as early as possible in life so that it does not have to be maintained for over a year before its infertility is recognized. For this reason, tests have been developed in order to identify chimeras. One way this can be done is to test the erythrocytes of an animal in order to determine whether they are homogeneous or composed of a mixture of cells of different blood groups. The technique is known as differential hemolysis. Thus, antibodies and complement acting against blood group antigens present on only a portion of the red cell population will never be able to cause more than partial hemolysis of the blood, whereas if the antigens are present on all cells, total hemolysis will result. By using a battery of different antisera for testing, it is usually possible to determine whether the red cell population is homogeneous or comprises two antigenically different populations. If the latter is the case, then the animal is a chimera, and if it is also a female calf born with a male twin, then it is also likely to be a freemartin.

Parentage Testing

Under some circumstances it is necessary to confirm the parentage of an animal. This may be accomplished by examining the erythrocyte antigens of an animal and its alleged parents (Example 2). This method is based on the principle that since blood group factors are inherited, they must be present on the erythrocytes of one or both parents. If a blood group factor is present in a tested animal but absent from both its putative parents, then parentage must be reassigned. Similarly, if one parent is known to be homozygous for a particular blood group factor, then this factor must also appear in the offspring. It must be recognized, however, that blood tests can only exclude parentage, never prove parentage.

Type II Hypersensitivity Reactions to Drugs

Red cells may be destroyed in drug hypersensitivities by three mechanisms. First, the drug and antibody may combine directly and activate complement; red cells will be destroyed in a bystander effect as activated complement components bind to nearby cells.

Second, some drugs may bind firmly to cells, especially those in the blood. For example, penicillin, quinine, L-dopa, aminosalicylic acid and phenacetin may adsorb onto the surface of erythrocytes. Since these cells are then modified, they may be recognized as foreign and eliminated by an immune response, resulting in the occurrence of hemolytic anemia. Sulfonamides, phenylbutazone, aminopyrine, phenathiazine and possibly chloramphenicol may cause agranulocytosis by binding to granulocytes, and phenylbutazone, quinine, apronalide (Sedormid), chloramphenicol and sulfonamides may provoke thrombocytopenia. If the cells from animals suffering

Example 2. The Use of Blood Groups in the Identification of Paternity. In this case, the technique was used to identify the sire of a litter of pups. (Courtesy of Mr. D. Colling.)

	Erythrocyte Groups				
	A_1	A_2	J	N	O
Putative sire 1	+	+	−	+	−
Putative sire 2	+	+	−	−	+
Dam	−	−	+	+	−
Puppy 1	+	+	−	−	−
2	+	+	−	+	−
3*	−	−	−	+	+
4	−	−	+	+	−

*Since Puppy No. 3 possesses O antigen, it cannot be derived from Sire No. 1.

from these reactions are examined by means of a direct antiglobulin test, antibody may be demonstrated on their surface. If these antibodies are eluted, they can be shown to be directed not against the blood cells but against the offending drug.

Third, drugs such as the cephalosporins may modify red cell membranes in such a way that the cells passively adsorb antibodies and are then removed by phagocytic cells.

Type II Hypersensitivity in Infectious Diseases

Just as drugs can adsorb to erythrocytes and render them immunologically foreign, so also can bacterial antigens such as the *Salmonella* lipopolysaccharides, viruses such as equine infectious anemia virus and Aleutian disease virus, rickettsia such as *Anaplasma* and protozoa such as the trypanosomes and *Babesia*. These altered red cells, being regarded as foreign, are either lysed by antibody and hemolytic complement or phagocytosed by mononuclear phagocytes. Clinically severe anemia is, therefore, characteristic of all these infections.

ADDITIONAL SOURCES OF INFORMATION

Animal Genetics is a journal that covers the most recent developments in the areas of animal blood groups and histocompatibility antigens. This journal was originally called Animal Blood Groups and Biochemical Genetics.

Auer L, Bell K and Coates S. 1982. Blood transfusion reactions in the cat. JAVMA 180, 729–730.

Bailey E. 1982. Prevalence of anti-red blood cell antibodies in the serum and colostrum of mares and its relationship to neonatal isoerythrolysis. Am. J. Vet. Res. 43 1917–1921.

Becht JL. 1983. Neonatal isoerythrolysis in the foal. Part 1. Background, bloodgroup antigens and pathogenesis. Comp. Cont. Ed. Pract. Vet. 5 591–599.

Bell K. 1983. The blood groups of domestic mammals. *In* Agar NS and Board PG. (eds.) Red Blood Cells of Domestic Mammals. Amsterdam, Elsevier Science Publishers, pp 133–164.

Cain GR and Suzuki Y. 1985. Presumptive neonatal isoerythrolysis in cats. JAVMA 187 46–48.

Colling DT and Saison R. 1980. Canine blood groups. I. Description of new erythrocyte specificities. Anim Blood Groups Biochem. Genet. 11 1–12.

Dimmock CK, Webster WR, Shiels IA and Edwards CL. 1982. Isoimmune thrombocytopenic purpura in piglets. Aust. Vet. J. 59 157–159.

Kallfelz FA, Whitlock RH and Schultz RD. 1978. Survival of ^{59}Fe-labeled erythrocytes in cross-transfused equine blood. Am. J. Vet. Res. 39 617–620.

Killingsworth, CR. 1984. Use of blood and blood components for feline and canine patients. JAVMA 185 1452–1454.

Linklater K. 1977. Post-transfusion purpura in a pig. Res. Vet. Sci. 22 257–258.

Pichler ME and Turnwald GH. 1985. Blood transfusions in the dog and cat: Part I. Physiology, Collection, Storage, and indications for whole blood therapy. Part II. Administration Adverse Effects and Component Therapy. Comp. Cont. Ed. Pract. Vet. 7:64–71, 115–122.

Scott AM and Jeffcott LB. 1978. Hemolytic disease of the newborn foal. Vet. Rec. 103 71–74.

Stormont C. 1977. The etiology of bovine neonatal isoerythrolysis. Bovine Pract. 12 22–27.

Symons R and Bell K. 1985. The occurrence of feline A blood group antigens on lymphocytes. Ani. Blood Groups Biochem. Genet. 16 77–84.

Wagner R, Oulevey J and Thiele OW. 1984. The transfer of bovine J blood group activity to erythrocytes: evidence of a transferable and of a non-transferable J in serum. Anim. Blood Groups Biochem. Genet. 15 223–225.

22

Type III Hypersensitivity: Pathological Consequences of Immune Complex Deposition

The formation of immune complexes through the combination of antibody with antigen is the initiating step in a number of biological processes. One of the most significant of these processes is the complement cascade. When complement-activating immune complexes are deposited in tissues, the subsequent generation of chemotactic factors leads to a local accumulation of neutrophils. These neutrophils release hydrolytic enzymes normally contained within their granules, and these enzymes, in turn, cause tissue destruction. Lesions generated in this way are classified as type III or immune complex-mediated hypersensitivity reactions.

CLASSIFICATION OF TYPE III HYPERSENSITIVITY REACTIONS

The site, severity and significance of type III hypersensitivity reactions depends, as might be expected, upon the amount and site of deposition of immune complexes. Two major forms of reaction are recognized. One form is a local reaction, which occurs when antigen and, hence, immune complexes are deposited locally within tissues. Local type III reactions may be induced in any tissue to which antigen can gain access.

The second form of type III hypersensitivity reaction results from the formation of large quantities of immune complexes within the circulation. This can occur, for example, when antigen is administered intravenously to a hyperimmune recipient. Complexes generated in this way are deposited in the walls of blood vessels. Local activation of complement then leads to neutrophil accumulation and the development of a vasculitis. Circulating immune complexes are also deposited within glomeruli; therefore, the occurrence of a glomerulonephritis is also characteristic of this type of hypersensitivity. If the complexes bind to blood cells, anemia, agranulocytosis or thrombocytopenia may also occur.

It might reasonably be pointed out that the combination of antigen with antibody inevitably results in the generation of immune complexes. It seems, however, that the occurrence of clinically significant type III hypersensitivity reactions is related to the formation of very large amounts of immune complexes. For instance, several grams of antigen may be needed to sensitize an animal such as a rabbit in order to produce experimental type III reactions. It is also apparent that minor immune complex-mediated lesions arise relatively frequently following the normal immune responses to many antigens without giving rise to clinically significant disease.

Local Type III Hypersensitivity Reactions

If antigen is injected subcutaneously into an animal that possesses circulating antibody capable of precipitating that antigen, then an acute inflammatory reaction will develop within several hours at the site of injection. This reaction is called an Arthus reaction after the scientist who first described it. The reaction starts as an erythematous, edematous swelling; eventually local hemorrhage and thrombosis occur and, if severe, culminate in necrosis.

Histologically, the first changes observed following antigen injection are neutrophil adherence to vascular endothelium, followed by emigration through the walls of small blood vessels, especially venules. By six to eight hours, when the reaction has reached its great-

est intensity, the injection site is densely infiltrated by very large numbers of these cells (Fig. 22–1). As the reaction progresses, severe destruction of blood vessel walls occurs, resulting in hemorrhage and edema. Platelet aggregation and thrombosis are also associated with this vascular destruction. By eight hours, mononuclear cells may be observed within the lesion, and by 24 hours or later, depending on the amount of antigen injected, they become the predominant cell type. Eosinophil infiltration is not a significant feature of this type of hypersensitivity.

The fate of the injected antigen may be followed using a direct fluorescent antibody test. It can be shown that antigen diffuses away from the injection site through tissue spaces. When small blood vessels are encountered, the antigen will diffuse into the vessel walls, where it comes into contact with circulating antibody. Consequently, immune complexes are generated and deposited between and beneath vascular endothelial cells. If these immune complexes activate complement, then neutrophil chemotaxis and accumulation follow (Fig. 22–2).

Neutrophils are attracted by C5a and C567, both products of the complement cascade. Because the neutrophils have C3b receptors they will adhere to immune complexes containing this component and promptly phagocytose them. Eventually, the immune complexes are eliminated. During this process, however, large quantities of neutrophil hydrolytic enzymes are released into the tissues. These enzymes mediate the tissue damage seen in the Arthus reaction.

Neutrophil hydrolytic enzymes are normally stored within the primary and secondary granules. The enzymes may be released into tissues through a number of processes, the most obvious of which is cell death; however, other release mechanisms are probably of greater importance in the Arthus reaction. For example, when neutrophils attempt to phagocytose immune complexes attached to a structure that is not phagocytosable, such as a basement membrane, they secrete their granule contents directly into the surrounding tissues. Neutrophils may also release their enzymes into the phagosome before the im-

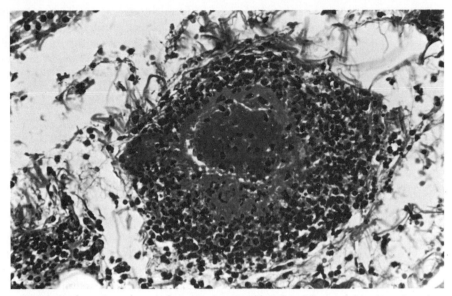

Figure 22–1. Histological section of an Arthus reaction in rabbit skin. The vessel is thrombosed, and fibrinoid material is deposited in its wall. Neutrophil infiltration is extensive. (From Thomson R. G. 1978. General Veterinary Pathology. WB Saunders Company, Philadelphia. Courtesy of Dr. Thomson.)

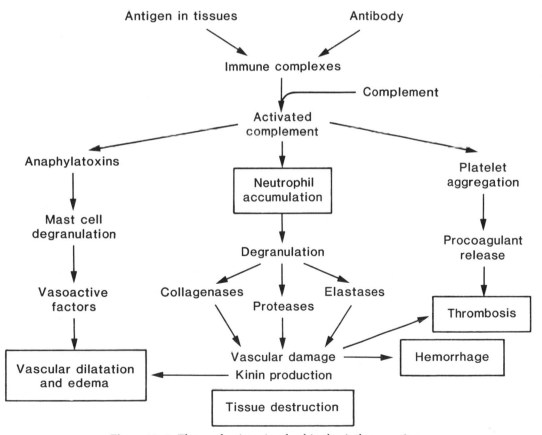

Figure 22–2. The mechanisms involved in the Arthus reaction.

mune complexes are completely enclosed. As a result, the enzymes escape into the surrounding tissues.

The enzymes released by neutrophils in this way include collagenases that disrupt collagen fibers, neutral proteases that destroy ground substances and basement membranes and elastases that destroy elastic tissue. Other enzymes released by neutrophils may degranulate mast cells or generate kinins, prostanoids and reactive oxygen metabolites. As a result of this enzyme release, destruction of tissues, especially blood vessel walls, occurs, resulting in the development of the edema, vasculitis and hemorrhage characteristic of the Arthus reaction.

In addition to causing neutrophil accumulation, complement activated by immune complexes may also make platelets clump and release procoagulants (Chapter 10). This, in conjunction with the severe vascular damage, may result in extensive thrombosis. Finally, the production of anaphylatoxins (C3a and C5a) and the C2 kinin as well as the release of kininogens from neutrophils and vasoactive amines from neutrophils, platelets and mast cells all contribute to the development of a severe local inflammatory response.

The antibodies involved in the Arthus reaction must be both precipitating and complement-activating and are therefore usually of the IgG isotype. Some studies have suggested that horse antibodies are relatively poor in provoking this reaction and give a considerably less severe response than an equivalent amount of rabbit antibody.

Although the "classic" direct Arthus reaction is produced by local administration of antigen to hyperimmunized animals, any technique that permits immune complexes to be deposited in tissues will stimulate a similar response. A "reversed" Arthus reaction can therefore be produced if antibody is administered intradermally to an animal with a high level of circulating antigen. Injected preformed immune complexes, particularly those containing a moderate excess of antigen, will provoke a similar reaction, although, as might be anticipated, there is less involvement of blood vessel walls and the reaction is less severe. A "passive" Arthus reaction can be produced by giving antibody intravenously to a nonsensitized animal followed by an intradermal injection of antigen, and real enthusiasts can produce a "reversed passive" Arthus reaction by giving antibody intradermally followed by intravenous antigen.

Naturally Occurring Local Type III Hypersensitivity Reactions

As mentioned previously, it is unusual for hypersensitivity reactions of only a single type to occur under natural conditions. Nevertheless, there exist a number of relatively common hypersensitivities in the domestic animals in which type III reactions play a major role. The classic Arthus reaction is usually produced in the skin, since that is the most convenient site in which to administer the antigen. Local reactions of this type can, however, occur in many tissues, the precise site depending upon the location of antigen.

Blue-Eye

Blue-eye is a condition seen in a small proportion of dogs that have been either infected or vaccinated with live canine adenovirus type 1 (see Figs. 16–6 and 16–7). The lesion in blue-eye is an anterior uveitis, leading to corneal edema and opacity. The cornea is infiltrated by neutrophils, and, by means of immunofluorescence, virus-antibody complexes may be detected in the lesion. Blue-eye develops around one to three weeks after the onset of infection and usually resolves spontaneously as virus is eliminated.

Hypersensitivity Pneumonitis

Local type III hypersensitivity reactions may occur in the lungs when highly sensitized animals inhale antigen. For example, cattle housed during the winter are usually exposed to dust from hay. Normally, these dust particles are relatively large and are deposited in the upper respiratory tract, trapped in mucus and eliminated. However, if hay is stored when damp, bacterial growth and metabolism will result in heating. This warmth allows thermophilic actinomycetes to grow. One of the most important of these thermophilic actinomycetes is *Micropolyspora faeni*, an organism that produces very large quantities of extremely small spores (1 μm in diameter). On inhalation, these spores can penetrate as far as the alveoli. If cattle are fed moldy hay for long periods, constant inhalation of *M. faeni* spores will result in sensitization and in the development of high titered precipitating antibodies to *M. faeni* antigens in serum. Eventually, inhaled spore antigen may encounter antibody within the alveolar walls, and the resulting immune complex formation and complement activation may result in the development of an interstitial pneumonia, the basis of which is a type III hypersensitivity reaction.

The lesion of this "hypersensitivity pneumonitis" consists of an acute alveolitis together with some vasculitis and exudation of fluid into the alveolar spaces (Fig. 22–3). The alveolar septa may be thickened, and the entire lesion is infiltrated with inflammatory cells. Since many of these cells are eosinophils and lymphocytes, it is obvious that the reaction is not a pure type III reaction. Nevertheless, examination of the lungs of affected cattle by immunofluorescence demonstrates the presence of deposits of immunoglobulin, complement and antigen. In animals exposed to low levels of antigen over a long period of time, a proliferative bronchiolitis and fibrosis may be observed. Clinically, hypersensitivity pneumonitis presents as a pneumonitis occurring between 5 and 10 hours after exposure to grossly moldy hay. The animal may be severely dyspneic and may cough repeatedly. In chronically affected animals dyspnea may be continuous. The most effective method of treating this condition is by removing the source of antigen. The administration of steroids may also be beneficial.

A hypersensitivity pneumonitis due to exposure to *M. faeni* spores also occurs in farmers chronically exposed to dust from moldy hay and is known as farmer's lung. Many other syndromes in man have an identical pathogenesis and are usually named after the source of the offending antigen. Thus pigeon breeder's lung arises following exposure to the dust from pigeon feces, mushroom grower's disease is due to hypersensitivity to inhaled spores from actinomycetes in the soil used for growing mushrooms and librarian's lung results from inhalation of dust from old books! Heaves in

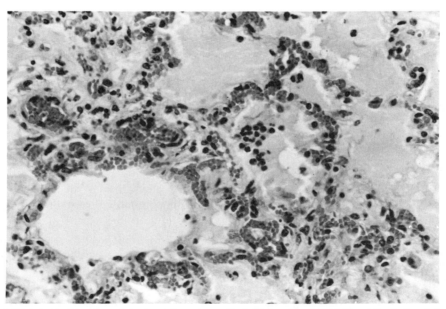

Figure 22–3. Histological section of the lung from a cow that died suddenly 24 hours after being fed moldy hay. The acute alveolitis is probably due to a hypersensitivity reaction to inhaled actinomycete spores. × 400. (Courtesy of Dr. B. N. Wilkie.)

horses (chronic obstructive pulmonary disease) is a pneumonitis of complex origin involving both type I and type III hypersensitivities (see page 294). The offending antigens in this case are probably derived from molds in dusty hay. Hay sickness is a form of hypersensitivity pneumonitis seen in horses in Iceland that is probably an equine equivalent of farmer's lung.

Although hypersensitivity pneumonitis as a distinct syndrome occurs in response to inhaled antigens, it should be remembered that the immune response to pneumonia-causing micro-organisms such as *Pasteurella* may also contribute to the development of pathological lesions through a similar mechanism.

Staphylococcal Hypersensitivity

Staphylococcal hypersensitivity is a pruritic pustular dermatitis of dogs. Skin testing with staphylococcal antigens suggests that type III hypersensitivity may be involved, as do the histological findings of neutrophilic dermal vasculitis. It may be treated with antibiotics.

Generalized Type III Hypersensitivity Reactions

If antigen is administered intravenously to animals with a pre-existing high level of circulating antibodies, then immune complexes form within the circulation. Most of these complexes, especially the large ones, are removed by the cells of the mononuclear-phagocytic system. However, some complexes, particularly those formed with excess antigen, are soluble and hence poorly phagocytosed. In addition, alternate pathway complement components are capable of inserting themselves into and solubilizing large immune complexes. These soluble complexes may activate complement and stimulate platelet aggregation and release of vasoactive amines, thus increasing the permeability of the vascular endothelium. Consequently, immune complexes may be deposited in the walls of blood vessels, especially medium-sized arteries and in vessels where there is physiological effusion of fluid—for example, glomeruli, synovia and the choroid plexus (Fig. 22–4).

Acute Serum Sickness

Many years ago, when the use of antisera for passive immunization was in its infancy, it was observed that individuals who had received a very large single dose of equine anti-tetanus serum developed characteristic side effects about 10 days later. These side effects consisted of a generalized vasculitis with erythema, edema and urticaria of the skin, neutropenia, lymph node enlargement, joint swelling and proteinuria. The reaction was usually of short duration, subsiding within a few days, and was known as serum sickness.

A similar reaction can be produced experimentally in rabbits by administration of a single, large intravenous dose of antigen. The development of lesions can be shown to coincide with the formation of large amounts of immune complexes in the circulation as a result of the immune response to circulating antigen (Fig. 22–5). Two types of lesion develop, a glomerulonephritis and an arteritis.

The nature of the glomerulonephritis varies with the size of immune complexes formed. Relatively large complexes in slight antigen excess can penetrate the vascular endothelium but not the basement membrane, and so become deposited in the subendothelial region, where they stimulate endothelial swelling and proliferation (Figs. 22–6 and 22–7). In contrast, if very small complexes are formed, as occurs in gross antigen excess, then these can penetrate both the vascular endothelium and the basement membrane. They are therefore deposited on the epithelial side of the basement membrane where they stimulate epithelial swelling and proliferation. Neutrophils do not normally accumulate within these glomeruli; nevertheless, damage does occur and results in the development of proteinuria. The precise mechanism of this damage is not clear, but it is probably due to the vasoactive properties of activated complement.

The most important of the arterial lesions is an Arthus-type reaction—neutrophil infiltration, disruption of the internal elastic membrane and medial necrosis—that occurs in medium-sized muscular arteries as a result of local deposition of immune complexes. Although the mechanisms of this deposition are not clear, it is probable that a transient type I

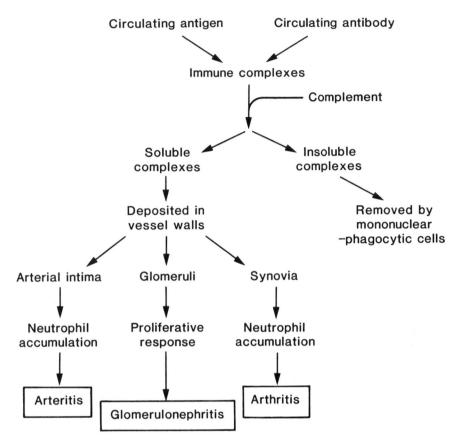

Figure 22–4. Mechanisms involved in the pathogenesis of acute serum sickness.

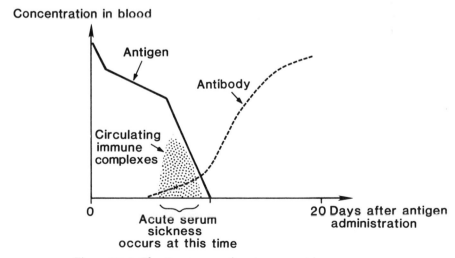

Figure 22–5. The time-course of acute serum sickness.

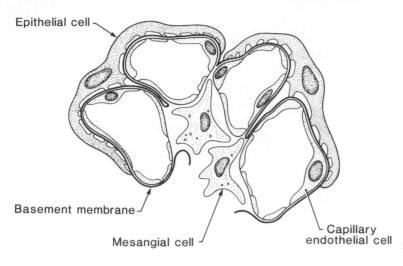

Epithelial cell

Basement membrane

Mesangial cell

Capillary endothelial cell

Figure 22–6. The structure of a glomerulus.

hypersensitivity reaction increases endothelial permeability and permits immune complexes to gain access to the arterial wall.

Chronic Serum Sickness

If, instead of a single high dose of antigen, an animal is given repeated injections of small doses of antigen over a long period of time, then two other types of glomerular lesion may develop. Continued deposition of immune complexes on the subepithelial surface of the glomerular basement membrane leads to an increase in its thickness, forming the so-called wire loop lesion or membranous glomerulopathy. Alternatively, the immune complexes

may be deposited in the mesangial region of glomeruli. Mesangial cells are a form of mono-nuclear-phagocyte; as such they possess Fc and complement receptors and are phagocytic. They respond to these immune complexes by proliferation (Fig. 22–8). Normally, this proliferation has little effect on glomerular function unless the mesangial cells expand to completely surround the glomerular capillaries. By immunofluorescence it can be shown that "lumpy-bumpy" aggregates of immune complexes are deposited in capillary walls and on the epithelial side of the glomerular basement membrane (Fig. 22–9). Arteritis is not a significant feature of experimental chronic serum sickness.

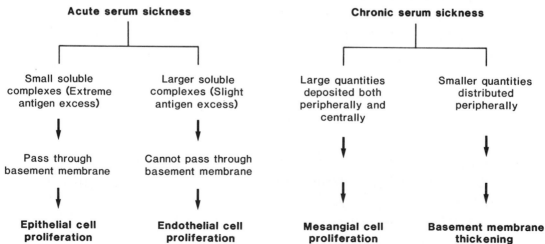

Figure 22–7. The different forms of immune complex–mediated glomerulonephritis. Remember, however, that more than one type of lesion may be present in an animal at the same time.

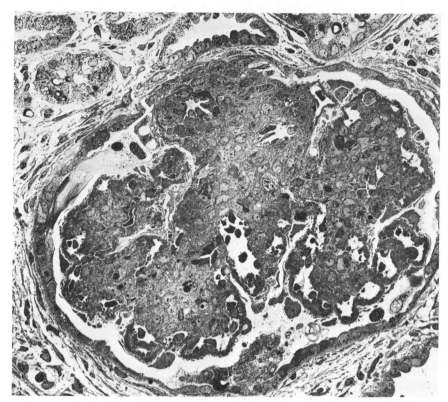

Figure 22–8. A thin section of a glomerulus from a Finnish-Landrace lamb suffering from an immune complex–mediated glomerulonephritis. The primary lesion in this case is mesangial proliferation with some basement membrane thickening. (From Angus K. W. et al. 1974. J. Comp. Pathol. 84 319–330. Used with permission.)

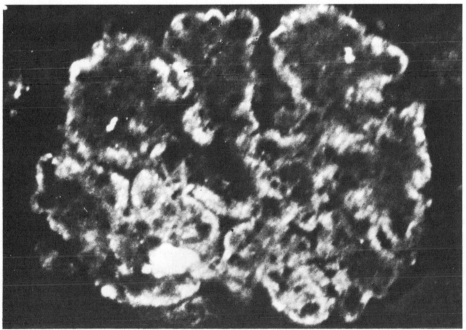

Figure 22–9. Fluorescent micrograph of a section of glomerulus from a Finnish-Landrace lamb with immune complex–mediated glomerulonephritis. The labeled antisheep globulin reveals the presence of "lumpy-bumpy" deposits characteristic of immune complex deposition. (From Angus K. W. et al. 1974. J. Comp. Pathol. 84 319–330. Used with permission.)

Table 22–1 INFECTIOUS DISEASES WITH A SIGNIFICANT TYPE III
HYPERSENSITIVITY COMPONENT

Organism or Disease	Major Lesion
Erysipelothrix rhusiopathiae	Arthritis
Mycobacterium johnei	Enteritis
Streptococcus equi	Purpura
Staphylococcus aureus	Dermatitis
Canine adenovirus I	Uveitis, glomerulonephritis
Feline leukemia	Glomerulonephritis
Feline infectious peritonitis	Peritonitis, glomerulonephritis
Aleutian disease	Glomerulonephritis, anemia, arteritis
Hog cholera	Glomerulonephritis
Bovine virus diarrhea	Glomerulonephritis
Equine viral arteritis	Arteritis
Equine infectious anemia	Anemia, glomerulonephritis
Dirofilaria immitis	Glomerulonephritis

CLINICAL ASPECTS OF IMMUNE COMPLEX-MEDIATED GLOMERULAR DISEASE

Immune complex-mediated glomerular lesions occur when prolonged antigenemia persists in the presence of antibodies. Glomerulonephritis, therefore, is characteristic of chronic viral diseases such as equine infectious anemia, Aleutian disease of mink and African swine fever (Table 22–1). Immune complex glomerulonephritis has also been reported to occur in dogs suffering from pyometra, chronic pneumonias, distemper encephalitis, acute pancreatic necrosis, bacterial endocarditis, systemic lupus erythematosus (Chapter 25) and certain malignant tumors, especially lymphosarcomas and mastocytomas. It may also arise in the absence of an obvious predisposing cause. The most common pathological lesion is mesangial proliferation, but diffuse membranous thickening is occasionally seen.

The presence of immune complexes within glomeruli leads to an increase in their permeability to protein, and as a result plasma proteins are lost in the urine. The major protein lost is albumin, since it is a relatively small molecule. This loss of protein, if severe, may exceed the ability of the body to replace it. As a result, the animal becomes hypoalbuminemic, the plasma colloid osmotic pressure falls, fluid passes into tissue spaces and the animal may become edematous and ascitic. The loss of fluid into tissues results in a reduction of blood volume, a compensatory increase in secretion of antidiuretic hormone, increased sodium retention and accentuation of the edema. The decreased blood volume will also result in a drop in renal blood flow, reduction in glomerular filtration, retention of urea and creatinine, azotemia and hypercholesterolemia. Although all these may occur as a result of immune complex deposition within glomeruli, the development of this nephrotic syndrome is not inevitable. In fact, the clinical course of these conditions is extremely unpredictable; some animals show a progressive deterioration in renal function whereas others show spontaneous remissions. Many animals may be clinically normal in spite of the presence of immune complexes within their glomeruli. Immune complexes are not uncommonly observed in old, apparently healthy dogs, horses and sheep. Because of the unpredictable occurrence of spontaneous remissions, it is difficult to judge the effects of treatment on this condition. It is usual to treat affected animals with corticosteroids and immunosuppressive drugs, but the rationale for this treatment is open to question. The glomerular lesion is not inflammatory, and although the lesion in primary immune complex glomerulonephritis contains immunoglobulin, there is no evidence to suggest that the condition occurs as a result of hyperactivity of the immune system. In addition, steroid treatment of rabbits with experimental immune complex disease has been shown to exacerbate the condition.

Finnish-Landrace Glomerulonephritis

Some lambs of the Finnish-Landrace breed die when about 6 1/2 weeks of age as a result of a glomerulonephritis. The glomerular lesions are similar to those seen in chronic serum sickness, with mesangial cell proliferation and basement membrane thickening (see Fig. 22–8). In extreme cases, epithelial cell proliferation may result in filling of the Bowman's capsule by an epithelial crescent. Neutrophils may be present in small numbers within glomeruli, and the rest of the kidney may exhibit diffuse interstitial lymphoid infiltration and necrotizing vasculitis. Deposits containing IgM, IgG and C3 are found within the glomeruli (see Fig. 22–9) and in the choroid plexus, and serum C3 levels are low. The lesions are, therefore, probably produced as a result of immune complex deposition within these organs, although the nature of the inducing antigen is unknown.

OTHER IMMUNE COMPLEX-MEDIATED LESIONS

Immune Vasculitis

Two types of immune vasculitis have been described in animals, namely polyarteritis nodosa and leukocytoclastic vasculitis.

Polyarteritis Nodosa. This condition is seen in man, swine, dogs and cats. It is characterized by a widespread, focal necrosis of the media of small and medium sized muscular arteries. The lesions are found in many organs, especially in the kidney. Vessels in the skin are rarely involved.

Leukocytoclastic Vasculitis. On occasion, focal vascular lesions characterized by neutrophil infiltration may develop in small blood vessels throughout the body, but especially in skin. Affected dogs have mucocutaneous ulcers, bullae, edema, polyarthropathy, myopathy, anorexia, intermittent fever and lethargy.

The causes of polyarteritis nodosa and leukocytoclastic vasculitis are unknown. The histology of both conditions suggests that they are forms of type III hypersensitivity reac-

tions, perhaps due to the presence of an infectious agent. Immunosuppression with steroids, possibly together with cyclophosphamide, has given good results in treating leukocytoclastic vasculitis in dogs. Polyarteritis nodosa is usually detected as an incidental finding on autopsy, although ocular defects may present clinically if the arteries of the eye are involved.

Dietary Hypersensitivity

If antigenic milk replacer, for example, soy protein, is fed to very young calves prior to the development of ruminal function, the foreign antigen may be absorbed and stimulate antibody formation and a type III hypersensitivity. As a result, the calves become unthrifty and begin to lose weight. The precise pathogenesis of this condition is, however, unclear. A small proportion of calves develop an IgE response and a type I hypersensitivity.

Purpura Hemorrhagica

Horses recovering from an acute streptococcal infection such as strangles occasionally suffer from an acute purpura. Immune complexes containing *Streptococcus equi* antigen may be found in the blood stream at that time. These immune complexes may be deposited in the kidneys, causing a mesangial and membranous glomerulonephritis with resulting proteinuria and azoturia.

Tumors

In some animals bearing tumors, large quantities of antigen may be shed into the blood stream and give rise to a glomerulonephritis. This is a very important feature of feline leukemia infection. It has also been reported in lymphosarcomas, osteosarcomas and mastocytomas.

Drug Hypersensitivities

In the previous chapter, it was pointed out that if a drug attached itself to a cell such as an erythrocyte, then the immune response against the drug could lead to the elimination of the cell. A similar reaction may occur through type III hypersensitivity reactions if immune complexes bind directly to host cells. In this case, the cells are recognized as being opsonized and are removed by phagocytosis. There are obviously only minor differences in mechanism between antibody binding to antigen-coated cells and antibody-antigen complexes coating cells directly, and it is therefore usually very difficult to distinguish between the two. As might be predicted, if immune complexes bind to erythrocytes, anemia results; if they bind to platelets, thrombocytopenia and purpura result; if they bind to granulocytes, agranulocytosis and, consequently, recurrent infection occur. In many cases, however, it is difficult to distinguish between the toxic effects of a drug and type III hypersensitivity unless specific antibodies can be eluted from affected cells.

Dirofilariasis

Some dogs that are heavily infected with the heartworm *Dirofilaria immitis* develop glomerular lesions and proteinuria. The lesions include thickening of the glomerular basement membrane with minimal endothelial or mesangial proliferation. Since "lumpy-bumpy," IgG1–containing deposits may be found on the epithelial side of the basement membrane, it has been suggested that immune complexes formed by antibodies to helminth antigens provoke these lesions. Other investigators dispute the immune complex nature of this condition and claim that the lesions develop in response to the physical presence of microfilariae within glomerular blood vessels. The fact that infected dogs may develop amyloidosis (Chapter 19) suggests strongly that they mount a significant immune response to the worms.

ADDITIONAL SOURCES OF INFORMATION

Angus KW and Gardiner AC. 1979. Mesangio-capillary glomerulonephritis in Dorset-Finnish-Landrace cross lambs. Vet. Rec. *105* 471.

Arthur JE, Lucke VM, Newby TJ and Bourne FJ. 1984. An immunohistological study of feline glomerulonephritis using the peroxidase-antiperoxidase method. Res. Vet. Sci. *37* 12–17.

Asmundsson T, Gunnarsson E and Johannesson T. 1983. "Haysickness" in Icelandic horses: precipitin tests and other studies. Equine Vet. J. *15* 229–232.

Drazner FH. 1978. Renal amyloidosis and glomerulonephritis secondary to dirofilariasis. Canine Pract. *5* 66–68.

Krakowka S. 1978. Glomerulonephritis in dogs and cats. Vet. Clin. North. Am. (Small Anim. Pract.) *8* 629–639.

Littlejohn A. 1979. Chronic obstructive pulmonary disease in horses. Vet. Bull. *49* 907–917.

McPherson EA and Thomson JR. 1983. Chronic obstructive pulmonary disease in the horse. 1. Nature of the disease. Equine Vet. J. *15* 203–206.

Schatz M, Patterson R and Fink J. 1979. Immunologic lung disease. N. Engl. J. Med. *300* 1310–1320.

Scott DW, MacDonald JM and Schultz RD. 1978. Staphylococcal hypersensitivity in the dog. J. Am. Anim. Hosp. Assoc. *14* 766–779.

Slauson DO and Lewis RM. 1979. Comparative pathology of glomerulonephritis in animals. Vet. Pathol. *16* 135–164.

Targowski S. 1982. Determination of immune complexes in sera of dogs with various diseases by mastocytoma cell assay. J. Clin. Microbiol. *15* 64–68.

Theofilopoulos AN and Dixon FJ. 1979. The biology and detection of immune complexes. Adv. Immunol. *28* 89–220.

Weissman G, Smolen JE and Korchek HM. 1980. Release of inflammatory mediators from stimulated neutrophils. N. Engl. J. Med. *303* 27–34.

Wright NG, Mohammed NA, Eckersall PD and Nash AS. 1985. Experimental immune complex glomerulonephritis in dogs receiving cationized bovine serum albumin. Res. Vet. Sci. *38* 322–328.

23

Cell-Mediated (Type IV) Hypersensitivity

When certain antigens are injected into the skin of sensitized animals, an inflammatory response, taking many hours to develop, may occur at the injection site. Since this "delayed hypersensitivity" reaction cannot be transferred from sensitized to normal animals by serum, but only by lymphocytes, it is clearly a cell-mediated reaction. Delayed hypersensitivity reactions of this type are classified as type IV hypersensitivity and occur as a result of the interaction between the injected antigen and sensitized T lymphocytes. An important example of a delayed hypersensitivity reaction is the tuberculin response, the reaction mediated in a tuberculous animal as a result of an intradermal injection of tuberculin—an antigenic extract derived from the tubercle bacillus.

TUBERCULIN REACTION

Tuberculin is the name given to extracts of *Mycobacterium tuberculosis*, *Mycobacterium bovis* or *Mycobacterium avium*, which are employed as antigens when skin testing animals in an effort to identify those suffering from tuberculosis. Several types of tuberculin have been employed for this purpose. The most important of these is purified protein derivative (PPD) tuberculin, which is prepared by growing organisms in synthetic medium, killing them with steam and filtering. The PPD tuberculin is precipitated from this filtrate with trichloracetic acid, washed and finally resuspended in buffer ready for use.

When PPD tuberculin is injected intradermally into a normal animal, there is no significant local inflammatory response. On the other hand, if it is injected into animals sensitized by infection with the tubercle bacillus, a delayed hypersensitivity response will occur. Following injection of tuberculin into such an animal, no changes are detectable either grossly or histologically for several hours. Later, however, vasodilation and increased vascular permeability occur, as a result of which erythema and swelling are observed.

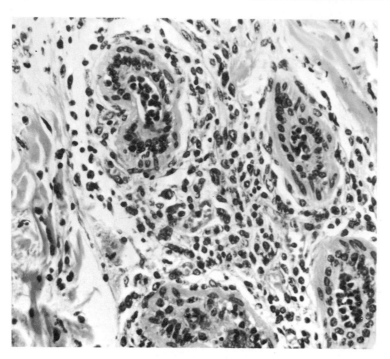

Figure 23–1. Histological section of a positive tuberculin reaction in bovine skin. Note the perivascular mononuclear cell infiltration and the lack of neutrophils and edema. (From Thomson, R. G. 1978. General Veterinary Pathology. WB Saunders Company, Philadelphia. Courtesy of Dr. Thomson.)

This swelling is characteristically indurated (hard). On histological examination, the lesion differs from the classic acute inflammatory response in that the infiltrating cell population consists largely of mononuclear cells (macrophages and lymphocytes) (Fig. 23–1), although a transient neutrophil accumulation also occurs in the early stages of the reaction. The reaction reaches its greatest intensity by 24 to 72 hours after injection and may persist for several weeks before gradually fading. In very severe reactions, necrosis may occur at the injection site.

The tuberculin reaction is an immunologically specific reaction mediated by T cells. It develops in two stages. It is believed that circulating antigen-sensitive T cells first encounter the injected antigen and respond by causing nearby mast cells to degranulate and release vasoactive factors such as serotonin. The resulting increase in vascular permeability and the opening up of interendothelial gaps in capillaries permit more T cells to migrate from the blood into the tissues. In the second stage of the reaction, these migrating T cells encounter antigen presented to them by Langerhans cells, divide, differentiate and release lymphokines (Fig. 23–2). The lymphokines involved and the order in which they act are unclear, but it is thought that macrophages accumulate at the site through the release of macrophage chemotactic factors and that their emigration from this site is then inhibited by migration inhibitory factors (IFNγ). The vascular changes are probably mediated through the release of ill-defined inflammatory mediators and lysosomal enzymes from macrophages. The macrophages ingest and eventually destroy the injected antigen, permitting the tissues to return to normal.

Cutaneous Basophil Hypersensitivity

Some antigens may elicit a different form of delayed inflammatory response in skin. In these cases, the lesion is infiltrated with large numbers of basophils as well as mononuclear cells. This reaction, called cutaneous basophil hypersensitivity (CBH), can be transferred between animals with antibody, purified B cells or T cells. It is, therefore, a very heterogeneous phenomenon that probably arises through a number of different mechanisms. CBH is observed in chickens in response to intradermal Rous sarcoma virus, in rabbits in response to schistosomes and in humans in allergic contact dermatitis and renal allograft rejection.

Tuberculin Reactions in Cattle

Because the tuberculin reaction occurs only in animals that have or have had tuberculosis, it may be employed to identify animals affected by this disease. Indeed, this test has provided the basis for all tuberculosis eradication schemes that involve the detection and subsequent elimination of infected animals.

Tuberculin testing of cattle may be performed in several ways. The simplest of these is the single intradermal (SID) test. In this test, 0.05 ml of PPD tuberculin derived from either *M. tuberculosis* or *M. bovis* is injected into one anal fold, and the injection site is examined 72 to 96 hours later. A comparison is easily made between the injected and the uninjected folds, and a positive reaction consisting of a diffuse, indurated swelling at the injection site is readily detected.

In the United States two injections are made, one into the mucocutaneous junction of the vulva and the other into an anal fold; in other countries the injection is normally made into the skin on the side of the neck. The neck site is more sensitive than the anal folds, but restraint of the animal may be more difficult, and good injection technique is critical.

The advantage of the SID test is its simplicity; its disadvantage is that by using this test it is not possible to distinguish between infection with the different species of mycobacteria, including *M. avium*, *M. paratuberculosis* and the related *Nocardia* group of organisms. A second disadvantage is the relatively high prevalence of animals that react positively to the test but on necropsy do not have detectable lesions of tuberculosis. The reasons for this are not clear but may involve inapparent infection with nonpathogenic mycobacteria.

False-negative SID tests may occur in animals with advanced tuberculosis, in animals with very early infection, in animals that have calved within the preceding four to six weeks, in very old cows and in animals tested within the preceding 1 to 10 weeks. The anergy seen in advanced cases of tuberculosis is also observed in clinical Johne's disease and appears to be due to the presence of a blocking factor in the serum of these animals, perhaps an antibody that prevents T cells from reacting with antigen; there is also, however, evidence

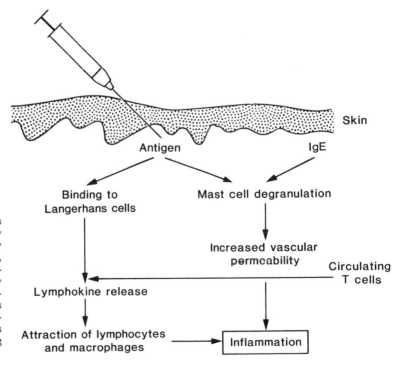

Figure 23–2. The pathogenesis of the delayed hypersensitivity reaction. It is an inflammatory reaction involving lymphocytes, mast cells and macrophages. Increased vascular permeability caused by mast cell derived factors permits circulating T cells to enter the tissues and encounter antigen. It eventually results in elimination of the inducing antigen.

Table 23–1 SOME TUBERCULIN TESTS USED IN CATTLE

Test	Usage	Advantages	Disadvantages
Single intradermal (SID)	Routine testing	Simple	False positives; poor sensitivity
Comparative	When much avian TB or Johne's disease is present	More specific than SID	More complex than SID
Short thermal	Use in post-partum animals and in advanced cases	High efficiency	Time consuming; potential risk of anaphylaxis
Stormont	Use in post-partum animals and in advanced cases	Very sensitive and accurate	Three visits required; leads to a long desensitization period

for the development of suppressor cells in this condition. Because of these defects in the SID, several modifications of this test have been developed (Table 23–1). The comparative test, for example, employs both avian and bovine tuberculins. Each of these is injected into the side of the neck at separate sites, and these sites are examined 72 hours later. In general, if the avian tuberculin site shows the greatest reaction, the animal is considered to be infected with *M. avium* or *M. paratuberculosis*. On the other hand, if the *M. bovis* site shows the greatest reaction, then it is felt that the animal is infected with either *M. tuberculosis* or *M. bovis*. Therefore, this test is useful when a high prevalence of avian tuberculosis or Johne's disease is anticipated, and it has been used with success in the United Kingdom. PPD from *M. bovis* is more specific in cattle than *M. tuberculosis*, giving less cross-reaction with *M. avium* as well as being more appropriate for use in cattle and is therefore preferred.

Other modified tuberculin tests include the short thermal test, in which a large volume of tuberculin solution is given subcutaneously and the animal examined for a rise in temperature between four and eight hours later. (Presumably, the tuberculin acts on T cells that then release lymphokines that provoke the release of interleukin 1 from macrophages.) The Stormont test relies on the increased sensitivity of a test site, which occurs after a single injection; it is performed by giving two doses of tuberculin at the same injection site seven days apart. Both these

tests are relatively sensitive and may be used in postpartum cows as well as for the testing of heavily infected animals.

Tuberculin Reactions in Animals Other Than Cattle

Tuberculin testing has never been a widely employed procedure in domestic animals other than cattle, so information on these is scanty. Nevertheless, it appears that the ability of different species to mount a classic tuberculin reaction varies greatly. In the pig and cat, for example, the tuberculin test is unreliable, being positive for only a short period following infection. In the pig and dog, the best test is an SID test given behind the ear, whereas in the cat the short thermal test is probably the best. In sheep, goats and horses the antigen is usually given in the caudal fold, but the results also tend to be highly erratic in these species. In birds, good reactions may be obtained by inoculating tuberculin into the wattle or wing web.

Johnin Reactions

Animals infected with *M. paratuberculosis* may exhibit a delayed hypersensitivity to an antigenic extract of this organism known as johnin. Johnin can be used in a single intradermal test but, like tuberculin, generally gives a negative result in animals with clinical disease. An intravenous johnin test may be a preferable alternative to the SID test. In this test the antigen is administered intravenously and the animal's temperature noted at intervals thereafter. A rise in temperature of 1°C or a neutrophilia after six hours is considered a positive result. These tests are probably of limited usefulness in individual animals but may be used for the identification of infected herds.

Other Skin Tests Involving Type IV Hypersensitivity

Positive delayed hypersensitivity reactions may be obtained in any infectious disease in which cell-mediated immunity plays a significant role. Thus, various extracts of *Brucella abortus* have been used from time to time in attempts to diagnose brucellosis. These include "brucellin," a filtrate of a 20-day broth culture, and "brucellergen," a nucleoprotein extract. Because these preparations may stimulate production of antibody to brucella, they must not be employed in areas where eradication is monitored by serological tests. In glanders of horses, a culture filtrate of the organism *Pseudomonas mallei*, termed mallein, is used for skin testing. Mallein can be used either in a short thermal test or an ophthalmic test. An ophthalmic test, also occasionally employed in tuberculosis, is performed by dropping the antigen solution into an eye. A transient conjunctivitis develops if the test is positive. Another and perhaps preferable hypersensitivity test for glanders is the intrapalpebral test, in which mallein is injected into the skin of the lower eyelid, where a positive reaction causes swelling and ophthalmia.

Skin tests are also employed in the diagnosis of many fungal diseases; thus, "histoplasmin" is used for histoplasmosis, "coccidioidin" in coccidioidomycosis and so on. In these cases, the tests are not very specific and the test procedure may effectively sensitize the tested animal, causing it to become serologically positive. This problem also arises when "toxoplasmin" is used in attempts to diagnose toxoplasmosis (Chapter 17).

PATHOLOGICAL CONSEQUENCES OF TYPE IV HYPERSENSITIVITY

Tubercle Formation

Although the intradermal tuberculin reaction is artificial in that antigen is administered by injection, a similar host response occurs if living tubercle bacilli lodge in tissues. However, *M. tuberculosis* is resistant to intracellular destruction until a cell-mediated immune response has developed (Chapter 15), and dead organisms are very slowly removed because they contain large quantities of poorly metabolized waxes. As a result of this, the delayed hypersensitivity reaction to whole organisms tends to be prolonged, and, consequently, macrophages accumulate in very large numbers. Many of these macrophages attempt to ingest the bacteria and die in the process, whereas others fuse to form multinucleated giant cells. The lesion that develops around invading tubercle bacilli therefore consists of a mass of necrotic material containing both living and dead organisms surrounded by a layer of macrophages, which in this location are known as epithelioid cells (Chapter 2). The entire lesion is known as a tubercle (Fig. 23–3). Persistent tubercles may become relatively well organized and develop a fibrous tissue capsule, resulting in the formation of a granuloma. (Interleukin 1 stimulates collagen production by fibroblasts and hence contributes to this process.) Granuloma formation is a frequent result of persistent chronic inflammation. This inflammation may be of immunological origin, as in tuberculosis or brucellosis in some species, but it may also occur as a result of the presence in tissues of other chronic irritants (Fig. 23–4). For example, granulomas may arise in response to the prolonged irritation caused by talc or asbestos particles.

In chronic interstitial nephritis (CIN) of dogs associated with leptospiral infection, it has been suggested that the organisms persisting in the kidney may induce a chronic inflammatory reaction in which delayed hypersensitivity as well as local antibody produc-

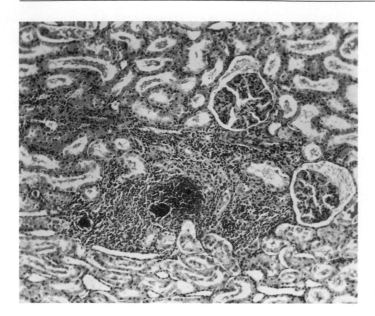

Figure 23–3. Histological section from the kidney of a black buck showing a small tubercle. ×250. (From a specimen kindly provided by Dr. R. G. Thomson.)

tion plays a role. Certainly, the histology of CIN shows a remarkable resemblance to that of chronic renal allograft rejection in the dog.

Allergic Contact Dermatitis

If reactive chemicals are painted onto the skin, they will bind to Langerhans cells in the dermis through the formation of protein-chemical complexes. These altered Langerhans cells form an antigenic focus for specifically sensitized lymphocytes. The sensitized lymphocytes attempt to destroy and remove the altered cells and give rise to a condition known as allergic contact dermatitis.

The chemicals that induce allergic contact dermatitis are usually relatively simple; they include such compounds as formaldehyde, picric acid, aniline dyes, plant resins and oils, organophosphates and salts of metals such as nickel and beryllium (Table 23–2). Thus, allergic contact dermatitis can occur on pathologists' fingers as a result of exposure to formaldehyde, on the foot pads and ventral abdomen of dogs on exposure to some carpet dyes, on parts of the body exposed to the oils (urushiol) of the poison ivy plant (*Rhus radicans*) and around the neck of animals as a result of exposure to dichlorovos (2,2–dichlorovinyldimethyl phosphate) in flea collars. Allergic contact dermatitis involving the muzzle of dogs has been reported to occur as a result of sensitivity of components of plastic food bowls. Some dogs, instead of developing the more usual type I hypersensitivity to pollen proteins, suffer from allergic contact dermatitis as a result of a type IV hypersensitivity to pollen resins. It is unusual for allergic contact dermatitis to severely affect the haired areas of the skin unless the allergen is in a liquid.

The lesions of allergic contact dermatitis generally vary greatly in severity, ranging

Table 23–2 SOURCES OF COMPOUNDS KNOWN TO CAUSE ALLERGIC CONTACT DERMATITIS IN ANIMALS

Insecticides
  in flea collars
  in sprays
  in dips
Wood preservatives
Floor waxes
Carpet dyes
Some pollens
Dermatological drugs (creams, ointments)
Leather products
Paints
House plants

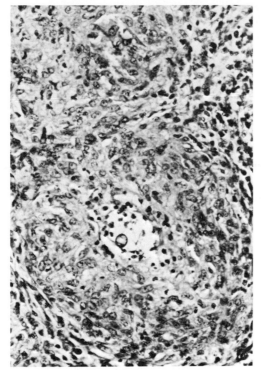

Figure 23–4. Granulomatous inflammatory reaction with *Coccidioides immitis* in the lymph node of a dog. ×250. (Courtesy of Dr. L. G. Adams.)

from a mild erythema to severe erythematous vesiculation. Because of the intense pruritus, however, self-trauma, excoriation, ulceration and secondary pyoderma often mask the true nature of the lesion. In chronic lesions, hy-

perkeratosis, acanthosis and dermal fibrosis may be produced. Histologically, the lesion is marked by a mononuclear cell infiltration and vacuolation of skin cells under attack by cytotoxic T cells (Table 23–3).

Diagnosis is made by removal of the suspected antigen and by patch testing. In patch tests, a small area of skin is shaved and covered with a patch of tissue or cloth impregnated with the suspected allergen. After 24 to 48 hours the patch may be removed, a positive reaction is indicated by local erythema and vesiculation. Patch tests tend to be impractical in dogs and cats. An alternative procedure is to simply rub the suspected allergen into shaved normal skin and examine the area daily for five days. Treatment makes use of steroids as well as antibiotics to control secondary infections.

THE MEASUREMENT OF CELL-MEDIATED IMMUNITY

Although diagnostic immunology is based largely upon the detection of antibodies, measurement of cell-mediated immune responsiveness in animals may be desirable under some circumstances. Currently, three major groups of techniques are widely used.

The simplest is the intradermal skin test described earlier in this chapter. The resulting

Table 23–3 COMPARISON OF THE TWO MAJOR FORMS OF ALLERGIC DERMATITIS

	Atopic Dermatitis	**Allergic Contact Dermatitis**
Pathogenesis	Type I hypersensitivity	Type IV hypersensitivity
Clinical signs	Hyperemia, urticaria, intense pruritus leading to self-mutilation	Spotty hyperemia, occasional vesiculation, erythematous alopecia, pruritus
Distribution	Face, nose, eyes, feet, perineum	Hairless areas, usually ventral abdomen, feet, nose
Major allergens	Foods and pollens, commonly seasonal; occasionally arthropod-associated	Reactive chemicals only after prolonged contact with skin
Diagnosis	Rapid erythematous response to intradermal and patch testing; commonly, other signs of allergy; eosinophilia or eosinophilic infiltration of lesions	Delayed (24 to 48 hr) response to patch test; mononuclear infiltration of the lesions
Treatment	Antihistamines, steroids, hyposensitization therapy	Steroids

inflammatory response may be considered cell-mediated, provided that it has the characteristic time-course and histology of a type IV reaction. Intradermal skin tests are not always convenient, and injection of antigen into an animal may effectively sensitize it. In addition, there is good evidence to suggest that widespread tuberculin testing may promote the spread of infections such as bovine leukosis between animals. For these reasons, *in vitro* tests may be more appropriate. The *in vitro* tests are designed to measure either the proliferation of T lymphocytes in response to antigen or their production of lymphokines.

In order to measure T cell proliferation in response to antigen, a suspension of purified peripheral blood lymphocytes from the animal to be tested is mixed with antigen and cultured for 48 to 96 hours. Twelve hours before harvesting, thymidine labeled with the radioactive isotope tritium is added to the cultures. Normal, nondividing lymphocytes do not take up thymidine but dividing cells do, because they are actively synthesizing DNA. Thus, if the T cells are proliferating, they will take up the tritiated thymidine and the radioactivity of the washed cells will provide a measure of the degree of proliferation. The greater the response of the cells to antigen, the greater the radioactivity. The ratio of the radioactivity in the stimulated cultures to the radioactivity in the controls is called the stimulation index.

The measurement of lymphokine release by T cells is a much more complicated procedure. One of the most common techniques involves incubating a purified lymphocyte suspension with antigen. After 24 to 48 hours, the supernatant fluid of the culture is removed and assayed for MIF (migration inhibitory factor) activity. This may be done by measuring the ability of the supernatant to inhibit the migration of macrophages out of a capillary tube (see Fig. 7–5).

It is sometimes useful to measure the ability of an animal to mount cell-mediated immune responses in general. One way to do this is to surgically graft the animal with allogeneic skin and measure its survival time. A much simpler technique is to paint the animal's skin with a sensitizing chemical such as dinitrochloroben-

zene. The intensity of the resulting contact dermatitis provides a rough estimate of the animal's ability to mount a cell-mediated immune response.

An alternative *in vitro* technique is to measure the response of lymphocytes to mitogenic lectins such as phytohemagglutinin, concanavalin A or pokeweed mitogen (Chapter 5). The intensity of the lymphocyte proliferative response, as measured by tritiated thymidine uptake, provides an estimate of the reactivity of an animal's lymphocytes (see Fig. 26–4). In addition, if phytohemagglutinin is injected intradermally, it provokes a reaction with many of the features of a delayed hypersensitivity response. This is a very convenient and rapid method of assessing an animal's ability to mount a cell-mediated response without the need for first sensitizing the animal to an antigen. However, the response to phytohemagglutinin is nonspecific and its interpretation may be difficult.

None of the currently available techniques to measure cell-mediated immunity, with the possible exception of intradermal testing, lends itself readily to use by any but investigators in well-equipped laboratories. The measurement of cell-mediated immunity has become an increasingly important feature of the analysis of immune reactivity, however, and refined and much simpler techniques are expected to become available in future.

ADDITIONAL SOURCES OF INFORMATION

Angus K and Young TJ. 1978. Lymphocyte response to phytohemagglutinin: temporal variation in normal dogs. J. Immunol. Methods 21 261–269.

Askenase PW and Van Loveren M. 1983. Delayed-type hypersensitivity: activation of mast cells by antigen-specific T-cell factors initiates the cascade of cellular interactions. Immunol. Today 4 259–264.

Chambers WH and Klesius PH. 1983. Direct bovine leukocyte migration inhibition assay: standardization and comparison with skin testing. Vet. Immunol. Immunopathol. 5 85–95.

Dixon JB, Allan D and West CR. 1979. Hematological correlates of phytohemagglutinin-induced lymphocyte transformation in horses. Res. Vet. Sci. 26 59–65.

Grant DI and Thoday KL. 1980. Canine allergic contact dermatitis: a clinical review. J. Small Anim. Pract. 21 17–27.

Halliwell REW and Longino DJ. 1985. IgE and IgG antibodies to flea antigen in differing dog population. Vet. Immunol. Immunopathol. 8 215–224.

Knox S and Shifrine M. 1980. Cell-mediated immunity in the dog in relation to disease: a review. Comp. Immunol. Microbiol. Infect. Dis. 2 405–514.

Kristensen F, Kristensen B and Lazary S. 1982. The lymphocyte stimulation test in veterinary immunology. Vet. Immunol. Immunopathol. 3 203–277.

Legendre AM, Mallman VII and Michel RL. 1977. Migration-inhibition response of peripheral leukocytes to turberculin in cats sensitized with *Mycobacterium bovis* (BCG). Am. J. Vet. Res. 38 819–822.

Lens JW, Drexhage HA, Benson W and Balfour BM. 1983. A study of cells present in lymph draining from a contact allergic reaction in pigs sensitized to DNFB. Immunology 49 415–422.

Scherba G, Gustafson DF, Kanitz CL and Sun IL. 1978. Delayed hypersensitivity reaction to pseudorabics virus as a field diagnostic test in swine. JAVMA 173 1490–1493.

Schultz KT and Maguire HC. 1982. Chemically induced delayed hypersensitivity in the cat. Vet. Immunol. Immunopathol. 3 585–590.

Toews GB, Bergstresser PR, Streilein JW and Sullivan S. 1980. Epidermal Langerhans cell density determines whether contact hypersensitivity or unresponsiveness follows skin painting with DNFB. J. Immunol. 124 445–453.

V

IMMUNOLOGICAL DISEASES

24

Autoimmunity: General Principles

It was once believed that normal healthy animals lacked the ability to mount any immune response against self-antigens as a result of self-tolerance. It is now clear, however, that animals are able to produce autoantibodies relatively easily when their immune system is appropriately stimulated. Thus, a small number of lymphocytes, reactive to normal tissue antigens, are always present in lymphoid organs. Stimulation of these cells by nonspecific mitogens such as bacterial endotoxin provoke the transient appearance of autoantibodies in serum. These autoantibodies are directed against some very common autoantigens, DNA, IgG, phospholipids, erythrocytes and lymphocytes, for example. These antibodies can react with normal tissues but usually have no adverse effects. On occasion, the regulation of the autoreactive cells may break down. When this happens, clones of normally quiescent lymphocytes may grow and generate high levels of autoantibodies or autoreactive T cells.

It has been generally assumed that autoimmune responses are bad and cause disease. This is now known to be untrue. It is recognized that certain autoimmune responses have important physiological functions and are therefore essential for the normal functioning of the body.

PHYSIOLOGICAL AUTOIMMUNITY

Three autoimmune processes serve major physiological roles in the body. These are the recognition of self MHC antigens, the recognition of self idiotypes and the recognition of senescent cells.

Recognition of Self MHC by T Cells

In Chapters 7 and 8 it was described how the cell-surface proteins, coded for by genes in the major histocompatibility complex, regulate cell-cell recognition and interaction. Class I histocompatibility antigens found on all nucleated cells serve to identify a cell as a normal body constituent. Recognition of these antigens is an essential prerequisite for the identification and destruction of virus-infected or tumor cells. Proteins coded for by class II histocompatibility genes are found on macrophages, B cells and activated T cells. These antigens must be recognized by cells of the immune system in order for effective cell cooperation to occur and for an immune response to be initiated. These antigens are recognized by the T4 or T8 components of the T cell antigen receptor. The T4 protein recognizes class II antigens while the T8 component recognizes class I antigens. It is believed that this dual recognition system assists in directing the effects of the T cell toward more efficient and more precise cell interactions.

Recognition of Self Immunoglobulins by Anti-Idiotypes

In Chapter 9, the way in which the antigen binding sites (idiotypes) on immunoglobulin molecules function as epitopes and provoke the production of autoantibodies (anti-idiotypes) was discussed. These newly formed anti-idiotypes also possess their own characteristic epitopes and so provoke anti–anti-idiotypes. This process can, in theory, continue indefinitely. Since each anti-idiotype response tends to exert a negative feedback on the preceding response, the net effect is to terminate an antibody response. Under some circumstances, anti-idiotype antibodies may also enhance some antibody responses. Thus, the idiotype–anti-idiotype network may serve a physiological function by regulating the level of the antibody response.

Removal of Senescent Cells

It has been known for many years that red cells are removed from the blood stream once they reach the end of their life span. This process is accomplished by autoantibodies. As red cells age, a cell membrane protein called band 3 is cleaved by cell-membrane enzymes, and a new epitope is exposed. This new epitope is recognized by an autoantibody of the IgG isotype, which attaches to the red cell and so causes its phagocytosis by macrophages in the liver and spleen. Band 3 protein is found on platelets, lymphocytes, neutrophils, hepatocytes and kidney cells. It may well be that the cleavage of band 3 in aged cells and the subsequent removal of those cells by antibodies constitutes a common mechanism for the elimination of senescent cells.

WITEBSKY'S POSTULATES

Because autoantibodies are commonly found in healthy normal individuals, their presence in a diseased animal does not automatically imply that an animal is suffering from an autoimmune disease. In order to establish firm criteria for the identification of a disease as autoimmune, the late Ernest Witebsky suggested that the following four postulates must be established. (1) The autoantibodies should be detectable in all cases of the disease. (2) The disease should be experimentally reproducible by some form of immunization with the antigen. (3) The experimental disease must show immunopathological lesions that parallel those seen in the natural disease. (4) The disease should be transferable from an affected animal to a normal animal by means of either serum or living lymphoid cells.

MECHANISMS OF INDUCTION OF AUTOIMMUNITY (Fig. 24–1)

Exposure of Previously Hidden Antigens

Some antigens may exist within the body in locations not normally visited by circulating

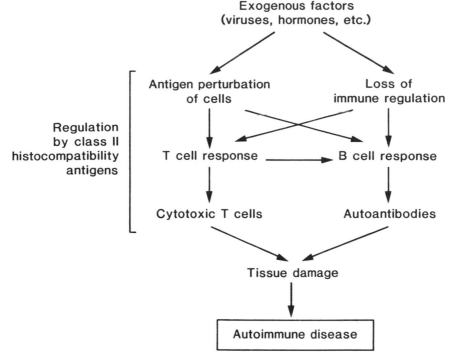

Figure 24–1. A simplified scheme for the pathogenesis of autoimmune diseases.

lymphocytes. Antigens may be hidden, for example, in the central nervous system and the testes, organs that are not drained by the lymphatic circulation. If the brain or testes is injured either by trauma or by infection, then the resulting breakdown in vascular barriers may permit antigens released by damaged cells to reach the general circulation, encounter antigen-sensitive cells and stimulate an immune response. Similar considerations apply to antigens that are normally found only within cells and to which tolerance may not be established. For example, after myocardial infarction autoantibodies may be produced against intracellular components such as mitochondria, although myocardial infarction is manifestly not an autoimmune disease. In diseases such as trypanosomiasis or tuberculosis in which widespread tissue damage occurs, autoantibodies to a wide range of tissue antigens may be detected at low titers in serum.

Exposure of Hidden Epitopes

The formation of autoantibodies may be provoked by the development of new epitopes on normal proteins. An excellent example of this type of antigen is the band 3 antigen on senescent red cells described earlier. Two other examples of autoantibodies generated in this fashion are rheumatoid factors and immunoconglutinins.

Rheumatoid factors (RF) are antibodies (largely IgM) that are directed against epitopes on other immunoglobulin molecules. When an immunoglobulin binds to an antigen, the Fab regions of the molecule are stabilized in such a way that new epitopes are exposed on the Fc region. These new epitopes stimulate rheumatoid factor formation. Rheumatoid factors therefore develop in diseases in which large quantities of immune complexes are generated, such as in rheumatoid arthritis and systemic lupus erythematosus (Chapter 25).

Immunoconglutinins (abbreviated to IK after the German spelling) are antibodies directed against epitopes on the activated complement components C2, C4 and C3. The most important of these is the IK directed against C3. The epitopes that stimulate IK formation are sites on the complement components newly revealed by complement activation. The level of IK in serum is a measure

of the amount of complement activation occurring, and this, in turn, is a measure of the
degree of antigenic stimulation to which an
animal is subjected. IK levels may, therefore,
be employed as nonspecific indicators of the
prevalence of infectious disease within a population. Their physiological role is unclear but
they may serve to enhance the opsonizing
function of C3.

Minor antigenic changes in normal body
components may also be generated artificially
and used to induce autoantibodies. For example, chemically modified thyroglobulin can
be used to stimulate the production of autoantibodies against normal thyroglobulin. It is
also possible to render normal tissues antigenic by injecting them together with
Freund's complete adjuvant.

Cross-Reactivity with Microorganisms

In porcine enzootic pneumonia, antibodies to
Mycoplasma hyopneumoniae cross-react with
pig lung, and in contagious bovine pleuropneumonia there is cross-reactivity between
Mycoplasma mycoides antigens and normal
bovine lung. It is not known to what extent
autoantibodies of this type contribute to the
pathogenesis of these diseases. Horses inoculated with some killed *Leptospira interrogans*
serovars may develop IgG(B) antibodies to
cornea and eventually develop corneal opaci-
ties.

Development of Suppressed Cells

Most autoimmune disorders probably occur as
a result of the development of cells that had
previously been suppressed by the normal
control mechanisms of the body. For example,
it can be shown that the severity of autoimmune thyroiditis in the OS strain of chickens
(see page 338) is increased following neonatal
thymectomy. It has been suggested that this
may be due to the removal of suppressor T
cells, which normally prevent the development of an immune response to normal thyroid antigens.

It is not uncommon to find autoimmune
disease associated with lymphoid tumors. For
example, myasthenia gravis may be associated
with the presence of a thymoma. In humans,
there is a fourfold increase in the incidence of
rheumatoid diseases in patients with malignant lymphoid tumors, and there is evidence
for a similar association in animals. The reasons for this are poorly understood, but since
many lymphoid tumors may arise as a result
of a failure in immunological control mechanisms, a simultaneous failure in self-tolerance
may also occur. Alternatively, some tumors
may represent the development of a "forbid-
den clone" of cells producing autoantibodies.
One other possibility that should be considered is that lymphoid tumors may arise as a
result of the chronic stimulation of the immune system by autoantigens.

Viruses as Inducers of Autoimmunity

A growing body of evidence has served to link
many autoimmune diseases to virus infections:
it has been suggested that viruses, particularly
those that infect lymphoid tissues, may be
capable of interfering with immunological control mechanisms and so permit autoimmunity
to occur. Thus, in New Zealand Black (NZB)
mice, persistent infection with a type C retrovirus leads to the development of autoantibodies against nucleic acids and erythrocytes.
Systemic lupus erythematosus (SLE) of dogs
and humans is a similar condition in which
the presence of autoantibodies to many different organs is possibly associated with either a
type C retrovirus or paramyxovirus infection
(Chapter 25). Mice infected with certain reoviruses will also develop an autoimmune
polyendocrine disease characterized by diabetes mellitus and retarded growth. These
mice develop antibodies against normal pituitary, pancreas, gastric mucosa, nuclei, gluca-
gon, growth hormone and insulin. It has been
suggested that the onset of type I diabetes in
children is associated with a viral infection.
No doubt, the potential for a similar condition
exists in domestic animals.

Histocompatibility Antigens and Autoimmune Disease

The class II histocompatibility antigens regulate an animal's ability to mount immune responses. As a result, they also influence resistance or susceptibility to diseases. Very few of these diseases are infectious, because infectious diseases tend to affect young animals prior to reaching reproductive age (Chapter 8.) Genes that predispose to susceptibility to infectious agents will be rapidly selected against; therefore, the class II genes that animals now possess have been selected for a rapid response to most pathogens.

Autoimmune diseases, in contrast, tend to affect older, postreproductive animals. As a result they generally do not offer a significant selective disadvantage. Studies of animal populations, especially humans, has shown that about 50 diseases are associated with the possession of certain class II haplotypes. They fall into two groups. There is one group of diseases associated with the intervertebral discs and sacroiliac joints that are very closely associated with the human class II antigen HLA B27. Thus 95 per cent of the individuals with ankylosing spondylitis have HLA B27.

The other associations are between a variety of class II antigens and many different autoimmune diseases, for example HLA DR4 is associated with juvenile rheumatoid arthritis, and HLA DR3 and DR4 are associated with juvenile onset diabetes. In chickens, possession of the histocompatibility antigens B[1] and B[4] is associated with increased severity of autoimmune thyroiditis. No doubt, many other associations will be found as our knowledge of the MHCs of the domestic animals increases.

MECHANISMS OF TISSUE DAMAGE IN AUTOIMMUNE DISEASE

Autoimmune Reactions Involving Type I Hypersensitivity

Milk allergy in cattle is an autoimmune disorder in which milk α casein, normally found only in the udder, gains access to the general circulation and so stimulates an immune response. This happens when milking is delayed and intramammary pressure forces milk proteins into the circulation. For some reason the immune response stimulated by α casein is of the IgE type, and affected cows show clinical signs of acute systemic anaphylaxis (Chapter 20). A similar condition is seen occasionally in other domestic animals such as the mare. Although antibodies in milk proteins are commonly found in human serum after rapid weaning, type I hypersensitivity is not a usual sequel.

Autoimmune Reactions Involving Type II Hypersensitivity

Autoantibodies directed against cell-surface antigens may cause lysis with the assistance of either complement or cytotoxic cells. If the autoantibodies are directed against erythrocytes, then autoimmune hemolytic anemia may result. If they are directed against platelets, thrombocytopenia will occur; and if they are directed against thyroid cells, thyroiditis will result. In one form of this reaction in humans with thyrotoxicosis, autoantibodies directed against thyroid stimulating hormone (TSH) receptors in the thyroid stimulate thyroid activity rather than mediate its destruction. This autoantibody is known as long acting thyroid stimulator (LATS). It is interesting to note that receptors are a common target of autoimmune attack. In addition to the TSH receptor in thyrotoxicosis, autoantibodies also attack the acetylcholine receptor in myasthenia gravis, the insulin receptor in some forms of diabetes in man and the β adrenergic receptor in some asthmatics.

Autoimmune Reactions Involving Type III Hypersensitivity

Autoantibodies will form immune complexes when bound to antigen, and these complexes may participate in type III hypersensitivity reactions. This occurs, for example, in systemic lupus erythematosus in the dog, a disease in which a wide variety of autoantibodies are produced, the most significant of which are those directed against nucleic acids. DNA-antibody complexes are formed in affected animals and are deposited in glomeruli to provoke the development of a membranous glomerulonephritis (Chapter 22). Similarly, in rheumatoid arthritis, immune complexes formed between rheumatoid factor (the antibody) and IgG (the antigen) are deposited in joints and, by fixing complement, contribute to the local inflammatory response.

Autoimmune Reactions Involving Type IV Hypersensitivity

Many lesions in autoimmune diseases are heavily infiltrated with mononuclear cells, and it is probable, therefore, that autosensitized T lymphocytes may contribute to the pathogenesis of disease of this type. Examples of such diseases include autoimmune thyroiditis, in which thyroid antigens may be shown to cause macrophage migration inhibition; experimental allergic encephalitis, in which cytotoxic T cells can cause demyelination; ulcerative colitis, in which cytotoxic T cells may destroy colon cells growing in culture; and dermatomyositis, in which cytotoxic T cells cause damage to striated muscle cells. Another example of a disease that may in some cases be due to a cell-mediated autoimmune response is juvenile diabetes mellitus in humans. In some cases of diabetes, lymphocytes have been shown to be cytotoxic for pancreatic islet cells.

Autoimmunity and Left-Handedness

It has been noticed in man that left-handed individuals are more likely to develop autoimmune diseases than right-handed individuals. Thus in one study, 11 per cent of left-handed individuals and 4 per cent of right-handed individuals suffered from autoimmune diseases—mainly autoimmune thyroiditis, ulcerative colitis and celiac disease. The reasons for this are very obscure. It has been suggested, however, that left-handedness and immune malfunction may both result from abnormal endocrine function in fetal life.

ADDITIONAL SOURCES OF INFORMATION

Fauci AS. 1980. Immunoregulation in autoimmunity. J. Allergy Clin. Immunol. *66* 5–17.

Hang L, Aguado MT, Dixon FJ and Theofilopoulous AN. 1985. Induction of severe autoimmune disease in normal mice by simultaneous action of multiple immunostimulators. J. Exp. Med. *161* 423–428.

Janeway C. 1982. Beneficial autoimmunity. Nature *299* 396–397.

Kahn CR. 1982. Autoimmunity and the etiology of insulin-dependent diabetes mellitus. Nature *299* 16–16.

Khansari N and Fudenberg MH. 1983. Immune elimination of autologous senescent erythrocytes by Kupffer cells *in vivo*. Cell. Immunol. *80* 426–430.

Lahita RG. 1984. Sex steroids and autoimmunity. Adv. Inflamm. Res. *8* 143–164.

Marx JL. 1982. Autoimmunity in left-handers. Science *217* 141–144.

Shoenfeld Y and Schwartz RS. 1984. Immunologic and genetic factors in autoimmune diseases. N. Engl. J. Med. *311* 1019–1029.

25

Autoimmunity: Specific Diseases

Autoimmune diseases may be divided into those affecting a single organ or tissue and those in which a wide variety of organs or tissues are affected.

ORGAN-SPECIFIC AUTOIMMUNE DISEASES

Autoimmune Thyroiditis

Dogs, humans and chickens suffer from a naturally occurring autoimmune thyroiditis. The disease in dogs is associated with the presence of autoantibodies against thyroglobulin, against thyroid follicular cell microsomes and against a thyroid colloid antigen. It is seen in Great Danes, Irish setters, beagles, and Old English sheepdogs. There is a major genetic component involved, and dogs related to affected animals commonly have anti-thyroid antibodies although they may be clinically normal. Affected dogs may also show a delayed hypersensitivity reaction to intradermally injected thyroid extract, suggesting that cell-mediated autoimmune mechanisms may also participate in the disease process. Histologically, the thyroid of affected animals is infiltrated with plasma cells and with large and small lymphocytes to such an extent that germinal center formation may occur (Fig. 25–1).

The clinical signs of autoimmune thyroiditis are those of hypothyroidism, that is, the animals are fat and inactive, they show patchy hair loss and they are relatively infertile. Tests of thyroid function such as plasma-bound-

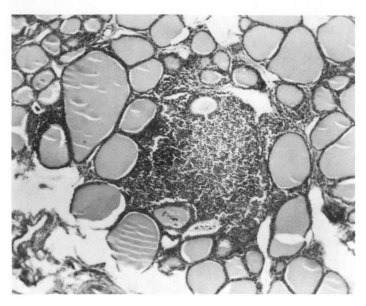

Figure 25–1. A lymphocytic nodule in the thyroid of a dog suffering from autoimmune thyroiditis. ×100. (From a specimen kindly provided by Dr. B. N. Wilkie.)

iodine levels tend to confirm the existence of hypothyroidism, but their usefulness depends upon the severity of the condition. In order to confirm the diagnosis of autoimmune thyroiditis, a thyroid biopsy must show the characteristic lymphocytic infiltration, and antithyroid antibodies must be detected in serum. These antibodies may be detected by a number of techniques. For example, a passive hemagglutination test using erythrocytes sensitized with thyroglobulin will detect antibodies to this hormone. A complement fixation test will detect antibodies directed against cytoplasmic antigens in thyroid follicular cells and an indirect fluorescent antibody test may detect antibodies to a thyroid colloid protein (not thyroglobulin). If none of these relatively sophisticated techniques is available to the clinician, an immunodiffusion test, in which the test serum is reacted against dog thyroid extract, may yield useful results. Appropriate negative controls should be incorporated in all these tests. Treatment of autoimmune thyroiditis involves replacement therapy with thyroxine or desiccated thyroid together with administration of steroids to suppress the immune response.

An autoimmune thyroiditis also occurs naturally in the OS (obese) strain of white Leghorn chickens. The thyroid tissue of these birds is heavily infiltrated by lymphocytes and plasma cells, which may organize to form germinal centers. Autoantibodies are directed against thyroglobulin, and affected birds are hypothyroid. These birds also possess antibodies against the adrenal gland, the exocrine pancreas and proventricular cells.

Avian autoimmune thyroiditis appears to

Diabetes Mellitus

Type I (insulin-dependent) diabetes mellitus in dogs is associated with marked atrophy of the pancreatic islets and a complete loss of beta cells. In some cases the islets may be infiltrated by lymphocytes. In man, this condition has been shown to be autoimmune in nature and associated with the development of islet cell autoantibodies. The situation in dogs remains very unclear. Thus, it has been possible to show positive immunofluorescence reactions on islet cell cytoplasm when the serum of many diabetic dogs is tested on sections of normal canine pancreas. Nevertheless, evidence suggests that these antibodies are not autoantibodies but are directed against the bovine or porcine insulin used to treat these dogs. The positive islet cell fluorescence may only be a cross-reaction between the antibodies to the foreign insulin and the insulin in the dog cells. It has not been possible to show anti-islet antibodies in the serum of untreated diabetic dogs.

result from the interaction of two genetically controlled lesions. First, there is a dysfunction of immune regulation. Thus, the B cells of these chickens make antithyroglobulin, a trait linked to the major histocompatibility complex. The T cells of these chickens also mature unusually early. As a result, autoimmune responses are stimulated before they can be prevented by suppressor cells. Second, these chickens have defective thyroid function in that they are refractory to thyroid stimulating hormone and they express class II MHC antigens on thyroid cells. Neonatal thymectomy prevents the development of lesions, but adult thymectomy may increase its severity by removing suppressor T cells, which presumably moderate the disease.

Autoimmune Encephalitis and Neuritis

Because brain antigens are normally sequestered behind the blood-brain barrier, it is relatively easy to induce an experimental autoimmune encephalitis. Known as experimental allergic encephalomyelitis (EAE), this condition may be produced by inoculating animals with brain tissue emulsified in Freund's complete adjuvant. After a few weeks, dogs or cats treated in this way develop erratic focal encephalitis and myelitis, possibly with paralysis; the brain lesions consist of focal vasculitis, mononuclear (lymphocyte and macrophage) infiltration associated with perivascular demyelination and some axon damage. It is possible to detect antibodies to brain tissue in the serum of these animals by means of a complement fixation test, although the lesion itself develops primarily as a result of a cell-mediated autoimmune response.

A clinically significant encephalitis, identical in many features to EAE, occurred following administration of older types of rabies vaccines containing phenolized brain tissue. The clinical signs of this postvaccinal encephalitis appeared between 4 and 15 days after vaccination. For this reason, suckling mouse brain tissue taken prior to myelination was used in the production of rabies vaccines. It is possible that postdistemper demyelinating leukoen-

cephalopathy is also of autoimmune origin (Chapter 16), although the production of antimyelin antibodies appears to be a frequent sequel to central nervous tissue destruction, regardless of its cause. In addition, the histopathology of postdistemper encephalitis is distinctly different from canine EAE.

Neurological diseases of autoimmune origin have been reported in horses, dogs and man. Equine polyneuritis (neuritis of the cauda equina) is an uncommon condition of horses in which a polyneuritis affects the sacral and coccygeal nerves. Affected horses show paralysis of the tail, rectum and bladder with a localized anaesthesia in the same region. Equine polyneuritis may also be associated with facial and trigeminal paralysis. Histologically, affected nerves are degenerate and infiltrated with mononuclear cells. Affected horses possess circulating antibodies to a protein found in peripheral myelin called P_2. This same protein has been shown to be able to induce experimental allergic neuritis in laboratory rodents (see following information). It is therefore believed that an autoimmune attack on peripheral myelin is involved in the pathogenesis of equine polyneuritis. However, equine adenovirus 1 has been isolated from lesions of equine polyneuritis; therefore, its etiology is probably complex.

Coonhound paralysis is an acute polyneuritis that affects dogs following a bite or scratch from a raccoon. Its onset is associated with an ascending symmetrical flaccid paralysis with mild sensory impairment. The disease is self limiting, and if respiration is not impaired, dogs may be expected to recover. Histologically, affected nerves show demyelination and axonal degeneration with macrophage infiltration.

Coonhound paralysis and equine polyneuritis both resemble Guillain-Barré syndrome in man. This is an autoimmune disease brought about by autoantibodies directed against peripheral nerve proteins.

If sciatic nerve tissue is used to immunize experimental dogs, it provokes a disease called experimental allergic neuritis (EAN) (Fig. 25–2). The development of EAN follows a latent period of 6 to 14 days before an ascending polyneuritis develops, which causes grad-

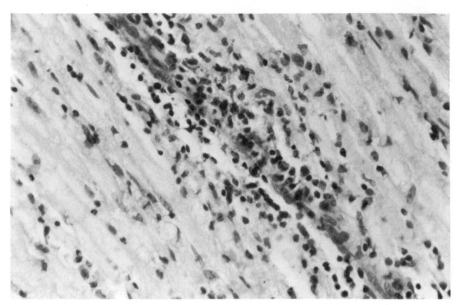

Figure 25–2. A section of rat sciatic nerve showing a mononuclear cell infiltration. This is the lesion of experimental allergic neuritis produced by inoculation of rat sciatic nerve in Freund's complete adjuvant. × 400. (Courtesy of Dr. B. N. Wilkie.)

ual paresis. EAN, therefore, resembles each of the diseases described previously. Treatment of Guillain-Barré syndrome in humans involves the use of steroids. It is logical to use them in the animal forms of the disease also.

Autoimmune Ocular Disease

The most common cause of blindness in horses is a condition called periodic ophthalmia. This disease arises as a result of recurrent attacks of an anterior uveitis (iridocyclitis). Each attack gets progressively more severe and gradually spreads to involve other eye tissues until complete blindness results. The lesions are infiltrated with lymphocytes and neutrophils, with extensive fibrin deposition. Affected horses can be shown to possess circulating antibodies to *Leptospira interrogans*. The titer of these antibodies tends to rise during a flareup of the lesion and drops while the lesion is in remission. If horses are inoculated with either equine cornea or with killed *L. interrogans* of certain serovars, they will develop corneal opacity. By means of gel diffusion it is possible to show partial antigenic identity between equine cornea and these *L. interrogans*

serovars. It is probable therefore that this disease is caused by an autoimmune attack on ocular tissues as a result of a cross-reactivity with *L. interrogans*.

Autoimmune Reproductive Diseases

Orchitis may be produced in animals such as bulls by administration of testicular extracts emulsified in Freund's complete adjuvant. Autoantibodies to sperm may also be detected in the serum of some animals, following injury to the testes or long-standing obstruction of the seminiferous ducts. A typical example of this occurs in male dogs infected with *Brucella canis*. These animals suffer from a chronic epididymitis and become sensitized by sperm antigens carried to the circulation after phagocytosis by macrophages. These sperm antigens stimulate the production of IgG or IgA autoantibodies. The autoantibodies agglutinate and immobilize sperm and, as a result, affected animals may be infertile. In cows, antibodies to sperm have been reported to arise as a result of the absorption through the vagina, uterus, fallopian tubes or peritoneum.

If these antibodies reach high levels, they may cause infertility. In certain lines of black mink, 20 to 30 per cent of the older males are infertile. This is associated with high levels of antisperm antibodies. The animals have a monocytic orchitis and extensive deposits of immune complexes along the basal lamina of the seminiferous tubules. Antisperm antibody can be eluted from the testes of these mink by the use of low pH buffer.

Dermatologists recognize an autoimmune dermatitis in which dogs develop a type I or type IV hypersensitivity to endogenous progesterone or estrogen. The condition is largely confined to intact female dogs and presents with pruritis, erythema and a papular eruption. Its development usually coincides with estrus or pseudopregnancy. Intradermal inoculation with the offending hormone may give rise to a local inflammatory response. Steroid treatment may have little effect, but testosterone may help.

If dogs are immunized with bovine or ovine luteinizing hormone (LH), then the antibodies produced may cross-react with canine LH and neutralize its activity. Similarly, it has proved possible to provoke autoantibodies that neutralize gonadotrophin releasing hormone in several species. As a result of both these procedures, the reproductive cycle is abolished in females and testicular, epididymal and prostatic atrophy occur in males, leading to sterility. This technique shows promise of becoming an effective immunological contraceptive method for animals.

In contrast, sheep immunized with polyandroalbumin (androstenedione-7, carboxyethyl thioester linked to human serum albumin) have about 23 per cent more lambs than untreated sheep. The ewes are given two doses of this prior to lambing. It is believed that this preparation stimulates the appearance of autoantibodies that reduce serum androstenedione levels.

Autoimmune Skin Diseases
(Fig. 25–3)

Dermatologists, unlike immunologists, have a tendency to use complicated terminology to describe relatively simple conditions. This is especially apparent in the nomenclature of the major autoimmune skin diseases. These diseases usually involve blister or vesicle formation in the skin, and dermatologists use the terms pemphigus or pemphigoid to describe them, after the Greek word *pemphix*, meaning a blister.

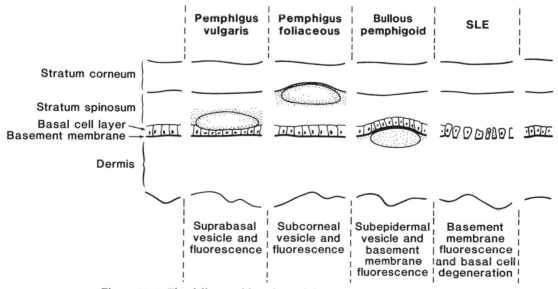

Figure 25–3. The differential histology of the autoimmune skin diseases.

Pemphigus

The term pemphigus applies to four rare skin diseases that occur in humans, dogs and cats. The most severe form is called pemphigus vulgaris. In this disease bullae (vesicles or blisters) develop around the mucocutaneous junctions, especially the nose, lips, eyes, prepuce and anus, and also on the tongue and the inner surface of the ear. These bullae are fragile and rupture readily, leaving weeping, denuded areas that may become secondarily infected. Histological examination of intact bullae shows a separation of the skin cells (acantholysis) in the suprabasal region of the lower epidermis (Figs. 25–4 and 25–5). Pemphigus vegetans is a very rare and mild variant of pemphigus vulgaris in which either bullae or pustules form, and papillomatous proliferation of the base of these occurs on healing.

Pemphigus foliaceous is a milder and more common disease than pemphigus vulgaris. It has been described in humans, dogs, cats, goats and horses. It, too, is a vesicular disease, but it is not confined so definitely to the mucocutaneous junctions, and it tends, at least in dogs, to present as a scaling eruptive der-

matitis. A high proportion of animals present with lesions on the head, ears or muzzle. Histological examination of the bullae reveals that the acantholysis and hence the vesicle formation occur superficially in the subcorneal region. The vesicles are very fragile and rarely persist. A milder variant of pemphigus foliaceous is known as pemphigus erythematosus. This may merely be an early stage of pemphigus foliaceous. The lesions in pemphigus erythematosus tend to be confined to the face and ears and are very similar to those of systemic lupus erythematosus.

All cases of pemphigus arise as a result of the formation of autoantibodies directed against intercellular cement in the skin. The correct diagnosis can only be arrived at by examination of histological sections. Immunofluorescence is of limited assistance in diagnosis because of the difficulties in locating the lesions precisely by this technique. The different location of the lesions of pemphigus vulgaris and pemphigus foliaceous is probably due to antigenic differences between intercellular cements in different regions of the skin. The autoantibodies, by binding to intercellular cement, induce nearby cells to release plas-

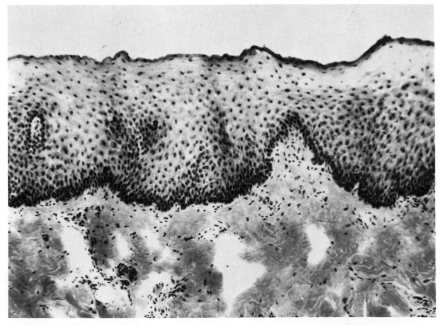

Figure 25–4. A section of normal canine squamous epithelium. Note the absence of clefts within the epithelium or between the epithelium and the underlying tissues. (From Bennett D. et al. 1980. Vet. Rec. *106* 497. Used with permission.)

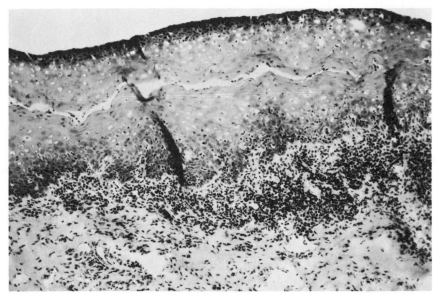

Figure 25–5. A section of an oral lesion of pemphigus vulgaris in a dog. Note the cleft formation at the base of the epidermis accompanied by extensive cellular infiltration. (From Bennett D. et al. 1980. Vet. Rec. *106* 497. Used with permission.)

minogen activator. This, in turn, causes the release of plasmin, which disrupts adhesion between cells to cause acantholysis and bulla formation. Direct immunofluorescent exami-

nation of skin lesions reveals immunoglobulins and complement deposited on the intercellular cement (Fig. 25–6).

It is important to differentiate between the

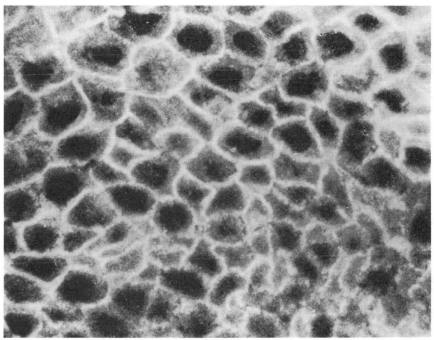

Figure 25–6. A direct immunofluorescent micrograph of a section of normal dog skin that has been incubated in serum from a dog suffering from pemphigus vulgaris. The intercellular cement is stained. (Courtesy of Dr. A. I. Hurvitz.) Compare this with Figure 11–6, which shows dog skin stained by the immunoperoxidase technique.

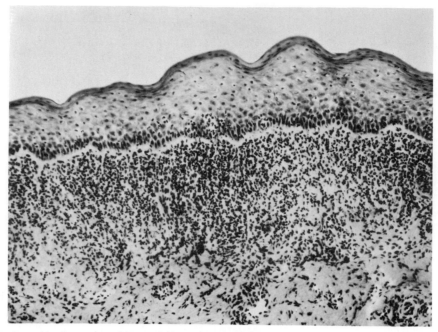

Figure 25–7. A section from an oral lesion of bullous pemphigoid in a dog. Note that the cleft is formed below the epidermis. Inflammatory cells are present in the superficial dermis as well as, to a lesser extent, the epithelium. (From Bennett D. et al. 1980. Vet. Rec. *106* 497. Used with permission.)

two major forms of pemphigus for prognostic reasons. Pemphigus vulgaris has a relatively poor prognosis; treatment tends to be unsatisfactory and the lesions are persistent. Owners of affected animals may become dissatisfied with the intractable disease and request euthanasia. In contrast, pemphigus foliaceous is milder, and the results of treatment may be more satisfactory. Treatment of either disease involves the use of large doses of corticosteroids with antibiotic cover. In refractory cases, cyclophosphamide, azathioprine or gold salts such as aurothioglucose may be of assistance. It may be necessary to continue the steroid treatment for a very long time, since the disease often recurs when treatment is stopped.

Bullous Pemphigoid

Bullous pemphigoid is a rare bullous skin disease in dogs and man. It resembles pemphigus vulgaris clinically. Multiple bullae develop around mucocutaneous junctions and in the groin and axillae. This disease differs from pemphigus vulgaris, however, in that the bul-

lae arise in the subepidermis (Fig. 25–7) and are therefore less likely to rupture. Bullae tend to be filled with fibrin as well as mononuclear cells or eosinophils, and they heal spontaneously. Bullous pemphigoid is associated with the presence of autoantibodies directed against the basement membrane of the skin and mucous membranes. The deposition of IgG (occasionally IgA) on the basement membrane may be demonstrated by immunofluorescent staining. The prognosis of bullous pemphigoid is usually poor, but some mild cases may recover after treatment with low doses of steroids. More commonly aggressive treatment is necessary. This requires high doses of prednisolone, supplemented, if necessary, with cyclophosphamide, azathioprine, chlorambucil or gold salts.

Dermatitis Herpetiformis

Another autoimmune skin disease that has been reported to occur in dogs is dermatitis herpetiformis. In this disease the autoantibodies are directed against antigens in dermal papillae and are usually of the IgA isotype.

Clinically, the lesions are pustular and papular, resembling pyoderma, although there are also eosinophil-filled subepidermal vesicles. Characteristically, the lesions involve the extensor surface of the limbs and are intensely pruritic. The drug dapsone is the specific treatment for this condition.

Alopecia Areata

Rounded spots of hair loss in the absence of obvious inflammation characterize this disease of man, dogs and cats. It may be autoimmune in origin, since the hair loss is associated with lymphoid infiltration into the hair follicles and C3, IgG or IgM may be detected in the follicles by immunofluorescence. Alopecia areata responds to corticosteroid treatment.

Autoimmune Nephritis

There are two immunopathogenic types of glomerulonephritis. In the immune complex type (type III hypersensitivity), immune complexes containing complement are deposited in a lumpy, granular fashion on glomerular basement membranes (GBM) (see Fig. 22–9). In contrast, if autoantibodies are produced against GBM antigens, they become deposited in a smooth, linear fashion. These anti-GBM antibodies may be produced experimentally in animals, but they may also arise spontaneously in a condition known as Goodpasture's syndrome in humans. In this condition, the autoantibodies react not only with the GBM but also with the basement membrane of pulmonary alveolar septae and capillaries. No condition exactly parallel to Goodpasture's syndrome has been observed to arise spontaneously in animals. However, horses may develop antibodies to GBMs, which may provoke a glomerulonephritis. Clinically, the condition is characterized by signs of renal failure. Immunofluorescent studies of the kidneys of affected animals show the basement membrane to be evenly coated with a smooth, linear deposit of immunoglobulin. As discussed earlier (Chapter 22), these deposits provoke a proliferative response in the glomerular epithelial cells, which, if severe, may result in epithelial crescent formation.

Autoimmune Hemolytic Anemia (AIHA)

Autoantibodies to erythrocytes will provoke erythrocyte destruction and thus cause an anemia. This destruction is due either to intravascular hemolysis mediated through complement or, much more commonly, to removal of antibody-coated erythrocytes by the macrophages of the spleen and liver. AIHA is not uncommon in dogs and cats and has been described in horses and cattle. It occurs more often in females by a 2:1 ratio. The average age of onset is around 4 to 5 years. German shepherds, Irish setters, Old English sheepdogs, miniature daschunds, Scottish terriers, Vizslas, and American cocker spaniels appear to have a relatively high susceptibility to the condition. There is good evidence for a genetic predisposition to the condition. It is commonly associated with other autoimmune disorders, such as systemic lupus erythematosus and autoimmune thrombocytopenia, and with lymphoid tumors such as feline leukemia. Its onset may be associated with obvious stress such as vaccination using modified live viruses, viral disease or hormonal imbalances such as pregnancy or pyometra. Usually, however, AIHA develops without any obvious predisposing cause.

Autoimmune hemolytic anemias may be divided into two major groups, depending upon whether the autoantibody is of the IgG or IgM isotype (Table 25–1).

AIHA Mediated by IgG Antibodies

AIHA mediated by IgG antibodies may present as an anemia of rapid or gradual onset. Affected dogs become weak, possibly jaundiced and hemoglobin may appear in the urine. Most cases of AIHA in dogs and cats are caused by IgG antibodies, which react optimally with red cells at 37°C. Since IgG antibodies are relatively small, they are unable to counteract the zeta potential of the red cells and therefore will usually not cause direct agglutination. In a very small proportion of cases, the IgG antibodies may cause direct agglutination, which may then be observed when the blood is withdrawn. Since IgG does

Table 25–1 COMPARISON OF THE MAJOR FORMS OF AUTOIMMUNE HEMOLYTIC ANEMIA

	IgG-Mediated	IgM-Mediated
Optimal temperature	37°C	4° or 37°C
Action of antibody	Incomplete (rarely direct agglutination)	Direct agglutination (4°C) Incomplete antibody (4°C) Hemolysis (37°C)
Fate of erythrocytes	Splenic phagocytosis	Hepatic phagocytosis Intravascular hemolysis
Major clinical findings	Progressive anemia	Necrosis of extremities Progressive anemia
Treatment	Steroids, cytotoxic drugs, splenectomy	Steroids, cytotoxic drugs
Prognosis	Fair to good	Poor

not activate complement efficiently, intravascular hemolysis is not a feature of this form of AIHA. The red cells, however, are destroyed by phagocytosis in the spleen. In very severe cases, a blood smear may show extensive erythrophagocytosis by neutrophils and monocytes, although jaundice is uncommon. Most of these animals also have hepatosplenomegaly and lymphadenopathy. IgG-mediated AIHA is diagnosed by demonstrating the presence of nonagglutinating (or incomplete) antibodies on the animal's red cells. This is done by means of a direct antiglobulin or Coombs' test (Chapter 11), which must be performed before the dog is treated with corticosteroids or false-negative results may result. The erythrocytes of the affected animal are first washed to remove free serum and then exposed to an antiglobulin serum. Erythrocytes coated with autoantibody will be agglutinated. If the antiglobulin serum possesses anticomplement (anti-C3) activity, it may give a false-positive reaction, since positive complement reactions of this type are not uncommon in canine internal diseases.

Treatment of AIHA involves specific management of the anemia and administration of corticosteroids to cause immunosuppression and to reduce erythrophagocytosis. The animal may respond within 24 to 48 hours. Once the animal's condition is stabilized, the dose of steroids should be reduced to as low a level as possible without permitting the patient to relapse. Steroid treatment may be supplemented with cyclophosphamide in acute cases. Splenectomy may be of assistance in refractory cases.

AIHA Mediated by IgM Antibodies

IgM autoantibodies mediate a different type of disease from that caused by IgG. Some IgM antibodies that act at 37°C activate complement and thus provoke intravascular hemolysis. Other IgM anti-erythrocyte antibodies cannot agglutinate red cells at body temperature but agglutinate them when the blood is chilled. These antibodies are then called cold agglutinins. As blood circulates through the extremities (tail, toes, ears, etc.) of an affected animal it may be cooled sufficiently to permit erythrocyte agglutination within capillaries. This can lead to vascular stasis, tissue ischemia and, eventually, necrosis. Affected animals may therefore present with necrotic lesions at the extremities of the body. Anemia may or may not be a significant feature. As might be anticipated, this form of AIHA is most severe during the winter.

Cold agglutinins can be detected by cooling a blood sample to below 20°C, at which point clumping will occur. The agglutination is reversed upon rewarming. Other cold-acting antibodies may combine with red cells when chilled but will not agglutinate them. These antibodies can only be identified by an antiglobulin test conducted at 4°C.

AIHA due to direct-acting agglutinins or to hemolysis is usually of acute onset, is rapidly progressive and has a poor prognosis. Steroids and cyclophosphamide may be used to treat the affected animal. Splenectomy is of little assistance in IgM-mediated AIHA, since the erythrocytes are largely destroyed in the liver.

Acute anemias have been observed in

horses following infection with *Streptococcus fecalis*, in sheep following leptospirosis and in pigs with eperythrozoonosis. In these cases cold agglutinins are produced that are capable of clumping erythrocytes from normal animals of the same species when chilled.

Hemoglobin itself may act as an autoantigen on occasion. Antihemoglobin antibodies are detectable in the serum of cattle severely infected with *Corynebacterium pyogenes*, perhaps as a result of bacterial hemolysis. The clinical significance of this is not clear.

Immune Suppression of Hematopoiesis

It has been demonstrated in humans, and surmised in dogs, that autoimmune responses may be directed against hematopoietic stem cells. For example, autoantibodies to erythroid precursors may give rise to red cell aplasia, and autoantibodies to myeloid precursors may provoke an immune neutropenia. These conditions can only be diagnosed by demonstrating these autoantibodies by immunofluorescence on bone marrow smears.

Autoimmune Thrombocytopenia

Autoimmune thrombocytopenia (AITP) may be induced by the development of antiplatelet autoantibodies. This condition has been reported in horses, dogs and cats. Affected animals usually present with a tendency to bleed from the skin and mucus membranes. Petechiae occur in the skin, gingiva and conjunctiva. If severe, epistaxis may occur and the dog may show melena and hematuria. Blood tests show a severe thrombocytopenia (<50,000/μl). The condition is very commonly observed in conjunction with AIHA, systemic lupus erythematosus, solid tumors and lymphoproliferative disorders.

Antibodies to platelets may be measured by several techniques, including agglutination, complement fixation, immunofluorescence on megakaryocytes and antiglobulin tests. However, the best test for this purpose is one that measures the release of factor 3 from platelets as a result of exposure to antibodies directed against the platelet membrane. This may be performed by incubating platelet-rich plasma with a globulin fraction of the serum being tested and then estimating the amount of procoagulant activity released into the supernatant fluid. In about 75 per cent of cases the antibodies are of the IgG isotype.

Steroids are used to treat AITP, since they lower the titer of antiplatelet antibody and reduce platelet sequestration by mononuclear phagocytes. As with AIHA, splenectomy or azathioprine treatment, or both, may be of assistance in the control of patients who do not respond to steroid therapy.

Sjögren's Syndrome

In Sjögren's syndrome, which has been described in both humans and dogs, autoimmunity develops against exocrine glands, most notably the lacrimal and salivary glands. As a result, the secretion of these glands is greatly reduced, and affected animals suffer from corneal dryness, leading to keratoconjunctivitis sicca and xerostomia (mouth dryness). These animals subsequently develop gingivitis, dental caries and excessive thirst.

Sjögren's syndrome is often associated with rheumatoid arthritis, systemic lupus erythematosus, polymyositis and autoimmune thyroiditis. The first two cases described in dogs were found in a colony maintained for investigations into canine systemic lupus erythematosus. Affected dogs develop antibodies to nictitating membrane epithelial cells and, less consistently, to lacrimal and salivary glands or to the pancreas, and these tissues may be extensively infiltrated with lymphocytes. A high proportion of affected animals are hypergammaglobulinemic and have antinuclear antibodies and rheumatoid factor. Many affected animals have other autoimmune conditions such as polyarthritis, hypothyroidism or glomerulonephritis. The triad of keratoconjunctivitis sicca, xerostomia and rheumatoid factor is considered to constitute classic Sjögren's syndrome. The condition may be treated by palliative dentistry and artificial tears. It would be logical to use immunosuppressive agents in refractory cases.

AUTOIMMUNE MUSCLE DISEASES

Myasthenia Gravis

Myasthenia gravis, a disease of humans, dogs and cats, is a disorder of skeletal muscle characterized by the occurrence of abnormal fatigue and weakness after relatively mild exercise. For example, a dog with myasthenia gravis will collapse exhausted after trotting for only a few yards. Myasthenia gravis occurs as a result of a blockage or deficiency of acetylcholine receptors on the motor end plate of striated muscle. In Jack Russell terriers, springer spaniels and fox terriers, a congenital form of the disease occurs as a result of an inherited deficiency of receptors. It is, therefore, a disease of young dogs. In adult dogs, however, an acetylcholine receptor deficiency occurs as a result of the production of autoantibodies to the receptor proteins and their accelerated destruction. It is possible to demonstrate the presence of these antireceptor antibodies by means of a radioimmunoassay. As a result of this destruction, the number of effective acetylcholine receptors is severely reduced (Fig. 25–8). Consequently, the end plate potentials induced at the neuromuscular junctions fall below threshold levels and fail to trigger the muscle to contract. Repeating the stimulus is ineffective, since the few available receptors are saturated with acetylcholine.

In some animals with myasthenia gravis, the thymus may show medullary hyperplasia, germinal center formation or even a thymoma. Since normal thymus tissue contains a population of "myoid" cells, striated muscle cells that possess acetylcholine receptors of their own, it is possible that the thymic changes result from immunological attack on myoid cells. Alternatively, since the thymic hormone thymopoietin is capable of neuromuscular blocking activity, thymoma-associated myasthenia may be due to excessive thymopoietin production. This is supported by the observation in humans that thymectomy usually, but not always, leads to significant remission of the disease.

Myasthenia gravis is a clinically obvious disease, and it is not normally necessary to resort to laboratory tests. Administration of a short-acting anticholinesterase such as edrophonium will lead to dramatic clinical improvement within seconds. The anticholinesterase, by permitting the acetylcholine to persist at the neuromuscular junction, enables the remaining receptors to be stimulated more effectively.

Myasthenia gravis is treated by means of long-acting anticholinesterase drugs such as pyridostigmine or neostigmine. In humans with myasthenia gravis, immunosuppressive therapy with corticosteroids, plasmapheresis and cyclophosphamide has been used with success. In dogs the disease tends to be self-limiting, unlike in humans. However, it is

Normal motor end plate
- ● Acetylcholine
- ◆ Acetylcholinesterase

In myasthenia gravis

Myasthenia gravis treated with anticholinesterase drugs

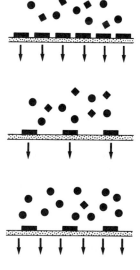

Figure 25–8. The mechanism of myasthenia gravis and its treatment. The destruction of acetylcholine receptors prevents effective neuromuscular transmission. Blockage of cholinesterase activity by anticholinesterase drugs permits acetylcholine to accumulate and so enhances neuromuscular transmission.

commonly complicated by a myositis, cytopenias, megaesophagus or myocarditis. Treatment with pyridostigmine and prednisolone is probably the preferred method of managing myasthenia gravis, and any thymoma should, of course, be removed.

Dermatomyositis

This is a disease of humans and collie dogs characterized by the presence of severe inflammatory lesions in skin and muscle. The cause of dermatomyositis is unknown, although it is conventionally regarded as being autoimmune in origin. The condition in collies is inherited.

The inflammatory lesions in muscle consist of multifocal accumulations of lymphocytes, plasma cells and macrophages. These lymphocytes can be shown in man to be cytotoxic for muscle cells *in vitro*. It is, therefore, assumed that the muscle lesions develop as a result of cell-mediated destruction. The severity of the disease is related to the level of circulating immune complexes and serum IgG levels. Although autoantibodies to muscle are not believed to play a direct role in the pathogenesis of the disease, the appearance of immune complexes prior to the development of lesions suggests that they contribute to their development. In severely affected dogs, circulating immune complexes remain at a high level while, in mildly affected dogs, the level of immune complexes tends to return to normal levels. Vaccination of puppies appears, in some cases, to provoke the onset of disease.

AUTOIMMUNE ARTHRITIS

Rheumatoid Arthritis

Rheumatoid arthritis is a common, crippling disease in humans that is also seen in domestic animals, especially dogs. Although, as its name suggests, it typically involves the joints, other body systems are commonly affected. Dogs with rheumatoid arthritis may present with depression, anorexia and pyrexia in addition to lameness, which tends to be most severe after inactivity (for example, immediately after awakening in the morning) and mainly affects peripheral joints, which show swelling and stiffness. The joint swelling is often symmetrical. Rheumatoid arthritis tends to pursue a progressive course and eventually leads to severe joint destruction and deformities. In advanced cases the joints may even fuse as the result of the formation of bony ankyloses. Radiological findings are variable, but the swelling is generally seen to involve soft tissues only, and there may be subchondral rarefaction, cartilage erosion and narrowing of the joint space.

The disease commences as a synovitis characterized by extensive infiltration by neutrophils. As the disease progresses, the synovia begin to swell and proliferate. Outgrowths of this proliferating synovia extend into the joint cavities, where they are known as pannus. Pannus consists of fibrous vascular tissue, that, as it invades the joint cavity, releases proteolytic enzymes that erode the articular cartilage and the neighboring bony structures. As the arthritis progresses, the infiltrating neutrophils may be partially replaced by lymphocytes, which can form lymphoid nodules and germinal centers. Another feature of rheumatoid arthritis that is commonly encountered is the development of subcutaneous nodules—necrotic foci surrounded by fibrous connective tissue containing lymphocytes and plasma cells. In addition, amyloidosis, disseminated arteritis, glomerulonephritis and lymphatic hyperplasia are occasional complications.

The immediate cause of rheumatoid arthritis is unknown. It is probably due to the chronic deposition of immune complexes in synovia. The offending antigen has not been identified, but there are two prime suspects, IgG and collagen.

The development of autoantibodies to IgG is characteristic of rheumatoid arthritis. These IgM autoantibodies, called rheumatoid factors, are directed against epitopes on the C_H2 domains of antigen-bound IgG. Rheumatoid factors are found not only in rheumatoid arthritis but also in systemic lupus erythematosus (SLE) and other conditions in which extensive immune complex formation occurs.

Rheumatoid factors may be detected by allowing them to agglutinate antibody-coated particles. In humans, latex beads coated with

IgG are used for this purpose. In dogs, it is easier to make a canine antisheep erythrocyte serum and to coat sheep erythrocytes with this in a subagglutinating dose. After washing, these erythrocytes will agglutinate when mixed with positive dog serum. In humans this technique is known as the Rose-Waaler test.

Although rheumatoid factors are of great diagnostic importance, their clinical significance is unclear. Rheumatoid factors can be found in joint fluid, where their titer tends to correlate with the severity of the lesions, and the lesions themselves may be exacerbated by intra-articular inoculation of autologous immunoglobulins. Nevertheless, some individuals with rheumatoid arthritis may not have detectable rheumatoid factors, and it is not uncommon to find humans who have no arthritis despite the presence of rheumatoid factor in their serum.

Other evidence suggests that autoantibodies to collagen may contribute to the development of rheumatoid arthritis. Thus, affected humans develop a cell-mediated reactivity to denatured collagen II and III, and horses with chronic, nonsuppurative arthritis develop antibodies to horse collagens I and II. An experimental autoimmune disease that closely resembles rheumatoid arthritis is seen in rats immunized with type II collagen.

Rheumatoid arthritis also has an important cell-mediated component. Synovial fluid in these cases contains a variety of lymphocyte- and macrophage-derived products such as macrophage migration inhibitory factors and IL-1 as well as an arthritogenic lymphokine that produces an erosive proliferative synovitis when injected into joints.

Over many years, attempts have been made to associate rheumatoid arthritis with infectious agents. Mycoplasmas such as *Mycoplasma hyorhinis* and bacteria such as *Erysipelothrix rhusiopathiae* produce a chronic nonsuppurative arthritis in pigs with a histological picture very similar to that seen in rheumatoid arthritis in humans. In spite of this and occasional reports of the isolation of bacteria or mycoplasmas from rheumatoid joints, no definite evidence is yet available to substantiate an infectious basis for this condition.

Diagnosis of rheumatoid arthritis in animals (Table 25–2) is generally based on the criteria established for human rheumatoid arthritis. At least five of the major clinical features should be present and any one of the first five shown in Table 25–2 should have been present for at least six weeks. In addition, steps should be taken to exclude SLE (by testing for antinuclear antibody) and to exclude an infectious cause for the arthritis.

Nonsteroidal antiinflammatory drugs (NSAIDs) such as acetylsalicylic acid are the first choice in treating early, uncomplicated cases of rheumatoid arthritis. Steroids such as prednisolone should be reserved for late, severe cases in which salicylates have proved inadequate. Local injections into affected joints will produce rapid relief and clinical remission. However, the joints are still subjected to stress and the steroids delay healing. Continued use may therefore permit articular damage to proceed unabated. Steroids may also induce a synovitis. Immunosuppressive drugs such as cyclophosphamide may also be useful. In human medicine gold salts such as sodium aurothiomalate and aurothioglucose and antimalarials such as chloroquine are com-

Table 25–2 THE DIAGNOSTIC CRITERIA FOR CANINE RHEUMATOID ARTHRITIS

Any five of the following signs must be present. One of the first five features on the list must be present for at least six weeks, and ANA or LE tests must be negative.

   Morning stiffness
   Pain on moving a joint
   Soft tissue swelling
   Swelling of at least one other joint within a three-
      month period
   Symmetrical joint swelling
   Subcutaneous nodules
   Consistent radiographic findings
   Presence of rheumatoid factor
   Characteristic synovial histology
   Characteristic nodule histology
   Poor mucin production in synovial fluid*

*This diagnostic test involves treating a synovial fluid sample with glacial acetic acid. This causes the protein in the sample to clot. The clot from normal joint fluid forms a solid mass. The clot from rheumatoid joints tends to be loose and friable.

monly used with success. However experience with these in animals is limited.

Feline Chronic Progressive Polyarthritis

This disease of male cats is characterized by polyarthritis with either osteopenia and periosteal new bone formation, periarticular erosions and eventual collapse or subchondral erosions, joint instabilities and deformities closely resembling those of rheumatoid arthritis. Affected cats may be infected with feline syncytia-forming virus or feline leukemia virus, or both. It is described here because of suggestions that it is of immunological origin. These suggestions are based on the massive lymphocyte and plasma cell infiltration of affected joints and the presence of an immune complex type of glomerulonephritis. However, affected cats are rheumatoid factor- and ANA-negative, and their serum immunoglobulin levels tend to be close to normal.

Rupture of the Cruciate Ligament

A high percentage of the sera and synovial fluid from dogs with ruptured cruciate ligaments contain immune complexes. It is believed that this is a secondary phenomenon and not a cause of the condition.

DISEASES OF WIDE ORGAN SPECIFICITY ASSOCIATED WITH AUTOIMMUNE COMPONENTS

In addition to the organ-specific autoimmune conditions discussed so far, there exist a number of diseases that involve many organs throughout the body and that are, at least in part, autoimmune.

Systemic Lupus Erythematosus

Systemic lupus erythematosus (SLE) is a generalized immunological disorder that has been described in humans, dogs and cats. About 75 per cent of the reported canine cases have occurred in females. Collies and Shetland sheepdogs appear to be especially susceptible.

SLE occurs as a result of an increase in the production of polyclonal immunoglobulins above the background level. In some, but not all, cases this has been associated with defective suppressor cell function. As a result of this loss of control, affected animals make autoantibodies against a great range of normal organs and tissues. These multiple autoantibodies in turn give rise to a wide spectrum of pathological lesions and clinical manifestations.

One consistent feature of SLE is the development of autoantibodies against nucleic acids. About sixteen different nucleic acid antigens have been described, but little is known about their biological roles or significance. The most important of these are antibodies to DNA. These autoantibodies can cause damage by several mechanisms. They can combine with free DNA to form DNA–anti-DNA immune complexes. These immune complexes may be deposited in glomeruli, causing a membranous glomerulonephritis (Chapter 22) and giving rise to a "wire-loop" lesion in the glomerular tufts. The complexes may also be deposited in arteriolar walls, where they result in local fibrinoid necrosis and fibrosis, or in synovia, where they provoke arthritis. Antinuclear antibodies also bind to the nuclei of degenerating cells. In tissues this results in the presence of round or oval bodies of DNA bound to antibody. Known as hematoxylin bodies, these are found in the skin, kidney, lung, lymph nodes, spleen and heart. Within the blood stream these "opsonized" nuclei may be phagocytosed, giving rise to the structures known as lupus erythematosus (LE) cells (Fig. 25–9). LE cells are found mainly in bone marrow and, less commonly, in blood.

Although antibodies to nucleic acids are important features of SLE, a great variety of other autoantibodies are also produced. Autoantibodies to red cells, for example, commonly give rise to an antiglobulin-positive hemolytic anemia. Antibodies to platelets give rise to an immunologically mediated thrombocytopenia.

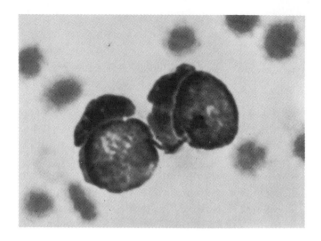

Figure 25–9. Two LE cells from a dog with SLE. × 1000. (From Quimby F. W. et al. Am. J. Vet. Res. 41 1662. Used with permission.)

Antilymphocyte antibodies may be present, and it is suggested that they may selectively destroy suppressor cells, thus enhancing the excessive immune reactivity. Antimuscle antibodies may provoke myositis, and antimyocardial antibodies may provoke myocarditis or endocarditis. Antibodies to skin components give rise to a bilaterally symmetrical dermatitis characterized by changes in the thickness of the epidermis, focal mononuclear cell infiltration, collagen degeneration and immunoglobulin deposits at the dermo-epidermal junction (see Fig. 25–3). These deposits form what is known as a "lupus band" and are seen in many other autoimmune skin disorders in addition to SLE. The lesions are commonly restricted to the bridge of the nose and the area around the eyes, since they are exacerbated by sunlight.

The results of this grossly excessive immune reactivity are also reflected in a polyclonal hypergammaglobulinemia, enlargement of lymph nodes with medullary disruption and thymic enlargement with germinal center formation.

The great variety of autoantibodies produced in SLE can give rise to an equally great variety of clinical manifestations. Polyarthritis, fever, proteinuria, anemia and skin diseases are the most common abnormalities. However, pericarditis, myocarditis, myositis, lymphadenopathy and pneumonitis have all been reported. A simple diagnostic rule could, therefore, be stated as follows: Suspect SLE in an animal with multiple disorders such as those described previously and either a posi-

tive test for antinuclear antibodies or a positive test for LE cells (Table 25–3).

Antinuclear antibodies (ANA) are normally demonstrated by immunofluorescence (Fig. 25–10). Cultured cells or frozen sections of mouse or rat liver on a microscope slide are used as a source of antigen. Dilutions of a patient's serum are applied to this, and the material is incubated and then washed off. The binding of antinuclear antibodies to the cell nuclei is revealed by incubating the tissue in a fluorescein-labeled antiserum to canine or feline immunoglobulins and then rewashing. A variety of different nuclear staining patterns have been described for humans, and their clinical correlations have been analyzed. In animals, staining patterns have been less thoroughly investigated, and their significance is currently unclear. Evidence suggests, however, that a homogeneous staining pattern or staining of the nuclear rim is of greatest diagnostic significance but that nucleolar fluorescence is not. Some normal dogs, dogs undergoing treatment with certain drugs (e.g., griseofulvin, penicillin, sulfonamides, tetra-

Table 25–3 THE DIAGNOSTIC CRITERIA FOR SYSTEMIC LUPUS ERYTHEMATOSUS

Any two of the following:
  Characteristic skin lesions
  Polyarthritis
  Antiglobulin-positive hemolytic anemia
  Thrombocytopenia
  Proteinuria
and either
  A positive ANA test or a positive LE cell test

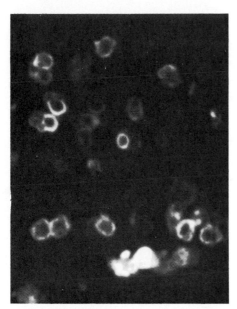

Figure 25–10. A positive ANA reaction (titer 1:160) showing rim fluorescence, from a dog with SLE. × 450. (From Quimby, F. W. et al. 1980. Am. J. Vet. Res. 41 1662. Used with permission.)

cyclines, phenytoin and procainamide) and some dogs with liver disease or lymphosarcoma may have detectable antinuclear antibodies, so this test must not be used as the only diagnostic test for SLE.

LE cells, as previously described, are polymorphonuclear neutrophils (PMNs) that have phagocytosed nuclei from dead and dying cells. They therefore look somewhat like binucleated cells (see Fig. 25–9). Their presence may be detected in the bone marrow and occasionally in buffy coat preparations from animals with SLE. It is usually necessary, however, to produce them *in vitro*. This can be accomplished by allowing the blood of an affected animal to clot and then incubating it at 37°C for two hours. During this time, normal PMNs will phagocytose the nuclei of any dying or damaged cells. The clot is then disrupted by pressing it through a fine mesh; the resulting cell suspension is centrifuged, and the buffy coat is smeared, stained and examined. The presence of LE cells is pathognomonic for SLE, but their absence does not disprove its diagnosis, since only 60 per cent of affected animals are positive in any one sample.

Pathogenesis of SLE (Fig. 25–11)

Although it is clear that SLE involves a loss of control of the specificity of the B cell response with resulting multiple autoimmune disorders, the initiating cause remains obscure. There is good evidence for a genetic predisposition in humans, dogs and mice. SLE is, for example, associated with the presence of certain class II histocompatibility antigens in man. Environmental factors also play an important role. For example, the skin lesions are aggravated by exposure to sunlight. Hormones clearly influence the development of the disease as shown by its tendency to occur in women and its exacerbation during pregnancy.

Virus infections may be responsible for initiation of the condition. Thus, individuals with SLE commonly have high titered antibodies to parainfluenza 1 and measles. Myxovirus-like structures have been observed within renal endothelial cells from SLE patients, and type C retroviruses have been isolated from SLE patients and associated with the disease.

When dogs affected by SLE are bred, the number of affected offspring is higher than can be accounted for genetically, suggesting that the condition may be vertically transmitted. Cell-free filtrates from asymptomatic but LE cell-positive dogs, when administered to newborn mice, have been reported to provoke the appearance of antinuclear antibodies and the development of some lymphoid tumors. Type C retroviruses have been isolated from these tumors, and antisera to these viruses may be used to demonstrate viral antigen on the lymphocytes and in the glomeruli of humans with SLE. Cell-free filtrates of these mouse tumors have also been reported to induce the formation of antinuclear antibodies and the production of LE cells in newborn puppies.

Treatment of SLE

SLE usually responds well to corticosteroids (prednisolone) accompanied if necessary by cyclophosphamide, azathioprine or chlorambucil. Levamisole (Chapter 27) has also been used with success. However, more drastic

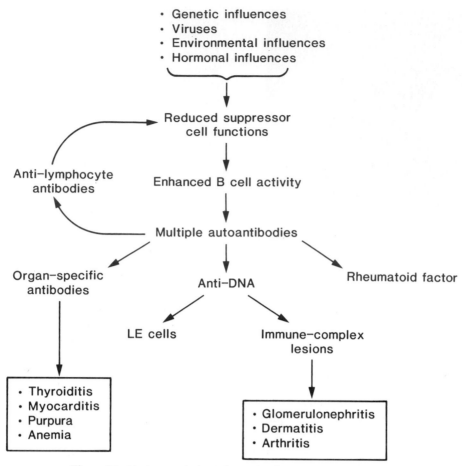

Figure 25–11. A speculative scheme for the pathogenesis of SLE.

measures such as plasmapheresis may be needed in refractory cases.

Discoid Lupus Erythematosus

Discoid lupus erythematosus is a mild, uncommon variant of SLE characterized by the occurrence of facial skin lesions and by the absence of other pathological lesions as well as negative ANA and LE tests. The most common abnormality in affected dogs is a nasal dermatitis with depigmentation, erythema, erosion, ulceration, scaling and crusting. Occasionally the feet may be affected, and some dogs may have ulcers in the oral cavity. Immunofluorescence tests may detect C3, IgA, IgG and IgM in the skin basement membrane in a dense, granular pattern (the lupus band). The skin lesions may be infiltrated with mono-

nuclear and plasma cells. Discoid LE has been described in collies and collie crosses, German shepherds, Siberian huskys and Shetland sheepdogs. It may be treated with prednisolone. Since the lesions are exacerbated by sunlight, it is appropriate to use sunscreens and encourage the owner to keep the animal out of intense sunlight.

ADDITIONAL SOURCES OF INFORMATION

Allen WE and Patel JR. 1982. Autoimmune orchitis in two related dogs. J. Small Anim. Pract. 23 713–718.

Bennett D. 1984. Autoimmune disease in the dog. In Practice 6 674–679.

Dodds WJ. 1983. Immune-mediated diseases of the blood. Adv. Vet. Sci. Comp. Med. 27 163–196.

Fisher TM and Fisher DR. 1982. Canine autoimmune progesterone dermatitis. Vet. Med. (Small Anim. Clin.) 77 1093–1094.

Gosselin SJ, Capen CC, Martin SL and Krakowka S. Autoimmune lymphocytic thyroiditis in dogs. Vet. Immunol. Immunopathol. *3* 185–201.

Grindem CB and Johnson KH. 1983. Systemic lupus erythematosus: literature review and report of 42 new canine cases. J. Am. Anim. Hosp. Assoc. *19* 489–503.

Haines DM. 1986. A re-examination of islet cell cytoplasmic antibodies in diabetic dogs. Vet. Immunol. Immunopathol. *11* 225–233.

Helfand SC, Couto CG and Madewell BR. 1985. Immune-mediated thrombocytopenia associated with solid tumors in dogs. J. Am. Anim. Hosp. Assoc. *21* 787–794.

Ihrke PJ, Stannard AA, Ardans AA and Griffin CE. 1985. Pemphigus foliaceous in dogs: a review of 37 cases. JAVMA *186* 59–66.

Indrieri RJ, Creighton SR, Lambert EH and Lennon VA. 1983. Myasthenia gravis in two cats. JAVMA *182* 57–60.

Kadlubowski M and Ingram PL. 1981. Circulating antibodies to the neuritogenic myelin protein, P_2, in neuritis of the cauda equina of the horse. Nature *293* 299–300.

Kaswan RL, Martin CL and Dawe DL. 1985. Keratoconjunctivitis sicca: immunological evaluation of 62 canine cases. Am. J. Vet. Res. *46* 376–383.

Lisak RP. 1983. Myasthenia gravis: mechanisms and management. Hosp. Pract. *18* 101–109.

Medleau L and Miller WH. 1983. Immunodiagnostic tests for small animal practice. Comp. Cont. Ed. Pract. Vet. *5* 705–717.

Parma AE, Santisteban CG, Villalba JS and Bowden RA. 1985. Experimental demonstration of an antigenic relationship between *Leptospira* and equine cornea. Vet. Immunol. Immunopathol. *10* 215–224.

Pedersen NC, Pool RR and O'Brien T. 1980. Feline chronic progressive polyarthritis. Am. J. Vet. Res. *41* 522–535.

Scott DW, Manning TO and Lewis RM. 1983. Linear IgA dermatoses in the dog: bullous pemphigoid, discoid lupus erythematosus and a subcorneal pustular dermatitis. Cornell Vet. *72* 394–402.

Scott DW, Walton DK, Manning TO, Smith CA and Lewis RM. 1983. Canine lupus erythematosus. I. Systemic lupus erythematosus. J. Am. Anim. Hosp. Assoc. *19* 461–479.

Scott DW, Walton DK, Manning TO, Smith CA and Lewis RM. 1983. Canine lupus erythematosus. II. Discoid lupus erythematosus. J. Am. Anim. Hosp. Assoc. *19* 481–488.

Worthington JW and Brown MJ. 1982. Acute canine idiopathic polyneuropathy. A Guillain-Barré-like syndrome in dogs. J. Neurol. Sci. *56* 259–273.

26

Disturbances in Immune Function: Deficiencies and Tumors

This chapter considers disorders of the immune system that result in an immunological deficiency. These include deficiencies that may arise in animals as a result of inherited defects in the development of the immune system, of defects secondary to other causes, or tumors of the immune system.

Any failure of the immune system and its associated systems, such as the mononuclear-phagocytic system, usually becomes apparent as a result of the increased susceptibility of affected animals to infectious diseases. Because of the nature of medical care, these conditions have been investigated primarily in humans, as infants who would otherwise die are kept alive by intensive efforts and the nature of their deficiency thoroughly investigated. In veterinary medicine, individual animals are unlikely to either receive this amount of attention or be so thoroughly investigated. Nevertheless, on the basis of the immunodeficiency syndromes studied so far, it is apparent that the same types of inherited deficiencies occur in both man and domestic animals.

INHERITED DEFECTS IN ANTIGEN PROCESSING

Two major classes of congenital deficiency syndromes associated with phagocytic failure have been reported in humans. In one there is a failure of opsonization; in the other there is a failure of intracellular killing.

Failures in opsonization have so far not been recorded in the domestic animals. If such a deficiency is suspected, it is possible to measure the opsonic activity of a serum by a simple test in which bacteria, phagocytic cells (such as buffy coat cells) and serum are mixed and incubated. After incubation the cells may be fixed, stained and examined for the presence of phagocytosed bacteria. By comparing the phagocytic activity of cells from a normal animal in the presence of normal and suspect serum, a rough indication of the opsonic activity of the serum may be obtained.

Chronic Granulomatous Disease

The most important phagocytic deficiency syndrome of humans is known as chronic granulomatous disease. This has not yet been reported as occurring in domestic animals. Children affected with chronic granulomatous disease suffer from recurrent infections characterized by the development of septic granulomata in lymph nodes, lungs, bones and skin. Analysis of the defect reveals that the neutrophils of these children are less capable than normal cells of destroying organisms such as staphylococci and coliforms. It is probable that the specific defect is a failure to activate NADPH oxidase, probably as a result of an inherited abnormality in the oxidase itself. As a result of this, the generation of oxidizing radicals by the respiratory burst fails to occur (Chapter 2), and the bactericidal efficiency of the neutrophils is grossly impaired. This impairment may be detected by incubating the neutrophils of an affected individual in nitro-blue tetrazolium (a yellow dye). Normal cells degrade this to produce dark blue deposits in their cytoplasm, whereas defective cells do not.

Chédiak-Higashi Syndrome

Although chronic granulomatous disease has not yet been reported to occur in animals, four other phagocytic deficiency syndromes have. One, the Chédiak-Higashi syndrome, is an inherited disease of Hereford cattle, Aleutian mink, Persian cats, white tigers, killer whales and humans. It is associated with a defect in cell structure that results in the production of abnormally large granules in neutrophils, monocytes and eosinophils and in enlarged melanin granules. The enlarged granules in neutrophils arise as a result of the fusion of primary and secondary granules (Fig. 26–1). In other cells they appear to be abnormal lysosomes. The abnormal melanin granules give rise to a very pale coat color and light-colored irises (pseudoalbinism). Cats with this condition have a red fundic light reflection rather than the normal yellow-green. The leukocyte granules of affected animals are more fragile than those of normal animals, rupturing spontaneously and causing tissue damage such as cataracts. The leukocytes of these animals have defective chemotactic responsiveness and a reduced capacity for intracellular killing as a result of defective granule fusion and a deficiency of enzymes such as elastase. The Chédiak-Higashi gene also influences the development of natural killer cells, which may be reflected in an increased susceptibility to tumors and to some viruses such as the Aleutian disease agent. It is believed that the NK cells are present but have a reduced ability to kill their targets. Affected animals commonly succumb to recurrent pyogenic bacterial infections or to lymphoid tumors. The Chédiak-Higashi syndrome may be diagnosed either by examining a stained blood smear for the presence of grossly enlarged granules within leukocytes or by examining hair shafts for enlarged melanin granules.

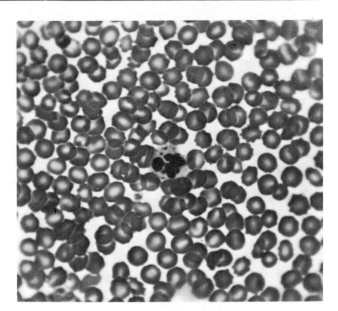

Figure 26–1. A neutrophil from an Aleutian mink. The large dark granules in this cell are abnormal and are characteristic of the Chédiak-Higashi syndrome. × 750. (From a specimen kindly provided by Dr. S. H. An.)

Canine Granulocytopathy Syndrome

The canine granulocytopathy syndrome is an autosomal recessive condition observed in Irish setters. Affected dogs suffer from recurrent severe bacterial infections, especially suppurative skin lesions, gingivitis and lymphadenopathy. They may have a pronounced leukocytosis, and their neutrophils are morphologically normal. In spite of this, the neutrophils are unable to kill opsonized *E. coli* or *Staph. aureus*. Closer examination of the neutrophils of these dogs has shown that their respiratory burst is depressed, as reflected by a decrease in glucose oxidation. Nevertheless, they are more effective than normal cells at reducing nitro-blue tetrazolium, implying that O_2^- is produced in greater quantities than normal. Further studies are clearly needed to clarify the precise nature of the defect in these cells.

Mac-1 Deficiency

Mac-1 is a glycoprotein found on the surface of macrophages, monocytes, granulocytes and large granular lymphocytes. It functions as a complement receptor so that phagocytic cells require Mac-1 for effective binding and ingestion of some complement-coated particles. Mac-1 is also required for the adherence of phagocytic cells to other surfaces. Several humans and one dog, an Irish setter, have been described as having an inherited deficiency of Mac-1. As a result of this, their phagocytic cells cannot bind to vascular endothelium and emigate from the blood stream into infected tissues. Thus, affected individuals suffer from severe recurrent bacterial infections. Neutrophils can be mobilized from the blood stream but are unable to migrate into tissues. The disease is, therefore, characterized by a very high neutrophilia, but neutrophils and macrophages are absent from infected areas. There is no pus formed in response to pyogenic infections. The Irish setter that suffered from this disease had severe intractible staphylococcal osteomyelitis. The mode of inheritance is unknown in dogs, although it is an autosomal recessive condition in man.

Gray Collie Syndrome

The fourth genetically determined neutrophil defect reported to occur in animals is the gray collie syndrome. This is a disease seen in collie dogs. It is associated with abnormal skin

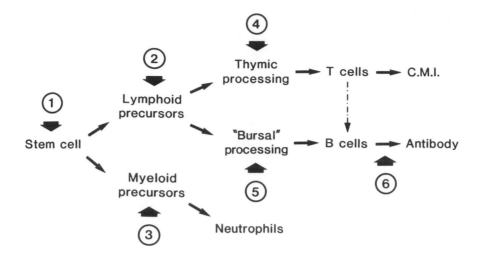

1 – Reticular dysgenesis
2 – Severe combined immunodeficiency
3 – Neutrophil defects
4 – Thymic aplasia
5 – Agammaglobulinemia
6 – Deficiencies in individual immunoglobulins

Figure 26–2. The points in the immune system at which development blocks may lead to immune deficiencies.

pigmentation, eye lesions and cyclical neutropenia. The loss of neutrophils occurs about every 11 days, and in their absence the animals become severely infected. They suffer from severe enteric disease, respiratory infections, bone disease and lymphadenitis. Immunoglobulin levels are somewhat elevated as a result of the recurrent antigenic stimulation but complement levels cycle in conjunction with the neutropenia. If affected animals are kept alive by aggressive antibiotic therapy, the continued stimulation of their macrophages may lead to the development of amyloidosis. The nature of the defect is not clear but appears to be due to a block in neutrophil maturation within the bone marrow and to a myeloperoxidase deficiency. Lithium carbonate appears to successfully "cure" this condition.

INHERITED DEFICIENCIES IN THE IMMUNE SYSTEM

The consequences of inherited immunological defects have served as excellent indicators of

the site of the genetic lesion and have confirmed the overall arrangement of the immune system, as outlined in Figure 26–2. For example, if both the cell- and antibody-mediated immune responses are defective, it may be assumed that the genetic lesion operates at a point prior to thymic and bursal cell processing—that is, it is a stem cell lesion. A defect that occurs only in thymic development will be reflected in an inability to mount a cell-mediated immune response, although antibody production will be normal. Similarly, a lesion restricted to the B cell system will be reflected in an absence of antibody-mediated immune responses.

Immunodeficiencies of Horses
(Fig. 26–3)

Horses are among the few domestic animals whose economic worth has permitted a thorough analysis of neonatal mortality. As a result, a significant number of primary immunodeficiency syndromes have been identified.

Combined Immunodeficiency

Probably the most important congenital equine immunodeficiency is the combined immunodeficiency syndrome (CID), which occurs in 2–3 per cent of Arabian foals. Affected foals fail to produce functional T or B cells. As a result, they are born with very few circulating lymphocytes. If they suckle successfully, they will acquire maternal immunoglobulins. Once these have been catabolized, however, the foal is unable to produce its own antibodies and eventually becomes totally agammaglobulinemic. Affected foals, therefore, are born healthy, but they sicken by two months of age. All are usually dead by four to six months as a result of overwhelming infection by a variety of low-grade pathogens. Organisms that have been implicated in these deaths include adenovirus, *Pneumocystis carinii* (an ill-defined protozoan-like organism), Cryptosporidium (a coccidian) and many different bacteria.

On necropsy, the spleens of affected animals are found to be devoid of both germinal centers and periarteriolar lymphoid sheaths. The lymph nodes lack lymphoid follicles and germinal centers, and there is cellular depletion in the paracortical zone. The thymuses of these animals are so hypoplastic that they may be difficult to find on necropsy.

CID is inherited in an autosomal recessive manner, and its occurrence indicates that both parents carry the offending gene. Accurate diagnosis is, therefore, of great importance, since it significantly reduces the economic value of the parent animals. The diagnosis of CID requires that at least two of the following three criteria be established: (1) very low (consistently below 1000/cumm) or no circulating lymphocytes, (2) histology typical of CID, that is, gross hypoplasia of the primary and secondary lymphoid organs and (3) an absence of serum IgM. IgM is synthesized by the normal equine fetus. As a result, normal newborn foals have about 160 μg/ml of IgM at birth. If the foal successfully suckles, it will obtain immunoglobulins of all the major isotypes from the mare's colostrum. However, the half-life of IgM is only about six days, so maternal IgM will disappear within a few days of birth. Thus a normal foal will have some IgM in its serum, a CID foal will have none.

If at all possible when diagnosing CID, it should be shown that the foal is unable to mount both cellular and humoral immune responses. The ability to mount a humoral immune response may be demonstrated by injecting a foal with sheep erythrocytes, since antibodies to these are not present in equine colostrum. Antibodies appear in normal foals two to three weeks after a single inoculation of sheep erythrocytes.

By using large quantities of blood it is possible to obtain sufficient lymphocytes from a CID foal and demonstrate that they are unreactive to mitogens such as phytohemagglutinin. A close study of these cells indicates

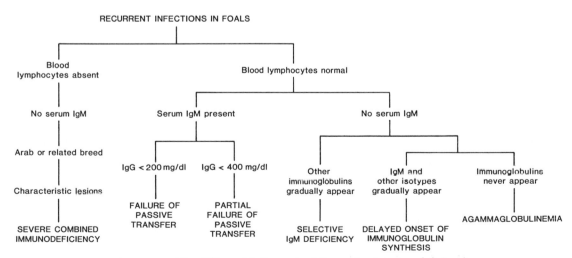

Figure 26–3. The differential diagnosis of the equine immune deficiencies.

that they are relatively large and contain cytoplasmic granules. They may well be NK cells. A type IV hypersensitivity reaction cannot be provoked by painting the skin with a contact allergen such as dinitrochlorobenzene or by inoculating the T cell mitogen phytohemagglutinin intradermally.

The precise biochemical lesion in CID is not known. However, fibroblasts from affected horses are more sensitive than normal fibroblasts to the growth inhibitory effects of adenosine. It may be that the defect lies in the transport or phosphorylation of adenosine. Successful attempts have been made to treat these foals using fetal marrow grafts. However, this is not very practical and if the detection of carriers becomes possible, then elimination of these animals would effectively eradicate the disease.

Agammaglobulinemia

At least two cases of primary agammaglobulinemia have been described in foals. The animals were devoid of identifiable B cells (cells with surface immunoglobulin) and were almost totally devoid of all immunoglobulins. Their lymphoid tissues had no primary follicles, germinal centers or plasma cells. Nevertheless, they possessed circulating blood lymphocytes that could respond to phytohemagglutinin and produce migration inhibitory factor. Intradermal inoculation of phytohemagglutinin caused a type IV delayed hypersensitivity reaction. Both animals suffered from recurrent bacterial infections but survived for 17 to 18 months.

Selective IgM Deficiency

Several cases of equine IgM deficiency have been described. The foals suffered from recurrent respiratory tract infections often involving *Klebsiella pneumoniae*. Their immune functions appeared to be normal in all respects except for very low or absent IgM.

Selective IgG Deficiency

A single case of putative IgG deficiency has been described in a three–month-old foal with salmonellosis. The animal had normal IgA and IgM but no germinal centers, lymphoid follicles, splenic follicles or periarteriolar lymphoid sheaths. Serum IgG was extremely low.

Transient Hypogammaglobulinemia

Between two and three months of age, some foals experience a transient episode of hypogammaglobulinemia as a result of a delayed onset of immunoglobulin synthesis. These animals may suffer from recurrent infections during the period when immunoglobulin levels are low.

The most important immunodeficiency in foals is not inherited but results from a failure to absorb sufficient colostral antibody from the mare (see Chapter 13). This may affect up to 10 per cent of all foals. Combined immunodeficiency occurs in 2 to 3 per cent of Arab foals (the gene is carried by 28 to 30 per cent of these horses) and is 10 times more common than selective IgM deficiency. Selective IgM deficiency is, in turn, 10 times more common than agammaglobulinemia.

Immunodeficiencies of Cattle

Trait A-46

Certain Black Pied Danish and Fresian cattle carry an autosomal recessive trait (trait A-46) of thymic and lymphocytic hypoplasia. Affected calves are born healthy, but by four to eight weeks they begin to suffer from severe skin infections. If untreated, they die a few weeks later, and none survive for longer than four months. Affected calves have exanthema, hair loss on the legs, and parakeratosis around the mouth and eyes. There is depletion of lymphocytes in the gut-associated lymphoid tissue and atrophy of the thymus, spleen and lymph nodes. It can be shown that these animals are deficient in T cells and have depressed cell-mediated immunity but normal antibody responses. Thus they have a normal response to tetanus toxoid but respond poorly to dinitrochlorobenzene or tuberculin. If these calves are treated by oral zinc oxide or zinc sulfate, they recover fully and acquire the ability to mount normal cell-mediated responses. If, however, the zinc supplementation is stopped, then the animals will relapse within a few weeks. The precise mechanisms are unknown, but it is probable that these animals have a reduced capacity to absorb zinc from the intestine. Zinc is an essential component of the thymic hormone thymulin (Chapter 5) and is therefore required for a normal T cell response.

Selective IgG2 Deficiency

IgG2 deficiency has been reported in Red Danish cattle. About 1 to 2 per cent of this breed are completely deficient in this immunoglobulin subisotype and as a result suffer from an increased susceptibility to pneumonias and gangrenous mastitis. In addition, up to 15 per cent of this breed have subnormal IgG2 levels, although they do not appear to suffer any ill effects in consequence.

Immunodeficiencies of Dogs

T Cell Deficiency with Dwarfism

A family of inbred Weimaraner dogs have been reported as suffering from immunodeficiency and dwarfism. The affected animals failed to grow after weaning and suffered from recurrent infections that eventually killed them. On necropsy their thymuses were atrophied and lacked a cortex. These animals had normal immunoglobulin levels, helper activity was unimpaired and their secondary lymphoid organs appeared normal. The lymphocytes of these dogs were unresponsive to phytohemagglutinin, concanavalin A and to pokeweed mitogen. Growth hormone treatment caused thymic cortical regeneration and clinical improvement. However, growth hormone did not restore responsiveness to mitogens. Thymosin fraction 5 also caused a clinical improvement but failed to improve the blastogenic response. The condition is almost certainly caused by a deficiency of growth hormone as a result of a lesion in the hypothalamus.

Combined Immunodeficiency

A case of combined immunodeficiency has been seen in a bassett hound. The patient was a male puppy that developed a pyoderma at 3-4 weeks of age. It also suffered from severe otitis and a gingivitis that was unresponsive to treatment. On examination the dog had no palpable lymph nodes, a very low white cell count, severe hypogammaglobulinemia and lymphocytes that were totally unresponsive to phytohemagglutinin. It died following administration of MLV distemper vaccine.

Because CID was suspected, its sire and dam were remated and eventually produced a litter of nine puppies. By three weeks of age pyoderma started in one of the puppies and eventually three males were affected. These three puppies failed to make IgG and IgA but their IgM levels were normal. Their blood lymphocyte counts were in the low normal range. The cells were unresponsive to phytohemagglutinin and pokeweed mitogen.

In the third litter of puppies produced by these parents, the lymphocytes from affected puppies were shown to be unresponsive to mitogens at five days of age. On necropsy the thymus and lymph nodes were absent. This condition is clearly a sex-linked disorder. It is apparent that the first affected puppy was a case of CID, but that the disease was different in subsequent generations. It is speculated that the lesion was due to a T cell defect in the control of the IgM to IgA or IgG switch.

Selective IgM Deficiency

A selective IgM deficiency has been reported in Doberman pinschers. These animals had raised IgA, low IgG and very low IgM. They suffered only a chronic nasal discharge, so the significance of this deficiency is in doubt.

Selective IgA Deficiency

Selective IgA deficiency was first detected when a group of beagles failed to be protected against kennel cough by vaccination and suffered from recurrent respiratory tract infections, eczema and otitis. Some affected dogs suffered from periodic seizures. Immunoelectrophoresis showed that the dogs had normal serum IgG and IgM levels but very little IgA (5 mg/dl, age matched controls had about 35 mg/dl). Their T and B lymphocyte numbers and their responses to mitogens were normal, and they responded normally to tetanus toxoid. Examination showed an absence of plasma cells secreting IgA. Affected puppies had no IgA while their sires and dams had very low IgA. The condition was not sex-linked. Four affected dogs had circulating anti-IgA antibodies. All affected puppies suffered from chronic recurrent respiratory disease due to *Bordetella bronchiseptica* and canine parainfluenza (SV5). It is believed that the defect lay in the ability of plasma cells to secrete IgA.

Transient Hypogammaglobulinemia

Transient hypogammaglobulinemia has been seen in a litter of Spitz puppies that suffered from recurrent respiratory infections. They had normal T cell function but had low immunoglobulin levels at six months of age. Immunoglobulins had risen to normal levels two months later. These puppies responded very weakly to tetanus toxoid when it was administered at four months.

Acrodermatitis

Acrodermatitis is an inherited disease of bull terriers. The animals suffer from growth retardation and develop severe dry, scaling skin lesions. They are severely immunosuppressed. Since their lymphocyte numbers are low, they fail to respond to mitogens such as phytohemagglutinin. On necropsy they have either no thymus or a very small one and a loss of T cells from the T-dependent areas of secondary lymphoid tissue. The disease is inherited as an autosomal recessive condition. Its pathogenesis is unknown, but it is very similar to trait A-46 of cattle described previously although it cannot be cured by a high zinc diet.

Immunodeficiencies of Chickens

Birds of the hypothyroid OS strain have a selective IgA deficiency. Birds of the UCD 140 line have a selective IgG deficiency known as hereditary dysgammaglobulinemia. These birds have normal immunoglobulin levels for about 50 days after hatching; then their IgG drops and their IgM and IgA rise. This is probably due to the development of specific suppressor cells. In addition to the hypogammaglobulinemia, UCD 140 strain birds show evidence of immune complex lesions; it has been suggested that this condition is mediated by a vertically transmitted virus.

Immunodeficiencies of Humans

A large number of well-characterized immunodeficiency syndromes have been reported in humans. It is anticipated that investigators will succeed eventually in identifying most of these syndromes in domestic animals as well.

The most severe immunodeficiency state in humans results from a defect in the development of primordial stem cells, as a result of which neither myeloid nor lymphoid cells develop. This condition, known as reticular dysgenesis, results in the very early death of affected individuals. An only slightly less severe disease occurs as a result of failure of the lymphoid stem cells to develop. The resulting lesion gives rise to combined immunodeficiency disease. In humans, some of these cases are due to a congenital deficiency of the enzymes adenine deaminase or purine nucleoside phosphorylase. Deficiency of adenine deaminase results in the accumulation of excessive deoxyadenosine phosphate within T cells. As a result, both effector and helper T cells are destroyed and both T and B cell functions are impaired. Deoxyadenosine phosphate also damages thymic epithelial cells and thus prevents T cell regeneration. A deficiency of purine nucleoside phosphorylase results in accumulation of deoxyguanosine phosphate in T cells. This affects only effector cells since it is selectively toxic for dividing T cells.

The most severe T cell defect in humans, DiGeorge's syndrome, results from a failure of the third and fourth thymic pouches to develop. It is therefore a congenital abnormality, not an inherited condition. In DiGeorge's syndrome, little or no thymic epithelial tissue develops and few, if any, cells populate the T-dependent areas of the secondary lymphoid tissues. Since these individuals have no functional T cells, they can neither mount a delayed hypersensitivity reaction nor reject allogeneic tissue grafts. The importance of the T cell system in providing protection against viral diseases is emphasized by the observation that individuals with DiGeorge's syndrome generally die from viral infections although they remain resistant to bacterial invasion.

A variety of other congenital T cell lesions have been described in man. Some are associated with a poorly developed thymus, lymphopenia and deficient cell-mediated immune responses. They may also be associated with hypogammaglobulinemia. They are differentiated on the basis of their mode of inheritance. Other immunodeficiency diseases may be associated with functional deficiencies such as the absence of class II antigens on monocytes or an absence of IL-1 or IL-2 receptors.

B cell deficiencies also occur in humans. The most severe of these, known as Bruton-type agammaglobulinemia, is an x-linked recessive condition; affected infants are devoid of all immunoglobulin isotypes. They suffer from recurrent infections due to organisms such as pneumococci, staphylococci and streptococci but are usually resistant to viral, fungal and protozoan infections. Inherited deficiencies of individual immunoglobulin isotypes have also been recorded in humans. As might be anticipated, there are many possible combinations of deficiencies in IgG, IgM, IgA and IgE and a tendency to give each a specific name leads to confusion. One of the most important of these is the Wiskott-Aldrich syndrome. In this disease, a selective IgM deficiency is associated with multiple infections, eczema and thrombocytopenia. Another such syndrome is ataxia-telangiectasia, in which serum IgA and IgE levels are extremely low or absent and cerebellar and cutaneous abnormalities exist. Affected children, lacking an effective surface immune system, suffer from recurrent bacterial respiratory tract infections. Ataxia telangiectasia is due to a defect in an individual's ability to repair DNA.

SECONDARY IMMUNOLOGICAL DEFECTS

Malnutrition and the Immune System

It has long been recognized that famine and disease are closely associated, and we tend to assume that malnutrition leads to increased susceptibility to infection. This is not necessarily true, since the effects of malnutrition on immune functions are complex. For example, malnutrition can include not only deficiencies, but also excesses or imbalances of individual nutrients. The clinical effects of malnutrition are greatest in animals with specific nutrient requirements, for example, very young or old animals or animals with severe infections.

In general, severe nutritional deficiencies reduce T cell function and therefore impair cell-mediated responses, at the same time sparing B cell function and humoral immunity. Thus starvation rapidly induces thymic atrophy and a reduction in the level of thymic hormones. Circulating T cell numbers drop and cells are lost from the T cell areas of secondary lymphoid tissue. As a result of this, delayed hypersensitivity reactions are reduced and graft rejection is delayed. Interferon production may also be impaired. In contrast, severe deficiencies have little effect on B cell functions. The B cell areas in lymphoid tissues and circulating B cell numbers remain unchanged. Serum immunoglobulin of all isotypes may remain normal or even rise. Secretory IgA levels commonly drop but secretory IgE may rise, suggesting abnormal immunoregulation. Starvation will, however, result in depressed complement levels and impairment of neutrophil and macrophage chemotaxis, the respiratory burst, release of lysosomal enzymes and microbicidal activity.

Specific nutritional deficiencies have a range of effects. Deficiencies of some B vitamins, vitamin A and polyunsaturated fatty acids can depress immunoglobulin levels through effects on regulatory T cells. Magnesium deficiency causes a similar effect by a direct action on B cells. Deficiencies of vitamin A, B_{12} and folic acid can depress cell-mediated immune responses. Zinc is especially critical for the proper functioning of the immune system. Zinc-deficient animals have depressed cytotoxic T cell activity, depressed B cell activity and depressed NK cell activity. Trait A-46, described previously, demonstrates the result of failure to absorb zinc in calves. Zinc can restore the responses of aged lymphocytes to normal. Indeed, if pregnant animals are deprived of zinc, their offspring have severely depressed immune function.

The effects of malnutrition may be reflected in altered resistance to infectious diseases. Because bacteria can readily survive and multiply in body tissues despite malnutrition of the host, malnutrition commonly increases the severity of bacterial diseases. Viruses, in contrast, usually require healthy host cells in which to replicate. Malnutrition, by rendering host cells unhealthy, can therefore increase resistance to viruses. Overnutrition can also influence susceptibility to viruses. For example, overfed dogs show an increased susceptibility to canine distemper and canine adenovirus 1. Parasites (especially intestinal helminths) usually compete with their host for nutrients. Should nutrition be reduced the parasite may also be adversely affected. Thus, the effects of malnutrition on parasitic infections can be very variable.

Vitamin E and the Immune Response

Of all the vitamins, vitamin E (alpha-tocopherol) appears to have the most significant effect on immune function. Vitamin E deficiency has variable effects, but it has been reported to cause a severe immunodepression in puppies. Vitamin E supplementation, at levels three to six times normal requirements, is claimed to stimulate immune reactivity. It specifically enhances IgG synthesis and promotes phagocytic activity.

For this reason, commercial IgE feed supplements are currently being promoted as immune stimulants. They are fed to calves, swine and poultry in an attempt to enhance disease resistance.

Virus-Induced Immune Disorders
(Table 26–1)

Viruses affecting the immune system may be divided into those that affect primary lymphoid tissues and those that affect secondary lymphoid tissues. For example, mice can be infected by a herpesvirus that causes massive necrosis of the cortex of the thymus. This "viral thymectomy" will naturally result in the development of immunological defects. In poultry, the virus of infectious bursal disease acts primarily on the lymphoid cells of the bursa of Fabricius to cause necrosis. This virus is not completely specific for the bursa, since it may also cause damage to the spleen and thymus. However, these tissues usually recover, whereas the bursa atrophies. The consequences of this infection, as might be predicted, are most evident in young birds infected immediately after hatching. These animals have a significantly reduced ability to make antibodies. If infection with the bursal disease virus is delayed for several weeks after hatching, then, again predictably, antibody production tends to be unaffected.

The most important virus-induced immunodeficiency disease is acquired immune deficiency syndrome (AIDS), a disease of man.

Table 26–1 VIRUSES THAT AFFECT LYMPHOID TISSUES OF ANIMALS

Viruses That Destroy Lymphoid Tissues
　Canine distemper
　Infectious bursal disease
　Newcastle disease
　Mouse thymus herpesvirus
　Feline panleukopenia
　African swine fever
　Bovine virus diarrhea
　Equine herpesvirus 1
　Simian AIDS virus
　Human immunodeficiency virus
Viruses That Stimulate Lymphoid Tissue Activity To An Unusual Extent
　Visna
　Aleutian disease
Viruses That Cause Lymphoid Neoplasia
　Marek's disease
　Feline leukemia
　Bovine leukemia
　Mouse leukemia
　Human T cell leukemia virus I

However, there are many viruses that cause similar lesions in animals. The one that resembles the human disease most closely is simian AIDS. Acquired immunodeficiency syndrome occurs in rhesus monkeys (*Macaca mulatta*) as a result of infection with a type D retrovirus transmitted by bites of carrier animals. The syndrome is associated with a profound drop in serum IgG and IgM levels and a severe lymphopenia. Monocyte function is unimpaired but the remaining lymphocytes do not respond to mitogens such as concanavalin A and phytohemagglutinin. On necropsy, the monkeys have a generalized lymphadenopathy, hepatomegaly and splenomegaly. Histologically there is a loss of lymphocytes from the T-dependent areas of the secondary lymphoid organs. B cell areas show an initial hyperplasia of the secondary follicles followed by the loss of these follicles and an absence of plasma cells. These histological changes are very similar to those seen in AIDS of man. About half the infected monkeys survive the disease; the others die as a result of septicemia or diarrhea with wasting. In many cases, normally inocuous agents such as Cytomegalovirus, Cryptosporidium and *Candida albicans* cause infection. Some affected monkeys develop tumors such as fibrosarcomas.

Other animal viruses are also capable of infecting and destroying secondary lymphoid organs. For example, canine distemper virus, although it can multiply in a wide variety of cells, has a predilection for cells of lymphatic tissues as well as for epithelia and nervous tissue. In experimentally infected dogs, the virus is found first in tonsils and bronchial lymph nodes, from which it spreads to the spleen, lymph nodes and bone marrow, where the virus replicates causing lymphoid destruction. The shedding of infected cells from these tissues enables the virus to reach epithelial tissues and the brain. While the virus has the ability to cause a lymphopenia and destroy lymphocytes, it can also depress the function of living macrophages and lymphocytes. Thus it depresses production of IL-1 and IL-2 while it also stimulates suppressor cell activity. As a result, lymphocyte blastogenesis is depressed, immunoglobulin levels may fall and immediate

hypersensitivity and skin graft rejection are suppressed. It has been suggested that this suppressive effect may be due to massive prostaglandin E_2 production by macrophages. The resulting immunosuppression accounts, in large part, for the clinical signs of canine distemper. If germ-free dogs are infected by virulent distemper virus, they suffer from a relatively mild disease, presumably because secondary infection cannot occur.

Depletion of lymphoid tissues is seen in feline panleukopenia, canine parvovirus infection, feline leukemia and African swine fever, where the virus tends to localize in germinal centers. Bovine virus diarrhea can cause a lymphopenia and destruction of both B and T lymphocytes in the lymph nodes, spleen, thymus and Peyer's patches. As in canine distemper, surviving B lymphocytes fail to make immunoglobulins. The destruction of the Peyer's patches causes local ulceration and permits secondary bacterial invasion. Bovine virus diarrhea also exerts a generalized immunosuppressive effect through stimulation of interferon production, and it is capable of depressing some neutrophil functions such as degranulation and antibody-dependent cellular cytotoxicity. Equine herpesvirus 1 causes a T cell lymphopenia in foals and, as a result, cell-mediated responses to antigens are depressed in these animals.

Parainfluenza 3 and infectious bovine rhinotracheitis viruses have long been known to interfere with alveolar macrophage function, inhibiting phagosome-lysosome fusion, and thus paving the way for secondary infections with pasteurella in stressed calves.

The results of virus-induced lymphoid tissue destruction are readily seen as a lymphopenia or as a depression in the ability of circulating lymphocytes to respond to mitogenic stimuli. For example, the response of peripheral blood lymphocytes to the plant lectin phytohemagglutinin is depressed in influenza, canine distemper, Marek's disease, Newcastle disease, bovine virus diarrhea and lymphocytic choriomeningitis. The immunosuppression observed in Newcastle disease infection is possibly due to the action of viral neuraminidase on lymphocyte membranes, which modifies their circulation pattern within the lymphoid organs. Destruction of lymphoid tissue may also be reflected in hypogammaglobulinemia or a depressed ability to respond to antigen either with humoral antibodies or by graft rejection.

The effect of some viruses on the immune system may be relatively complex or anomalous. In canine distemper, for instance, lymphocyte reactivity to phytohemagglutinin is depressed but graft rejection may be normal. In visna, a neurological disease of sheep caused by a retrovirus, cell-mediated immune reactions such as graft rejection are suppressed while B cell responses are enhanced. Some leukemia viruses can exert selective depressive effects, so that depression of the IgG response is greater than that of the IgM response. In equine infectious anemia, the IgG(T) response is variably depressed, whereas synthesis of the other immunoglobulin isotypes remains unaffected. It has been claimed that although chickens infected with Marek's disease show enhanced graft-versus-host reactivity (Chapter 18) they exhibit depressed graft rejection.

Thymic atrophy and lymphopenia are common manifestations of many viral infections, and before a congenital immunodeficiency syndrome is identified, rigorous steps must be taken to exclude the possibility that it is secondary to a viral infection. In addition, immunosuppression generally accompanies infestation with *Demodex*, *Toxoplasma* or trypanosomes, helminths such as *Trichinella spiralis* and bacteria such as *Pasteurella hemolytica*, the Actinobacilli, and some streptococci.

Toxin-Induced Immunosuppression

Many environmental toxins such as polychlorinated biphenyls, polybrominated biphenyls, iodine, lead, cadmium, methyl mercury and DDT have a suppressive effect on the immune system. Mycotoxins may be of importance in situations in which cattle are fed moldy grain. These include T2 toxin from *Fusarium* sp., which depresses the response of calf lympho-cytes to mitogens and decreases the chemotactic migration of neutrophils. T2 toxin also reduces IgM, IgA and C3 levels in cattle. Some of the aflatoxins may also be immunosuppressive and increase the severity of infections.

Other Secondary Immunodeficiencies

Immunoglobulin synthesis is generally very much reduced in animals suffering from absolute protein loss. Thus, immunosuppression occurs in the nephrotic syndrome, in heavily parasitized or tumor-bearing animals and following severe burns or trauma. Adult horses with chronic diarrhea are immunosuppressed, as reflected by a hypogammaglobulinemia A and reduced lymphocyte responses to phytohemagglutinin. It is debatable whether the immunosuppression is due to a protein-loosing enteropathy or the immunosuppression causes the diarrhea. By chilling newborn puppies for five to ten days, it is possible to provoke an immunodeficiency syndrome very similar in appearance to CID. Other stresses such as rapid weaning, prolonged transportation, crowding and trauma are all recognized as effective immunosuppressants. Destruction of lymphoid tissue leading to immunosuppression may occur in tumor-bearing animals, especially if the tumors themselves are lymphoid in origin (Fig. 26–4). Some endocrine disorders such as thyrotoxicosis and diabetes may also cause immunosuppression.

NEOPLASMS OF LYMPHOID CELLS

The immune response requires that antigen-sensitive cells stimulated by appropriate exposure to antigen respond in a controlled fashion by division and differentiation. Much of the complexity of the immune system outlined in earlier chapters is due to the need for rigid control of this cellular response. A failure in this control system may result in uncontrolled lymphoid cell proliferation. Surveil-

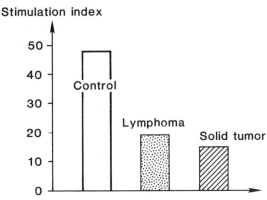

Figure 26–4. Immunosuppression in dogs suffering from lymphomas or solid tumors as compared with normal control dogs. The stimulation index is a measure of the response to lymphocytes to the mitogenic lectin phytohemagglutinin. (Data from Weiden P. L. et al. 1974. J Natl Cancer Inst 53 1053. Used with permission.)

lance was originally proposed as a function of the immune system when it was observed that immunosuppressed animals and humans suffered from an increased prevalence of tumors. Analysis of the types of tumors seen in these individuals, however, shows that an unusually high proportion of them are of lymphoid origin. It is not unlikely, therefore, that at least some of these lymphoid tumors in immunosuppressed individuals arise as a result of a failure in the immunological control systems rather than from a failure of surveillance.

Neoplastic transformation may occur in lymphoid cells of both branches of the immune system at almost any stage in their maturation

process. Providing that the tumor cells have not dedifferentiated as a result of very rapid growth (as in acute lymphatic leukemia of calves), it is possible to identify the cells present in a lymphoid tumor by means of surface markers. The presence of cell-surface immunoglobulin is considered characteristic of B cells; the ability to form rosettes with sheep erythrocytes is an identifying feature of T cells.

Lymphoid tumors usually cause immunosuppression (Fig. 26–4). As a broad generalization, it may be claimed that T cell tumors interfere with the cell-mediated immune system and B cell tumors interfere with the antibody-mediated immune system (Table 26–2).

Bovine Lymphosarcoma

Bovine lymphosarcoma is one of the most common neoplasms of cattle. It occurs in two main forms, an enzootic form and a sporadic form. The enzootic form of the disease is caused by infection with bovine leukemia virus (BLV). A related condition is a persistent lymphocytosis. This is not just a subclinical form of lymphoma but is a distinctly different condition. Bovine leukemia virus, the cause of these conditions, infects B lymphocytes primarily but some T cells can also be shown to contain the BLV provirus. Lymphosarcoma or persistent lymphocytosis are uncommon

Table 26–2 THE IMMUNOSUPPRESSIVE EFFECTS OF LYMPHOID TUMORS

Tumor	Cell Type	Evidence for Immunosuppression	Mechanism
Feline leukemia	T cell	Lymphopenia, Prolonged skin grafts, Increased susceptibility to infection, Lack of response to mitogens	Suppressive viral protein, p15E, Suppressor cells
Marek's disease	T cell	Lack of response to mitogens, Depressed cell-mediated cytotoxicity, Depressed IgG production	Suppressor macrophages
Avian lymphoid leukosis	B cell	Increased susceptibility to infection	Suppressor lymphocytes
Bovine leukosis	B cell	Depressed serum IgM	Soluble suppressor factor
Myeloma	B cell	Increased susceptibility to infection	Soluble tumor cell factor, Negative feedback
Canine malignant lymphoma	B cell	Predisposition to infection associated with autoimmune disorders	Unknown
Equine lymphosarcoma	T cell	Increased susceptibility to infection	Tumor of suppressor cells

sequels to infection with BLV. Animals with advanced bovine leukosis are usually immunosuppressed as a result of the presence in their serum of an ill-defined suppressor factor. This suppression is commonly associated with reduced numbers of T cells and lowered serum IgM levels. Occasionally, the neoplastic cell in bovine leukosis may be sufficiently differentiated to secrete immunoglobulin in a manner similar to that seen in myelomas.

Lymphomas in Other Species

In sheep, lymphomas are divided fairly evenly between T and B cell neoplasms, about 15 per cent are untypable (null cells). Some of these may be due to BLV infection. A B cell lymphoma inherited as an autosomal recessive condition is recognized in swine. Horses carrying lymphosarcomas are commonly immunosuppressed. This immunosuppression usually involves T cell functions, but B cell function may also be impaired. A case of a horse having a lymphosarcoma with suppressor cell activity has been described. The animal presented with signs of immunodeficiency and was found to be deficient in IgM. The tumor cells grew in the presence of interleukin 2, possessed many T cell markers and were noncytotoxic.

Lymphosarcomas account for 57 per cent of canine malignancies, and there is no evidence to suggest that these tumors are virus induced. They may be classified according to their apparent site of origin (e.g., multicentric, alimentary, anterior mediastinal, etc.) or by their cell type (e.g., histiocytic, lymphocytic, lymphoblastic or plasmacytic). The lymphocytic forms are usually of T cell origin.

Feline Leukemia

Cats probably have the highest incidence of lymphoid tumors of any animal. Most of these lymphoid tumors are due to the feline leukemia virus (FeLV). The response of cats to FeLV demonstrates many of the immunological problems encountered in response to viral infections. FeLV is an oncogenic retrovirus that can cause a number of different syndromes in cats, including both proliferative and degenerative conditions. The proliferative conditions caused by FeLV include lymphosarcoma, reticulum cell sarcoma, erythroleukemia and granulocytic leukemias. The degenerative conditions include immunosuppressive diseases, thymic atrophy, anemia, pancytopenia and thrombocytopenia, The lymphosarcoma caused by this virus is usually a T cell neoplasm, although FeLV grows in cells of many types and is not restricted to lymphoid tissues. Some FeLV alimentary lymphomas may be of B cell origin.

About 30 per cent of the cats exposed to FeLV fail to mount an adequate immune response against the virus and become persistently infected. About 40 per cent of exposed cats mount a strong immune response. These cats develop high titers of neutralizing antibodies to the virus, eliminate it and become strongly immune. The remaining 30 per cent of exposed cats become neither infected nor immune. Persistently infected cats remain viremic. This viremia may be readily detected either by a direct immunofluorescent test on a buffy coat smear using antibodies to group-specific antigen (see Fig. 16–8) or by an enzyme-linked immunosorbent assay (ELISA) on a whole blood sample. The latter test detects soluble viral antigen and may therefore detect infection prior to the development of viremia, since soluble virus antigens are shed into the blood stream.

Persistently infected cats show several interesting immune phenomena. For example, in FeLV infected cells a viral gene codes for a protein which is associated with the malignant transformation of the cell. This antigen is called feline oncornavirus cell membrane antigen or FOCMA. The presence of FOCMA on a cell membrane identifies the cell as an FeLV-induced tumor cell. FOCMA is not found on normal cat cells. Of those cats that fail to make neutralizing antibodies to FeLV and hence remain viremic, about 80 per cent develop antitumor activity by making antibodies against FOCMA. Thus, a cat that makes antibodies to FOCMA can usually destroy virus-induced tumor cells. Unfortunately, the possession of antibodies to FOCMA does not confer protection against the FeLV-induced degenerative diseases, and viremic cats that fail to produce anti-FOCMA antibodies are fully susceptible to all the FeLV syndromes, including lymphosarcoma.

Immune Dysfunction in FeLV-Infected Cats

Persistent FeLV infection is associated with two major immunopathological lesions: destruction of lymphocytes and interference with their function, leading to immunodeficiency and production of large quantities of immune complexes, leading to severe glomerulonephritis.

Some persistently infected cats suffer from a severe lymphopenia, neutropenia or both. The lymphopenia is primarily due to a loss of circulating T cells. B cell numbers may also be depressed, but this is variable. The numbers of B cells appear to depend upon the severity of secondary infections. Kittens infected with FeLV develop a runting syndrome associated with thymic atrophy and recurrent infections. Depending upon the severity of the secondary infections, either lymphoid atrophy or lymphoid hyperplasia may occur.

In cats without secondary infection, lymphoid atrophy is associated with a loss of cells from the T-dependent areas of lymph nodes. The changes in the spleens of these animals are less marked but may result in a reduction in the entire white pulp. As a result of this loss of T cells, FeLV-infected cats have depressed cell-mediated immune functions. The remaining T cells also show depressed reactivity toward the mitogen concanavalin A. This depression is probably due to the effects of p15E, the immunosuppressive envelope protein of the FeLV virus, which is produced in very large quantities from cells dying as a result of FeLV infection. It suppresses the responses of cats to FOCMA, suppresses lymphocyte blastogenesis and blocks the responses of T cells to interleukins 1 and 2. As a result of the activities of p15E, FeLV-infected cats may carry allogeneic skin grafts for about twice as long as normal cats (24 days as compared to 12). This immunosuppression also predisposes viremic cats to secondary diseases such as feline infectious peritonitis, hemobartonellosis, toxoplasmosis, septicemia and fungal infections. p15E also blocks the activity of bone marrow stem cells, preventing production of erythroid cells and causing a nonregenerative anemia.

In contrast to the severe T cell dysfunction, B cell activities in FeLV-infected cats are only mildly impaired. Thus infected cats have a reduced antibody response to low doses of sheep erythrocytes but their IgG levels in serum remain normal. Because B cell function and antibody production are relatively normal in cats chronically infected with FeLV, antibodies to the virus are produced in large quantities. These antibodies combine with circulating virus particles or soluble proteins to form immune complexes. These circulating immune complexes are deposited on the basement membranes in the renal glomeruli and cause severe glomerulonephritis, leading to hypoproteinemia, edema, uremia and death. If viral antigen binds to the cat's erythrocytes, the immune response can cause a severe antiglobulin-positive hemolytic anemia.

Immune complexes will also activate the classical complement pathway. As a result, complement will be consumed and disappear from the blood stream. Thus FeLV-infected cats may have very low levels of hemolytic complement. This loss of complement may play a role in reducing resistance to the tumor, since normal cat serum infused into leukemic cats may cause tumor regression.

A vaccine against FeLV has now been developed. It contains the supernatant fluid from a cell line persistently infected with FeLV. This fluid contains several of the major protein antigens of FeLV including gp70, the major capsid antigen. Resistance to disease is associated with a response to gp70, but the other antigens are also required for effective protection.

Avian Lymphoid Tumors

Marek's disease is a virus-induced tumor of T cell origin. Birds that suffer from this disease are usually immunosuppressed; their antibody responses, rejection of allografts and delayed hypersensitivity responses are all depressed. This depression results from several factors including virus-induced lymphoid destruction and the development of suppressor macrophages. These macrophages act to restrict the replication of the tumor cells but in doing so suppress the resistance of birds to other infections. Lymphoid leukosis is a tumor of B cell origin. Birds with avian lymphoid leukosis normally have a depressed antibody response and a defective response to phytohemagglutinin. Nevertheless, some cases of this disease may present with a hypergammaglobulinemia.

Myelomas

Malignant transformation of a single B cell may give rise to the development of a clone of immunoglobulin-producing tumor cells. The morphological features of these cells may vary, but they are usually recognizable as plasma cells (Fig. 26–5). Plasma cell tumors are known as myelomas or plasmacytomas. Because myelomas arise from a single precursor cell, they produce a homogeneous immunoglobulin product known as a myeloma protein or M protein (Fig. 26–6).

Myeloma proteins may belong to any im-munoglobulin isotype. For example, IgG, IgA and IgM myelomas have been reported in the dog and cat (Fig. 26–7). In humans, in addition to myelomas of the major immunoglobulin isotypes, rare cases of IgD and IgE myelomas have also been described. In general, the prevalence of the various immunoglobulin isotypes in myeloma proteins correlates well with their relative quantities in normal serum, suggesting that the condition arises as a consequence of a random mutation in a single B cell clone. Light chain disease is a condition in which light chains alone are produced or the production of light chains is greatly in excess of the production of heavy chains. Similarly, there is a very rare variant of this condition in which Fc fragments alone are produced. This condition is erroneously termed heavy chain disease.

Myelomas have been reported to occur in humans, mice, dogs, cats, horses, cows, pigs, ferrets and rabbits. The most common clinical manifestation in dogs is a bleeding problem that occurs as a result of a hyperviscosity syndrome as well as a thrombocytopenia and an effective loss of clotting components due to their binding to myeloma proteins. The hyperviscosity syndrome results from the presence in serum of abnormally large quantities

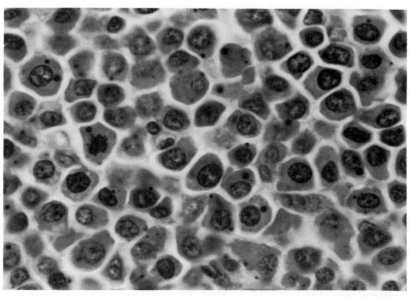

Figure 26–5. A section of a myeloma tumor mass in a dog. × 900. (From a specimen kindly provided by Dr. R. G. Thomson.)

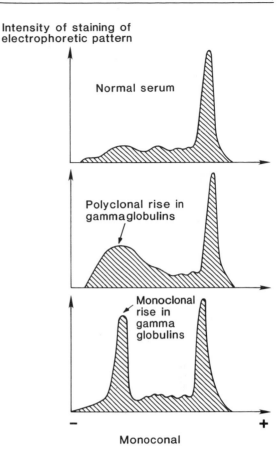

Intensity of staining of
electrophoretic pattern

Normal serum

Polyclonal rise in
gammaglobulins

Monoclonal
rise in
gamma
globulins

−   +

Monoconal

Figure 26–6. Serum electrophoretic patterns showing the normal pattern and the characteristic features of monoclonal and polyclonal gammopathies. Monoclonal gammopathies commonly occur as a result of the presence of a myeloma.

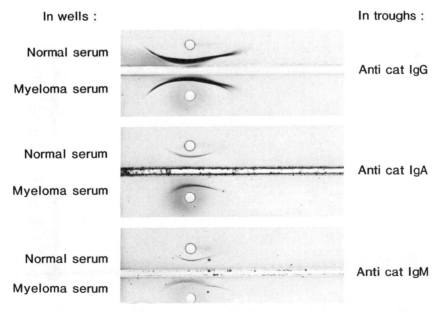

In wells :   In troughs :

Normal serum

Myeloma serum   Anti cat IgG

Normal serum

Myeloma serum   Anti cat IgA

Normal serum

Myeloma serum   Anti cat IgM

Figure 26–7. Immunoelectrophoresis of serum from a cat suffering from an IgM myeloma. Note that the line of precipitate formed by the reaction between anti cat IgM and the myeloma serum is distorted. The line is much thicker than the control and it forms two distinct joined arcs as a result of the presence of the IgM myeloma protein. (Courtesy of Dr. G. Elissalde.)

of immunoglobulins and is especially severe in animals suffering from an IgM myeloma (macroglobulinemia). As a result of the increase in blood viscosity, the heart must work harder and congestive heart failure, retinopathy and neurological signs may result. Because myeloma cells are also osteolytic, the presence of tumor masses in bone may lead to bone pain and to the development of multiple radiolucent osteolytic lesions and diffuse osteoporosis, both of which are readily observed by radiography. These lesions may also lead to the occurrence of pathological fractures. Light chains, being relatively small (22,000 daltons), pass through the glomerulus and are excreted in the urine. Unfortunately, these molecules are toxic for renal tubular cells and, as a result, myelomas may be associated with renal failure. These light chains may also be detected in urine by electrophoresis of concentrated urine or, in some cases, by heating the urine. Light chains may precipitate when heated to 60°C but redissolve as the temperature is raised to 80°C. Proteins possessing this curious property are known as Bence-Jones proteins, and their presence in urine is suggestive of a myeloma.

Because of the overwhelming commitment of the body's immune resources to the pro-

duction of neoplastic plasma cells as well as to the replacement of normal marrow tissue by tumor cells and to the negative feedback induced by elevated serum immunoglobulins, animals with myelomas are profoundly immunosuppressed. As a result of this, they commonly suffer from pyogenic bacterial infections. In humans, renal failure and overwhelming infection are the most common causes of death in this disease. On occasion, old dogs and humans may develop a monoclonal gammopathy in the absence of a myeloma. The cause is unknown, but the prognosis in these cases is good. Myelomas may be treated by plasmapheresis to remove the myeloma protein. The tumor itself can be treated with alkylating agents such as cyclophosphamide and melphalan.

Polyclonal Gammopathies

In contrast to monoclonal gammopathies, which are generally associated with myelomas, polyclonal gammopathies are observed in a wide variety of pathological conditions. The condition that most resembles a myeloma is Aleutian disease of mink (Chapter 16). Animals infected by the Aleutian disease virus show, in the progressive form of the disease, marked

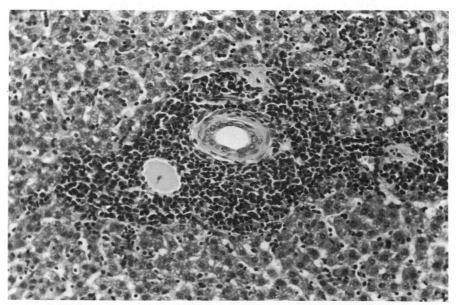

Figure 26–8. A section of liver from a mink infected by Aleutian disease. There is marked plasma cell and mononuclear cell infiltration. × 250. (From a specimen kindly provided by Dr. S. H. An.)

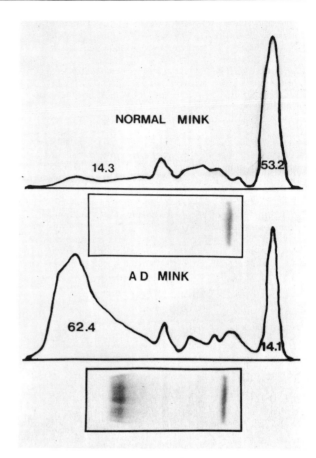

Figure 26–9. A comparison of the serum electrophoretic patterns seen in normal and Aleutian disease-infected mink. The serum of the infected animal shows a polyclonal gammopathy so that the gammaglobulins account for 62.4 per cent of the serum proteins in contrast to the normal level of 14.3 per cent. (Courtesy of Dr. S. H. An.)

plasmacytosis and lymphocyte infiltration of many organs and tissues (Fig. 26–8) as well as polyclonal (occasionally monoclonal) gammopathy (Fig. 26–9). As a result of the elevated immunoglobulin levels, affected mink suffer from blood hyperviscosity and are severely immunosuppressed.

Other causes of polyclonal gammopathy include autoimmune diseases such as systemic lupus erythematosus, rheumatoid arthritis and myasthenia gravis (Chapter 25); certain infections such as tropical pancytopenia of dogs (*Ehrlichia canis*) and African trypanosomiasis, in which B cells are polyclonally stimulated; and chronic bacterial infections such as pyometra and pyoderma, in which the prolonged antigenic stimulus leads to a hypergammaglobulinemia G. In horses heavily parasitized with *Stronglylus vulgaris*, IgG(T) levels rise significantly. Polyclonal gammopathy also occurs in viral infections such as feline infectious peritonitis and African swine fever and in conditions in which extensive liver damage occurs.

ADDITIONAL SOURCES OF INFORMATION

Boxer GJ, Curnette JT and Boxer LA. 1985. Disorders of Polymorphonuclear leukocyte function. Hosp. Pract. *20* 129–138.

Buntain B. 1981. IgG immunodeficiency in a half-Arabian foal with salmonellosis. Vet. Med. (Small. Anim. Clin.) *76* 231–234.

Dopson LC, Reed SM, Roth JA, et al. 1983. Immunosuppression associated with lymphosarcoma in two horses. JAVMA. *182* 1239–1241.

Hardy WD. 1981. The feline leukemia virus. J. Am. Anim. Hosp. Assoc. *17* 951–980.

Kelley KW, Osborne CA, Evermann JF, et al. 1982. Effect of chronic heat and cold stressors on plasma immunoglobulin and mitogen-induced blastogenesis in calves. J. Dairy Sci. *65* 1514–1528.

MacEwen EG, Patnaikak, Hurvitz AL, et al. 1984. Nonsecretory multiple myeloma in two dogs. JAVMA *184* 1283–1286.

Magnuson NS, Perryman LE, Wyatt CR, et al. 1984. Continuous cultivation of equine lymphocytes: evidence for occasional T cell-like maturation events in horses with hereditary severe combined immunodeficiency. J. Immunol. *133* 2518–2524.

McClure JJ, Addison JD and Miller RI. 1985. Immunodeficiency manifested by oral candidiasis and bacterial septicemia in foals. JAVMA *186* 1195–1197.

Medleau L, Crowe DT and Dawe DL. 1983. Effect of surgery on the *in vitro* response of canine peripheral blood lymphocytes to phytohemagglutinin. Am. J. Vet. Res. *44* 859–860.

Ohmann HB and Babiuk LA. 1986. Alteration of alveolar macrophage functions after aerosol infection with bovine herpesvirus type 1. Infect. Immun. *51* 344–347.

Olsen RG and Krakowka S. 1984. Immune dysfunctions associated with viral infections. Comp. Cont. Ed. Pract. Vet. *6* 422–430.

Osborn KG, Prahalada S, Lowenstine LJ, et al. 1984. The pathology of an epizootic of acquired immunodeficiency in Rhesus macaques. Am. J. Pathol. *114* 94–103.

Perryman LE, Buening GM, McGuire TC, et al. 1979. Fetal tissue transplantation for immunotherapy of combined immunodeficiency in horses. Clin. Immunol. Immunopathol. *12* 238–251.

Perryman LE and Magnuson NS. 1982. Immunodeficiency disease in animals. *In*: Desnick, RJ, Patterson, DF, and Scarpelli, DG, eds. Animal Models of Inherited Metabolic Diseases. Prog. in Clin. Biol. Res. Vol. 94. Alan R Liss Inc., New York, pp. 271–307.

Rosen FS, Cooper MD and Wedgewood RJP. 1984. The primary immunodeficiencies. N. Engl. J. Med. *311* 235–242 and 300–310.

Roth JA, Kaeberle ML, Grier RL, et al. 1984. Improvement in clinical condition and thymus morphologic features associated with growth hormone treatment of immunodeficient dwarf dogs. Am. J. Vet. Res. *43* 1151–1155.

Snyderman R and Cianciolo GJ. 1985. Immunosuppressive activity of the retroviral envelope protein p15E and its possible relationship to neoplasia. Immunol. Today *5* 240–244.

Targowski SP, Wlodzimiers K, Littledike ET and Hoy DL. 1985. Suppression of mitogenic response of bovine lymphocytes during experimental ketosis in calves. Am. J. Vet. Res. *46* 1378–1380.

Whitbread TJ, Batt RM and Garthwaite G. 1984. Relative deficiency of serum IgA in the German shepherd dog: a breed abnormality. Res. Vet. Sci. *37* 350–352.

27

Biological Response Modifiers

There are many situations in which it is desirable to either stimulate or suppress the immune system of an animal, and many different drugs or techniques are available to do this. Indeed, this area of immunology is a discipline in its own right, immunopharmacology.

SUPPRESSION OF THE IMMUNE SYSTEM

The approaches available for inhibiting immune responses may be classified into two main groups. The most widely employed techniques involve drugs or radiation that by inhibiting cell division in general serve to reduce the multiplication of antigen-sensitive cells upon encountering antigen. This approach is crude and dangerous, since other rapidly proliferating cell populations such as intestinal epithelium and bone marrow cells may also be severely depleted, with potentially disastrous consequences. Alternatively, it is possi-

ble to employ techniques that selectively eliminate T or B cells. This can be done by means of specific antiserum, by selective drugs or by thoracic duct drainage.

Nonspecific Immunosuppression

Radiation

X-radiation exerts its effects on cells by several different mechanisms. The simplest of these is through ionizing rays hitting an essential, unique molecule within the cell. The most important of these molecules are the nucleic acids, particularly DNA. A loss of even one nucleotide entails a permanent mutation of a gene, with potentially lethal effects on the progeny of the affected cell. Radiation also causes ionization and the formation of highly reactive free hydrogen and hydroxyl radicals in the environment of the cell. These free radicals can react with dissolved oxygen to form peroxides that have toxic effects on many cell processes, especially cell division. Although x-radiation is of some use in prolonging graft survival in many experimental animals, especially laboratory rodents, the amount of radiation required for effective prolongation of graft survival in the dog is usually lethal.

Corticosteroids

Although corticosteroids have been used as immunosuppressive agents for many years, their precise mode of action remains unclear. There are several reasons for this. One important factor is the differences between species. Species may be classified as corticosteroid sensitive or corticosteroid resistant on the basis of the ease with which they can be depleted of lymphocytes. Most of the laboratory rodents are much more sensitive to the immunosuppressive effects of corticosteroids than the major domestic animals; therefore, care should be taken not to extrapolate results from laboratory animals directly to other animals.

Corticosteroids act in four areas. They have effects on leukocyte circulation; they influence the immune effector mechanisms in lymphocytes; they modulate the activities of inflammatory mediators; and they modify protein, carbohydrate and fat metabolism.

The effects of corticosteroids on leukocyte circulation vary between species. In horses and cattle, the number of circulating eosinophils, basophils and lymphocytes declines abruptly when corticosteroids are administered. The number of neutrophils, on the other hand, increases as a result of a decreased adherence to vascular endothelium (margination) and reduced emigration into inflamed tissues (Table 27–1).

The effects of corticosteroids on cellular function all appear to have a common pathway. Thus corticosteroids are rapidly adsorbed into a cell, where they bind to a receptor in the cytoplasm. They are then transported to the cell nucleus, where they bind to the chromatin protein and the DNA. As a result of derepression of RNA transcription, new mRNA is formed and promotes new protein synthesis. These proteins are the mediators of the effects of corticosteroids. For example, a protein

Table 27–1 THE EFFECTS OF CORTICOSTEROIDS ON CELLS OF THE IMMUNE SYSTEM

Cell	Effect
Neutrophil	
	Neutrophilia
	Depressed chemotaxis
	Depressed margination
	Depressed phagocytosis
	Depressed ADCC
	Depressed bactericidal activity
Macrophages	
	Monocytopenia
	Depressed chemotaxis
	Depressed phagocytosis
	Depressed bactericidal activity
	Depressed IL-1 production
	Depressed antigen processing
Lymphocytes	
	Lymphopenia
	Depressed proliferation
	Depressed T cell responses
	Impaired T cell-mediated cytotoxicity
	Depressed IL-2 production
	Depressed lymphokine production

called macrocortin or lipomodulin is synthesized that blocks the activities of cell membrane phospholipase A2 and thus prevents the synthesis of prostanoids such as the leukotrienes and prostaglandins.

Corticosteroids act on T cells to depress their ability to produce interleukin 2 and thus interfere with their responses to mitogens such as concanavalin A and phytohemagglutinin. Lymphocyte proliferation in the mixed lymphocyte reaction is suppressed, suggesting that there is interference with the recognition of class II histocompatibility antigens. Corticosteroids also block production of lymphotoxin and monocyte chemotactic factors. Natural killer and some antibody-dependent cell-mediated cytotoxicity (ADCC) reactions may be refractory to corticosteroid treatment, and in cattle corticosteroids may increase serum interferon levels. The effects on antibody responses occurring during corticosteroid therapy may be variable and depend on the time of administration and on the dose given. In general, B cells tend to be corticosteroid resistant and enormous doses are usually required to depress antibody synthesis.

Neutrophil, monocyte and eosinophil chemotaxis are suppressed by corticosteroids, but neutrophil random migration is enhanced. Corticosteroids suppress the phagocytic ability of neutrophils and their ability to mediate ADCC reactions. However, these results do seem to depend on the concentration and type of corticosteroid involved. Macrophage production of prostanoids and interleukin 1 is also diminished.

The synthetic glucocorticoids are able to suppress the major features of the acute inflammatory response. They inhibit the increases in vascular permeability and vasodilation. As a result, they prevent edema formation and fibrin deposition. At the same time, corticosteroids block the emigration of leukocytes from the capillaries. One way this is accomplished is by depressing cellular metabolism in neutrophils and macrophages, thus inhibiting the release of lysosomal enzymes and impairing antigen processing by macrophages. Corticosteroids can also inhibit the effects of phospholipases and so prevent the production of leukotrienes and prostaglandins. These effects of corticosteroids may mask the signs of tissue damage. In the later stages of inflammation, they inhibit capillary and fibroblast proliferation (perhaps by blocking interleukin 1 production) and enhance collagen breakdown. Corticosteroids, therefore, delay wound and fracture healing. The effects of corticosteroids on complement activities are variable.

When corticosteroid therapy is initiated, prednisolone is usually the agent selected for treatment of small animals, whereas betamethasone and dexamethasone are commonly employed in large animal practice. This treatment is not without risks, since it has the potential to suppress the pituitary adrenal axis and induce Cushing's syndrome. Corticosteroids may also, by suppressing inflammatory responses and phagocytic cell function, render an animal highly susceptible to infection.

Cytotoxic Drugs

The major immunosuppressive drugs, having been designed to inhibit cell division, act on various stages of nucleic acid synthesis and activity. The four major drugs currently used are cyclophosphamide, azathioprine, methotrexate and cyclosporine (Fig. 27–1).

The alkylating agents are a major group of immunosuppressive drugs that act by crosslinking DNA helices, preventing their separation and thus inhibiting template formation. The most important of these is cyclophosphamide. Cyclophosphamide is toxic for resting and dividing cells, especially for dividing immunocompetent cells. It impairs both B and T cell responses, especially the primary immune response. It blocks mitogen- and antigen-induced blastogenesis and the production of soluble mediators such as MIF (IFN-γ). Early in therapy cyclophosphamide tends to destroy more B cells than T cells. In chronic therapy it has a similar effect on both cell populations. It also suppresses macrophage function and therefore has an anti-inflammatory effect. Cyclophosphamide may be administered parenterally or orally; it is inactive until biotransformed in the liver. It has a half-life of 4-6.5 hours and is largely excreted through the kidney. It is of interest to note that corticosteroids tend to enhance the metabolism of cyclophosphamide and thus render it less potent. Because cyclophosphamide is such a toxic drug, its value as an immunosuppressant is reduced. The main toxic effect is bone marrow suppression, leading to leukopenia with predisposition to infection. However, thrombocytopenia and anemia may also be induced. Cyclophosphamide can also damage the urinary tract, especially the bladder. Other alkylating agents such as chlorambucil and busulfan may be employed in a similar fashion.

Purine analogs may also be used as immunosuppressive agents. The most widely employed of these is azathioprine. Unlike cyclophosphamide, azathioprine affects only proliferating not resting lymphocytes and is therefore a less potent immunosuppressant. It can suppress both primary and secondary antibody responses if given after antigen exposure. Azathioprine has a significant anti-inflammatory action as a result of its ability to inhibit the production of macrophages. It has no effect on the production of soluble mediators by lymphocytes, and it affects both T and B responses equally. Like cyclophosphamide, the major toxic effect is bone marrow depression, which tends to affect leukocytes rather than platelets or red cells. The only other

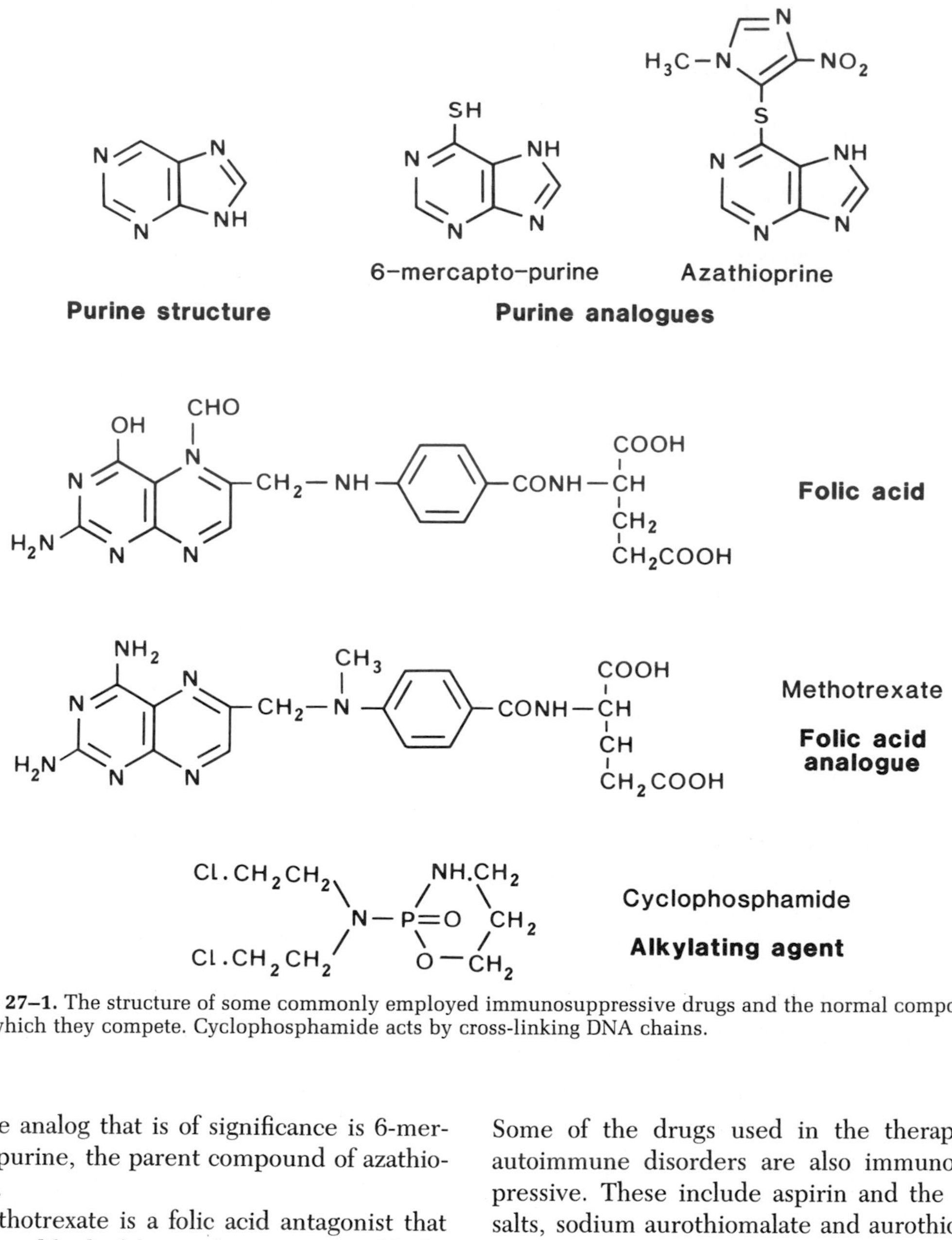

Figure 27–1. The structure of some commonly employed immunosuppressive drugs and the normal compounds with which they compete. Cyclophosphamide acts by cross-linking DNA chains.

purine analog that is of significance is 6-mer-capto-purine, the parent compound of azathioprine.

Methotrexate is a folic acid antagonist that binds to dihydrofolate reductase and so blocks the synthesis of tetrahydrofolate, leading to failure to synthesize thymidine and purine nucleotides. It can suppress antibody formation and its side effects are similar to those seen with cyclophosphamide and azathioprine.

Less commonly used drugs include the alkaloids, vincristine and vinblastine, which bind to tubulin and prevent mitosis; hydroxyurea, which blocks DNA synthesis; and 5-fluorouracil, which is a pyrimidine analog.

Some of the drugs used in the therapy of autoimmune disorders are also immunosuppressive. These include aspirin and the gold salts, sodium aurothiomalate and aurothioglucose, which depress antigen-induced blastogenesis.

Specific T Cell Destruction

Cyclosporine

Cyclosporine is a cyclic polypeptide derived from the fungus, *Tolypocladium inflatum*. It acts as a specific suppressor of the T cell response by blocking the response of T cells to interleukins 1 and 2. It also interferes with the production of IL-2, IL-2 receptors, IL-3 and IFN-γ by blocking the transcription of lymphocyte genes. Since corticosteroids have a similar effect, the combination of corticosteroids and cyclosporine is especially potent. The net effect of the action of cyclosporine is blockage of the T cell response without affecting nonresponding lymphocytes. Unfortunately, several patients receiving cyclosporine have developed B cell lymphomas. If it were not for this problem and the drug's nephrotoxicity, cyclosporine would be an almost perfect immunosuppressive agent.

Depletion of Lymphocytes

Because of the many adverse side effects of the nonspecific immunosuppressive agents (not the least important of which is an increased predisposition to infection) a considerable effort has been made to establish more specific alternative immunosuppressive procedures. One relatively simple technique that largely depletes T cells is to administer an antiserum specific for T lymphocytes. Antilymphocytic serum (ALS) can be made by inoculating a recipient of a different species with a purified lymphocyte suspension. The antiserum produced must be refined to ensure that it is specific for lymphocytes. Thus, it is usual to attempt to remove antibodies for the other blood elements by repeated absorption. ALS suppresses the cell-mediated immune response and leaves the humoral immune response relatively intact. Theoretically, it is, therefore, a great improvement on other immunosuppressive techniques. In practice, however, ALS has proved to be of variable efficiency. In experiments in mice, ALS-treated animals have been shown to accept rat xenografts, whereas clinical use of ALS in humans has not been universally accepted as being useful. Being a foreign antigen, ALS induces an immune response against itself, a feature that prevents prolonged therapy and increases the risks of anaphylaxis and serum sickness. Finally, since ALS is a suppressor of all cell-mediated immune functions, it may render treated animals susceptible to viral infections, permitting, for instance, the development of distemper and hepatitis in vaccinated dogs.

STIMULATION OF THE IMMUNE SYSTEM

There are many situations in veterinary medicine in which it is desirable to enhance the immune response. These include the potentiation of the normal immune response in order to enhance protection, and the treatment of immunosuppressive conditions.

Several different categories of immunopotentiators exist. They vary according to their origin, their mode of action and the way in which they are used.

Adjuvants

Materials that promote the immune responses when administered with antigens are called adjuvants. A large variety of compounds have been employed as adjuvants, although in many cases their mode of action is unclear. The simplest adjuvants are those that function by slowing the release of antigen into the body. As described in Chapter 9, the immune system is antigen-driven. The system responds to the presence of antigen but ceases to respond once antigen is eliminated. It is possible to slow the rate of antigen elimination and thus prolong an immune response by first mixing the antigen with an insoluble adjuvant to form a "depot." Examples of depot-forming adjuvants include aluminum salts such as aluminum hydroxide, aluminum phosphate and alum (potassium aluminum sulfate). The antigen is adsorbed onto the salt crystals prior to inoculation. Upon injection the salt-antigen mixture forms a small nodule in the tissues. The antigen within this nodule slowly leaks into the body and so provides a prolonged antigenic stimulus. Antigens that normally persist for only a few days may be retained in the body for several weeks by means of this technique. These adjuvants influence only the primary immune response and have little effect on secondary reactions. Other adjuvants that also form a local depot and stimulate antibody formation through slow release include beryllium sulfate, silica, kaolin and carbon.

Another very potent adjuvant consists of a mixture of mineral oil, emulsifier and killed mycobacteria and is known as Freund's complete adjuvant (FCA). Antigen in aqueous solution is emulsified with this adjuvant and the resulting water-in-oil emulsion is injected into an animal. The presence of the oil stimulates a local inflammatory response and granulomatous tissue formation around the site of the inoculum, while the antigen is slowly leached from the aqueous phase of the emulsion. Although Freund's complete adjuvant is a potent stimulator of the immune response, it has some adverse side effects. The presence of the mineral oil causes severe local irritation and granulomatous reactions. The adjuvant also renders its recipients tuberculin positive because of the mycobacteria present. Freund's complete adjuvant cannot, therefore, be used in the large domestic animals but is used extensively in laboratory rodents. The mechanism of action of this adjuvant is poorly understood. The emulsion probably serves as a depot, permitting the very slow release of antigen into the tissues. The presence of mycobacteria probably serve to enhance interleukin 1 production thus promoting effective presentation of antigen to T and B cells.

FCA promotes IgG production over IgM, inhibits tolerance induction, favors delayed hypersensitivity reactions and accelerates graft rejection as well as tumor immunity. FCA is required to induce some experimental autoimmune diseases such as experimental allergic encephalitis and thyroiditis (Chapter 25). It also stimulates macrophage activity, promoting phagocytosis and cytotoxic activity.

Freund's incomplete adjuvant is a simple emulsion of aqueous antigen solution in mineral oil. It is a relatively poor adjuvant.

Immunostimulants

In contrast to adjuvants, immunostimulants need not be administered together with antigen in order to enhance an immune response.

They are generally given to induce a nonantigen-specific enhancement of the immune system.

Bacteria and Bacterial Products

A wide variety of bacteria have been employed as immunostimulants. The most potent of these is BCG, the live, attenuated vaccine strain of *Mycobacterium bovis*. BCG produces a generalized enhancement of both B and T cell-mediated responses, of phagocytosis, of graft rejection and of resistance to infection. Fractionation of BCG has resulted in the isolation of several active constituents. Trehalose dimycolate (cord factor) is one of these. It promotes specific immunity against several bacterial infections and may provoke regression of some experimental tumors. Muramyl dipeptide (MDP), another active factor from mycobacteria, enhances antibody production, stimulates polyclonal activation of lymphocytes and activates macrophages. In addition, MDP does not sensitize animals to tuberculin. Because MDP is rapidly excreted in the urine, its biological activity is greatly enhanced by incorporation into liposomes. The immunostimulant effects of MDP can also be enhanced by polymerization and conjugation with glycopeptides or synthetic antigens.

Anaerobic coryneforms, especially *Propionobacterium acnes* (*Corynebacterium parvum*) promote antibody formation when administered as a killed suspension. This material has a complex activity since it stimulates macrophages and the antibody response to thymus-dependent antigens but has a variable effect on the response to thymus-independent antigens. As a result, these organisms have a general immunostimulating action, leading to enhanced antibacterial and antitumor activity. Nocardia derivatives are structurally related to mycobacteria and have similar properties to mycobacterial fractions. They stimulate both humoral and cell-mediated immune responses. Staphylococcal cell walls, some streptococcal components, products from *Bordetella pertussis*, *Brucella abortus*, *Bacillus subtilis* and *Klebsiella pneumoniae* all have complex immunomodulating activity.

Endotoxins from gram negative bacteria enhance antibody formation if given at about the same time as the antigen. They have no effect on delayed hypersensitivity but they can break tolerance, and they have a general immunostimulatory activity reflected in a nonspecific resistance to bacterial infections. Endotoxins act as polyclonal B cell mitogens (Chapter 15), stimulating them to divide while they activate macrophages, and promote the release of interleukin 1. Endotoxins may also enhance immune reactivity by promoting the release of interferons from cells (Chapter 16)

Yeast and Fungal Derivatives

Certain derivatives of yeasts, namely zymozan, glucans and lentinans have the ability to increase phagocytic abilities by activating macrophages. They may thus function as adjuvants and potentiate resistance to infectious agents. Two fungal derivatives named statolon and bestatin also function as immune stimulants, being potent enhancers of interferon production.

Thymic Hormones and Other Immune Mediators

Several of the soluble factors extracted from the thymus have significant effects on the immune system. Thus, thymic humoral factor enhances T helper activity, promotes IL-2 release and stimulates cytotoxic T cell activity. Alpha 1 thymostimulin enhances IFN-γ production, and thymosin fraction 5 promotes the regression of some viral infections.

The soluble proteins that mediate interactions between the cells of the immune system—interleukin 1, interleukin 2 and interferon—have also been administered to animals in attempts to modify immune function. Because this form of treatment is still being investigated, it is difficult to make specific comments about the appropriate use of any individual factor. Interleukin 1 will probably have similar effects to endotoxin, since endotoxin seems to exert many of its immunostimulatory effects by promoting IL-1 release. Interleukin 2 has been used as an immunostimulant and has induced some remarkable improvements when administered to human

cancer patients. It is predicted that IL-2 will be useful in situations in which enhancement of T cell function is required.

It was predicted for many years that the interferons would prove to be very effective antiviral agents if they were made available in large quantities for animal treatment. This has proved to be an oversimplification. High doses of interferons are very toxic and cause severe fever, malaise and inappetance, and they seem to be relatively poor antiviral agents. Very low doses of interferons may be useful in treating retrovirus-induced immunosuppression such as occurs in feline leukemia.

Immunoenhancing Drugs

Several drugs are available that stimulate the immune system. The earliest of these was levamisole. A broad-spectrum anthelmintic, levamisole functions in a manner similar to the thymic hormone thymopoietin (Chapter 5); that is, it stimulates T cell differentiation and response to antigens. Thus, levamisole enhances bovine lymphocyte blastogenesis at suboptimal mitogen concentrations, it enhances interferon production and increases Fc receptor activity in bovine macrophages. It probably also enhances cell-mediated cytotoxicity, lymphokine production and suppressor cell function. Levamisole stimulates the phagocytic activities of macrophages and neutrophils. The effects of levamisole are greatest in animals with depressed T cell function, and it has little or no effect on the immune system of normal animals. Levamisole may therefore be of assistance in the treatment of chronic infections and neoplastic diseases, but it may exacerbate disease caused by excessive T cell function.

Other synthetic immunostimulants that may be useful in domestic animals include Isoprinosine and Avridine. Isoprinosine is a drug that enhances T cell function and macrophage activity. It possibly acts by stimulating IL-2 production. Avridine is a lipoidal amine that enhances neutrophil function when depressed. Polyribonucleotides consisting of double-stranded nucleic acids such as polyinosinic acid:polycytidilic acid (poly I:C) and polyadenilic:polyuridilic acid (poly A:U) act as immunostimulants on mature T and NK cells, probably by functioning as interferon inducers.

Dialyzable Leukocyte Extract

In order to demonstrate that an immune reaction is cell mediated, it is usually necessary to demonstrate that it can be transferred from a sensitized animal to a normal animal by means of washed lymphocytes. In humans, cattle, sheep and dogs, and to a lesser extent in rodents, successful and specific transfer may sometimes be achieved by means of lymphocyte extracts (Fig. 27–2). The activity in these extracts, known as dialyzable leukocyte extract (DLE) or transfer factor, will pass through a dialysis membrane and must therefore have a molecular weight of less than 10,000 daltons. A single injection of DLE may confer specific cell-mediated reactivity on a normal recipient, lasting for over a year in some cases. DLE contains several hundred different compo-

nents, many of which can influence immune function. These include prostaglandins, histamine and thymosin. The factors responsible for transferring cell-mediated reactions are polyribonucleopeptides. Their polypeptide segment probably regulates antigen specificity and may be a fragment of the T cell antigen receptor. The efficiency of transfer seems to depend upon the immune status of the recipient. Thus the effects of DLE may be transient in immunosuppressed recipients but may persist for years in normal recipients. DLE has been used therapeutically in humans to confer immunity toward antigens to which patients are unreactive. An example of this is the treatment of chronic mucocutaneous candidiasis. This is a disfiguring fungal infection that occurs in individuals who are unable to respond immunologically to the yeast *Candida albicans*. Administration of DLE from immune individuals permits recipients to mount a successful immune response and thus control the infection.

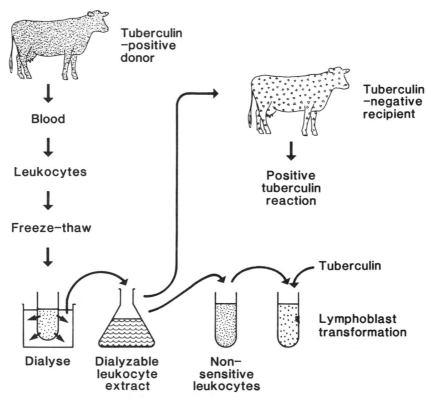

Figure 27–2. The production and use of dialyzable leukocyte extract. In this case it is used to transfer tuberculin reactivity from a tuberculin-positive cow to a tuberculin-negative one.

ADDITIONAL SOURCES OF INFORMATION

Bomford R. 1980. Comparative selectivity of adjuvants for humoral and cell-mediated immunity. Clin. Exp. Immunol. *39* 426–434.

Brunner CJ and Muscoplat CC. 1980. Immunomodulatory effects of levamisole. JAVMA *176* 1159–1162.

Gialdroni-Grassi G and Grassi C. 1985. Bacterial products as immunomodulating agents. Int. Arch. Allergy Appl. Immunol. *76* Suppl. 1 119–127.

Guelfi JF, Courdouhji MK, Alvinene M and Toutain PL. 1985. *In vivo* and *in vitro* effects of three glucocorticoids on blood leukocyte chemotaxis in the dog. Vet. Immunol. Immunopathol. *10* 245–252.

Guenounou M, Vacheron F and Nauciel C. 1985. Interleukin 1, a mediator of immunoadjuvant peptidiglycans. Comp Immunol. Microbiol. Infect. Dis. *8* 273–284.

Jenkins WL. 1984. Concurrent use of corticosteroids and antimicrobial drugs in the treatment of infectious diseases in large animals. JAVMA *185* 1145–1149.

Klesius PH. 1981. Modulation of cell-mediated responses with dialyzable leukocyte extract containing transfer factor. *In* Butler, JE Ed. The Ruminant Immune System. New York, Plenum Press, pp 293–323.

Klesius PH, Fudenberg HH and Smith CL. 1980. Comparative studies on dialyzable leukocyte extracts containing transfer factor. A review. Comp. Immunol. Microbiol. Infect. Dis. *3* 241–260.

Murray FA, and Chenault JR. 1982. Effects of steroids on bovine T-lymphocyte blastogenesis *in vitro*. J. Anim. Sci. *55* 1132–1138.

Roth JA, and Kaeberle ML. 1982. Effect of glucocorticoids on the bovine immune system. JAVMA *180* 894–901.

Schwartz RS. 1981. Therapeutic uses of immune suppression and enhancement. Hosp. Pract. *16* 93–101.

Spreafico F. 1985. Problems and challenges in the use of immunomodulating agents. Int. Arch. Allergy Appl. Immunol. *76* suppl 1. 108–118.

Thompson AW. 1983. Immunobiology of cyclosporin A— a review. Aust. J. Exp. Biol. Med. Sci. *61* 147–172.

Trainin N, Pecht M and Handzel ZT. 1983. Thymic hormones: inducers and regulators of the T-cell system. Immunol. Today *4* 16–21.

Wilson GB and Fudenberg HH. 1983. Is controversy about "transfer factor therapy" nearing an end? Immunol. Today *6* 157–161.

Index

Note: Numbers in *italics* refer to illustrations;
numbers followed by (t) indicate tables.